Fitness through Aerobics

Eighth Edition

JAN GALEN BISHOP
Central Connecticut State University

Benjamin Cummings

Boston Columbus Indianapolis New York San Francisco Upper Saddle River
Amsterdam Cape Town Dubai London Madrid Milan Munich Paris Montréal Toronto
Delhi Mexico City São Paulo Sydney Hong Kong Seoul Singapore Taipei Tokyo

Senior Acquisitions Editor: Sandra Lindelof
Development Manager: Barbara Yien
Associate Editor: Emily Portwood
Editorial Assistant: Brianna Paulson
Managing Editor: Deborah Cogan
Production Supervisor: Dorothy Cox
Production Management and Composition: Electronic Publishing Services Inc., NYC
Cover Designer: tani hasegawa
Cover Photographs: (top) Simon Bottomley; (bottom) Image Source
Manufacturing Buyer: Jeffrey Sargent
Marketing Manager: Neena Bali

All photos copyrighted by the author except for the following: p. 37: 4.2, 4.3; p. 54: 6.1; p. 58: 6.2a, 6.2b; p. 59: 6.4a, 6.4b; p. 60: 6.6a, 6.6b; p.61: 6.7c, 6.8; p.70: 7.2a, 7.2b; p.71: 7.3, 7.4, 7.5, 7.6, 7.7a, 7.7b; p. 72: 7.8, 7.9; p.73: 7.10a, 7.11a, 7.11b; p. 74: 7.12a, 7.12b; p. 75: 7.14; p. 76: 7.17a; p. 78: 7.21; p. 79: 7.22, 7.23, 7.24a; p. 80: 7.25; p. 81: 7.28c; p. 82: 7.29, 7.30b; p. 83: 7.32c; p. 86: 8.1; p. 87: 8.2; p. 88: 8.3; p. 111: 9.1, 9.2; p. 119: 10.1; p. 120: 10.2, 10.3b; p. 121: 10.5; p. 122: 10.6b, 10.7b; p. 123: 10.9; p. 125: 10.12b; p. 126: 10.13a; p. 127: 10.15, 10.16; p. 128: 10.17; p. 129: 10.20b, 10.21; p. 131: 10.25, 10.26, 10.27; p. 132: 10.28; p. 133: 10.29; p. 134: 10.32, 10.33; p. 135: 10.38; p. 136: 10.40, 10.41; p. 138: 10.46; p. 139: 10.47; p. 140: 10.48, 10.49; p. 141: 10.51; p. 142: 10.52, 10.53; p. 143: 10.54, 10.55, 10.56; p. 144: 10.57, 10.58; p. 145: 10.60, 10.61b, 10.62; p. 146: 10.64; p. 147: 10.65b, 10.66; p. 148: 10.67, 10.68a, 10.68b; p. 150: 10.71a, 10.71b, 10.71c; p. 151: 10.75; p. 151: 10.76; p. 153: 10.79a, 10.79b, 10.80; p. 153: 10.81; p. 154: 10.85; p. 155: 10.86, 10.87; p. 160: 11.2a, 11.2b; p. 161: 11.3; p. 162: 11.4, 11.5; p. 163: 11.6, 11.7, 11.8; p. 200: 14.1, p. 240: A, B. Copyright Pearson Education, Benjamin Cummings

Library of Congress Cataloging-in-Publication Data
Bishop, Jan Galen.
    Fitness through aerobics / Jan Galen Bishop. — 8th ed.
        p. cm.
    Includes bibliographical references and index.
    ISBN 0-321-67828-1 (paperbound)
    1. Aerobic exercises. 2. Physical fitness. 3. Health. I. Title.

RA781.15.B58 2011
613.7'1—dc22   2009052294

Benjamin Cummings
is an imprint of

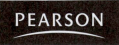

www.pearsonhighered.com

ISBN-13: 978-0-321-67828-7
ISBN-10:   0-321-67828-1
1 2 3 4 5 6 7 8 9 10—EB—14 13 12 11 10

Contents

Preface

Jackie Sorensen, inspired by Kenneth Cooper's ideas of aerobic fitness, set dance steps to music in the seventies and gave birth to aerobic dancing. Judy Shepard-Misset quickly followed with Jazzercise. Aerobic dance exploded in popularity. The eighties and Gin Miller brought a new challenge and more coed classes into the mix with step aerobics. Since then, aerobic dance exercise has continued to change and grow. Choreography used for classes has broadened from strictly dancelike steps to a wide variety of styles including kickboxing and boot camp. Recently one style, Zumba, has circled back to dance but in a less structured form. Muscle fitness, which started with body weight calisthenics accompanying the aerobic workout, now includes exercise bands, stability balls, and free weights. Some group fitness classes moved right off the dance floor and onto the machines (spinning, for example), while another trend has been the addition of mind–body exercises that draw on the techniques and exercises of pilates and yoga.

As classes continue to thrive with new and veteran exercisers, this enthusiasm for aerobic exercise has created a delightful dilemma. People who have never exercised before or who have had limited instruction in exercise are asking all kinds of questions about aerobics and muscular fitness. Instructors are faced with educating a gymnasium filled with people in an environment that demands movement and motivating music, not talk. A good instructor can educate as the class proceeds but is often severely limited by time and acoustics. This book was written to provide a solution. Students can read through vital information outside class; instructors can quickly clarify, reinforce, and supplement the information during class; and everyone has time to enjoy a full aerobic workout.

Therefore, the goal of the eighth edition of *Fitness Through Aerobics* is to provide the aerobic dance exercise participant with important information on the four health-related components of physical fitness: cardiorespiratory fitness, muscular fitness, flexibility, and body composition. Knowledge presented in this book will enhance the participants' ability to

(1) understand the important relationship between regular exercise, health, and wellness, (2) perform exercises correctly, (3) maximize the training effect of exercise, and (4) take control of planning and setting forth on a lifetime fitness plan.

NEW TO THIS EDITION

Aerobic exercise classes continue to grow in exciting new ways. To keep pace, a number of updates, additions, and improvements have been made to the eighth edition. Here is a preview of the most significant changes.

- **The 2008 Physical Activity Guidelines (USDHHS) have been infused into Chapters 1 and 5.** They are included in Chapter 1 because they reflect the latest standard for health and wellness promotion, and they are part of Chapter 5 because they have clear implications to setting goals.
- **Former Chapter 3 with information on how to select clothing and equipment has been condensed and is now Appendix 2.** Note that this change has renumbered the chapters that follow.
- **A discussion on how to use pedometers** to set goals, track activity (steps), and measure intensity (steps per minute) has been added to Chapter 5, and a worksheet to log goal tracking with a pedometer has also been added at the back of the book (Worksheet 8).
- **The muscular fitness Chapters 9 and 10 have been reorganized** so that Chapter 9 now addresses principles and concepts and Chapter 10 contains descriptions and explanations of how to perform all of the exercises. In previous editions, the exercises were grouped by the type of resistance being used (body weight, bands, balls, etc.). They are now organized according to the muscle or muscle group being worked. This means that one exercise (i.e., the squat) is shown using a variety of resistance methods.

This will make it easier for the reader to select an exercise of choice for a given body part and put together a personalized fitness workout. New artwork provided with the exercises allows students an immediate reference to which muscles are worked in a particular exercise and where they are located in the body.

- **Review questions have been added to the end of each chapter.** These questions, in sections titled "Think About It," can be used by the reader to review material and potentially can be used by the instructor as short-answer exam questions.
- **The bibliography that used to appear as one list at the end of the book has been broken up** to allow pertinent references to appear at the end of each chapter.

CHAPTER ORGANIZATION AND DESCRIPTIONS

The text opens with a discussion of wellness and how exercise, particularly aerobic dance exercise, can enhance personal wellness. Chapter 1 explains the importance of a lifetime habit of exercise, including the benefits of exercise to achieve mental, social, emotional, spiritual, and physical wellness. Guidelines, including the most recent 2008 Physical Activity Guidelines, are presented with a historical perspective to enhance understanding of why there are more than one set of guidelines and the implications for goal setting. The chapter concludes with a discussion of the many short- and long-range effects and benefits of exercise on the systems of the body.

Chapter 2 addresses the issue of tailoring "one-size-fits-all" exercise programs to meet individuals' needs. Guidelines are provided for conditions such as asthma, back and joint pain, pregnancy, diabetes, and obesity—conditions that may require an individual to adjust his or her exercise plan.

Chapter 3 covers foundational information about fitness components and exercise principles—information that is applied to aerobic fitness in Chapter 4, and again later in the book to flexibility and muscular fitness.

Chapter 4 focuses on how to set and monitor aerobic exercise intensity. This chapter also thoroughly examines the different guidelines for exercise in an effort to clarify the variety of published recommendations. The discussion provides guidance in interpreting the different guidelines to help the student design a personalized exercise program. The chapter also discusses a small change to the newer maximal heart-rate formula and how the change is also reflected on the accompanying worksheets.

Chapter 5 takes the next step to show the reader how to establish specific and attainable exercise goals. Logging worksheets for both aerobic workouts and pedometer counts are provided at the back of the book to make tracking goals easy.

Chapters 6 through 10 delve into the specifics of exercise technique using numerous photographs and detailed descriptions of exercises. Chapter 6 discusses postures important both in daily activities and in exercise performance. Alignment and back care are an integral part of this chapter, complete with self-tests for alignment and an introduction to core training. Chapter 7 educates students on how to stretch, warm up, develop flexibility, and cool down. Dynamic warm-ups and flexibility are discussed in addition to more traditional static stretching. A variety of rhythmic aerobics approaches are discussed in Chapter 8, including low-, high-, combination-, and moderate-impact, circuit, interval, step, and water aerobics. New trends on cardio equipment are also discussed, and the chapter introduces a wide variety of aerobic styles, such as salsa, martial arts, and funk aerobics. One section discusses how choreography is set to music. Understanding how music is organized and then how the steps are set to it will enable students to work with rhythmic movement more easily. Basic information to help students choreograph their own songs when instructors give them the opportunity is also included.

Chapters 9 and 10 focus on muscular fitness and how to add resistance to body weight exercises. Chapter 9 applies the fitness components and principles of exercise to muscular strength and endurance. Chapter 10 is filled with detailed descriptions of exercises and includes explanations of techniques, photographs, and icons highlighting the muscles used in each exercise. Those exercises that work the same muscle or muscle group are presented together. This allows students to see how they can challenge muscles using different positions and forms of resistance such as dumbbells, barbells, bands, and stability balls.

At this point, three important concepts have been addressed: (1) why exercise is important, (2) how best to optimize your benefits from exercise, and (3) how to exercise safely and effectively. Chapter 11 takes the next step by exploring the connection between the body and the mind and includes discussions on stress and strategies for managing stress. Pilates and yoga, two popular forms of group exercise, are introduced in this chapter, along with several techniques for relaxation and mental rehearsal.

Chapter 12 adds the crucial element of nutrition. Many exercisers list at least one goal that has to do with weight control. This chapter explains how exercise and diet are linked and how to use the power of both to obtain the results you want.

Chapter 13 provides information on how to stay injury free when participating in exercise. The chapter emphasizes injury prevention, focusing on common injuries and their symptoms. This knowledge will help prompt early detection and promote a speedier recovery if a problem should develop.

The final chapter (Chapter 14) encourages the reader to look beyond the immediate college course, take a fitness-for-life approach, and plan how and where to exercise in the future.

Each chapter opens with an overview and closes with a summary, a list of knowledge tips, review questions, and pertinent references. Key words, highlighted in bold throughout the book, are defined in a glossary at the back. Tear-out worksheets that allow the reader to apply the information presented in the chapters are also located at the back of the book. These worksheets include a health and fitness questionnaire, training heart-rate formulas, fitness tests, goal setting, a fitness log, a pedometer log, healthy weight assessments, and nutrition awareness exercises.

The information in this book is a synthesis of my experiences teaching at colleges, private clubs, instructor training/certification workshops, and conventions, plus knowledge and ideas I have gathered from instructors, professors, professional organizations, and, perhaps most important, students. These pages contain what I believe is the most pertinent, up-to-date information available. My hope is that this book will enable readers to more fully realize their exercise dreams.

ACKNOWLEDGMENTS

As the eighth edition emerges, I am struck by how many exceptional people have dedicated their talents to making this book an ever-evolving success over many years. Let me lead off by thanking the most recent team, including Sandy Lindelof, Emily Portwood, Dorothy Cox, and the production team at EPS. I would like to continue to thank the individuals who came before this team; it is upon their work that we build, and I thank all of you. Even though my book has long left the capable hands of the GSP staff, I'd like to express a continued debt of gratitude to Gay Pauley and Colette Kelly for seeing me through three and a half editions and for taking me into their hearts as a friend. I would also like to thank the Allyn & Bacon staff, who picked up and ran with the improved fourth edition. A special nod to Marret Kauffner, who added just the right touches and dealt beautifully with my eccentricities. Fifth edition appreciation goes to Benjamin Cummings' Susan Teahan, Wendy Earl, Anna Reynolds Trabucco, Cecelia Morales, and especially to Leslie Austin, who managed to chuckle every time I added another headache to her ace production efforts.

Valuable information has been provided in the form of reviews by colleagues and professional advisors. I couldn't have done it without Jennifer Morley (artistic director at Figments Dance Ensemble), who provided my Pilates education; my Central Connecticut State University colleagues, David Harackiewicz, PhD, who reviewed the nutrition chapter; Catherine Fellows, MS, and Susan Smith, MS, who helped with the yoga section; Frank Frangione, PhD, and Peter Moreno, PhD, who answered all my anatomy and physiology questions; and Patricia Gaedeke for keeping me up to date with the fitness club scene. Thank you to Ruth Sova, MS (founder and president of the Aquatic Therapy and Rehabilitation Institute, Inc.) and Kristie Romley (University of Arizona) for my education in water aerobics. The reviewers for this edition were Carol Hirsh (Austin Community College), Jane Curth (Georgia Perimeter), Lisa Chaisson (Houston Community College), Marcos Briano (University of Southern California), and Peggy Domingue (North Carolina State University).

Photographs bring the information alive; my thanks to the generous, kind, and very talented photographer Marc Regis. I would also like to acknowledge the work of previous edition photographers, many of whose photographs continue to appear in this edition: David Mager and his assistant, Elbaliz Mendez; Lisa Lake; Tony Neste; William G. Nelson and his assistant, Christopher St. Johns; Bob Pangrazi; and John Dice. Thanks also to Dave Neurath, whose illustration appears in the instructor's guide. A special thank you also to owners Jack Banks and Paul Carson for allowing us to shoot some of our photographs for previous editions at their Malibu Fitness & Powerhouse Gym in Farmington, CT.

Pictured in this book are some very special people—my models. You all have so effectively brought the information in this book alive: Omaris Journet, Chanhdy Ly, Dan Matthews, Shanley Fitzgerald, Cassie Stewart, Katie Wartonick, Ashley M. Hill, Doug Semenuk, Robert Kucharski, Sherrie Santangelo, Patricia Gaedeke, Amanda Lang, Jennifer Morley, Sean Callahan, Amanda K. Hilson, Anne M. Charter, Heather Snyder, Larry Holmes Jr., Eileen Sachs, Ashley Smith, Steven Cook, Brittany L. Auld, Kyle Dailey, Joanna Hollenback, Rebecca Rhodes, James Braswell, Jim Walczyk, Jessica Aman, Dara Elena Johnson, Teri So Dame, Patrick Decker, Ed Duclos, Richard Bishop, and our youngest models, Noah Ramon Bishop, Olivia Jean Bishop, and Marie Louisa Bishop.

Finally, I'd like to thank those closest to me—my neighbors, friends, and family—who have seen me through countless deadlines. Thank you, Dad, for encouraging me with a passion for healthy living; Mother, for your kitchen-counter editing and countless years of good advice; sister Melissa Bennie for your artistic eye and original shoe drawing; brothers Robert, Timur, and Derrick, who helped shape my active childhood; husband Rich for your loving support and unwavering faith in me; and my children, Noah, Olivia, and Marie, for making fitness a natural part of my life.

Jan Galen Bishop
Associate Professor
Central Connecticut State University

1

Aerobics, Wellness, and You!

"The only thing that ever sat its way to success was a hen."

SARAH BROWN

- What is aerobics?
- Why is doing aerobics important? What are the benefits?
- What is a wellness lifestyle and how do I achieve it?
- What should I expect an aerobic dance exercise class to be like?

AEROBICS

"Aerobics" has been a word for only about 30 years, but in its short history it has become a household term that has dramatically reshaped the public's approach to fitness. The adjective "aerobic" is much older and, according to *Merriam-Webster's Collegiate Dictionary,* 11th edition, means "living, active, or occurring only in the presence of oxygen." You and I are aerobic. We take in and use oxygen in combination with carbohydrates and fats to produce energy. In 1968, Dr. Kenneth Cooper, a researcher and flight surgeon for the U.S. Air Force, put the "s" on the end of the adjective "aerobic" and defined his new noun **aerobics** as any physical activity that requires oxygen for a prolonged period of time. Such activities, he argued, cause a training effect that will improve the pulmonary and cardiovascular systems—the key to good fitness. When Cooper published his little book, titled *Aerobics,* he began what has become a lifetime conversation with the public about the benefits of aerobic exercise. Cooper's research over the past 35 years—as well as that of many other notable researchers—has linked aerobic fitness to numerous health benefits and spurred many of us to think about exercise as preventive medicine and a way to a more fulfilling life.

Prior to the aerobics movement, physical fitness was often thought of in terms of muscle development. Individuals performed calisthenics, isometrics, and weight training. Jack Lalanne used television to lead millions in a series of calisthenics. Sports, particularly team sports, were also popular, primarily among young men. The idea of **aerobic exercise,** defined as any large-muscle, continuous, rhythmic activity, completely changed the focus. People who wanted health-related fitness started taking up aerobics-based activities such as jogging, cross-country skiing, rowing, cycling, and swimming.

The aerobics revolution, and evolution, was off and running—literally. At the same time as thousands took to the pavement to run, Jacki Sorensen, an Air Force wife stationed in Puerto Rico, was asked to develop a fitness television program for other Air Force wives at the base. Her background was in dance, but she was also familiar with Cooper's Air Force Aerobics Program. Based on her own fitness from dance and Cooper's concepts of aerobic fitness, she developed a set of vigorous dance routines set to lively music and gave birth to aerobic dancing. It became very popular, particularly among women. When she returned to the mainland in 1971 and started promoting her program, Jacki Sorensen started one of the most popular fitness movements ever seen. Many dance exercise professionals believe the number of people involved in aerobic dance today exceeds 24 million, although no one knows for sure. Although it was never meant to refer to only one kind of aerobic exercise, the word "aerobics" for many, especially women, became synonymous with aerobic dance.

Since aerobic dance began, it has been shaped and changed by many innovative and creative instructors. Judi Sheppard Missett used her dance background in the early 1970s to develop what is now widely known as Jazzercise. Gin Miller added step aerobics to the mix in the late 1980s. Today, aerobic dance includes high-, low-, and nonimpact styles influenced by jazz, hip-hop,

1

Latin American dance, modern dance, boxing, kick boxing and other martial arts, yoga, and many other styles of movement. In addition to regular aerobics classes, there are step, double step, aquatic step, slide, and water (aqua) aerobics classes. You can also get an aerobic workout on a rower, stair climber, elliptical trainer bike, slide board, or ski machine. Many clubs and some universities and colleges now offer group classes on stationary bikes, stair steppers, and treadmills, as well as traditional aerobics classes. **Group fitness** is the popular term to describe all the aerobic activities offered in a class or group setting. In this text, I will continue to use the phrase "aerobic dance exercise" to describe the floor- or land-based (as opposed to water- or cardio-machine-based) aerobics class with its many styles and variations.

Because the group setting is so important to motivation and having fun, instructors are challenged to lead an aerobic workout that fits the needs of a group of individuals who in many cases encompass a wide range of fitness levels. One of the best ways to meet this challenge is to educate participants on how to make movements easier or more challenging, so that they can perform a workout at their own fitness level. A good instructor will flow from one level to another, demonstrating different intensities and modifications of exercises. Step aerobics makes the job of individualizing exercise even easier: More highly fit participants challenge themselves with higher steps, while others use lower steps (or even no steps). Power moves and arm work can also add intensity. This particular style of aerobics appeals to both men and women and has increased the number of mixed-gender classes.

The wide variety of styles in aerobic dance exercise keeps it fresh and exciting and enables people of all ages and fitness levels to join in the fun. Innovative instructors and exercise-smart participants are riding the wave of wellness . . . and aerobic dance exercise is one of the popular ways they are doing it. Welcome back if you are experienced; welcome aboard if you are a newcomer!

WELLNESS AND YOU

You are the heart of the aerobics program. Your needs, your goals, your preferences—in short, your wellness—are what should determine your workout. And it can, if you take an active role in designing your fitness plan. How? By combining what you know about yourself with the expertise of the instructor. If you take a "one size fits all" program and tailor it to fit your needs, you will be more motivated to stay with your program and reach your goals.

In the 1960s and 1970s, rapid advancements in medicine lulled people into believing that they could lead any kind of life and medical science would bail them out if they became sick or injured. Individuals allowed the primary responsibility for their health to shift to doctors and other health care professionals; a "here I am, doctor—cure me" attitude evolved. But medicine is not a cure-all. Each year millions of people in the United States die prematurely from heart disease, cancer, stroke, and tobacco-related illnesses.

The good news is that you can substantially lower your risk of disease and premature death by adopting healthy lifestyle habits. Behaviors such as eating a low-fat, nutrient-rich diet, getting enough rest, managing stress, and exercising regularly put prevention on the front line and allow medicine to be an effective second line of defense. These are all things each of us can do for ourselves.

In the 1980s the idea of taking responsibility for your own well-being became the cornerstone of what is now popularly known as the **wellness** movement. There are two main tenets of wellness: (1) that you take control of your personal well-being by adopting and maintaining healthy lifestyle habits; and (2) that to be completely well, you must be more than physically healthy; you must also be socially, emotionally, mentally, and spiritually healthy. (Some wellness definitions include occupational and environmental wellness.) The following metaphor, the balloon theory, describes how the wellness concept works.

THE BALLOON THEORY

Imagine that you are standing on the ground holding on to five balloons.[1] Each balloon represents a part of you—the emotional, mental, social, spiritual, and physical parts. Your five balloons can inflate or deflate with helium, depending on what is happening in your life. Most of the time, the balloons have some helium in them, and you are pulled upward. A big date may have your social balloon tugging you to the stratosphere, whereas breaking up with someone could temporarily pop it, sending you back to earth. Your mental health balloon may be inflated by a compliment from a professor, whereas a problem with financial aid could weaken your emotional balloon.

Because all the balloons are connected, any upward or downward motion of one balloon will create a pulling effect on the others. If, for example, you abuse your physical health through sleep deprivation, poor

---

1. Portions of this section also appear in J. G. Bishop and S. G. Aldana, *Step Up to Wellness: A Stage-Based Approach*. Copyright © 1999 by Allyn & Bacon. Reprinted by permission of Pearson Education, Inc.

diet, chronic injury, or drugs, you will also be affected mentally, emotionally, socially, and spiritually. Similarly, prolonged or intense mental and emotional stress can result in physical ailments such as headaches or stomach upset. The reverse is also true. People with good social relationships have, on the average, longer, healthier lives.

Although all the balloons that encompass your life are loosely tied together, you do have control in that you can deliberately choose to deflate a balloon. Occasionally it may be good to let a balloon deflate while you attend to something else. For example, some religions celebrate holy days by fasting. The spiritual benefits of such rites may outweigh any temporary loss in physical health. Caring for a sick child, parent, or sibling, or helping a friend in crisis may detract from your ability to progress academically, but fulfilling this social role as a good friend or family member may be more important during critical times. These swings are okay as long as they do not come one right after another and no one balloon is neglected for a prolonged period. If you lead a fairly balanced life and consciously decide when to alter the balance, you will have the reserve needed to handle surprises and emergencies, and the energy to take advantage of opportunities. In new situations such as entering college or starting a new job, everything can look important, and it takes a little time to sort out priorities and find a balance. Problems occur most often when an imbalance lasts too long or the sacrifice is too large.

Learning to manage your balloons (your life) and taking responsibility for decisions that affect you describes a "wellness lifestyle." Consistent wellness lifestyle habits fill the balloons even when a sudden disturbance occurs. For example, individuals can lean on their spiritual faith, family, and friends when faced with a traumatic experience. This helps them stay emotionally and mentally stable; the spiritual and social balloons lift the others, thus preventing a total loss of self. There may be times when all your balloons are deflating. Sometimes this is the result of poor personal choices. Substance abuse, for example, can plummet you into disaster. In these cases, seeking help from friends, clergy, or physicians or other health care professionals may be necessary to get your balloons back in the air. You will weather lows better if you have built a good wellness network around you.

Occasionally, you will find that everything in your life is going just right. All the balloons are filled to their maximum, and it feels good. Take a deep, satisfying, relaxing breath, and admire the world around you. You are feeling very "well" indeed! These moments are to be savored. However, if you consider anything short of this a failure, then most of your life will be judged as such. Life is full of changes, and living a "well" life is not about having all the balloons filled all the time. Living a well life means keeping a positive attitude as you manage your balloons and successfully handle the changes that come your way.

Wellness does not assume that you are free of disease, disability, or other limitations. It does assume a proactive stance. People with a wellness attitude take actions to maximize their potential; they do not allow their limitations to control them. We are surrounded by inspirational people who do just that. For example, Muhammed Ali, his muscles weakened by Parkinson's disease, proudly lit the 1996 Olympic Torch, and Michael J. Fox educates us by allowing us to witness how he embraces life while suffering from the same disease. Christopher Reeve, paralyzed from the neck down, used his acting ability to speak out for the disabled at the 1994 Democratic Convention, and skater Ekaterina Gordeeva has retained her love of skating and has come back as a singles skater after tragically losing her husband (who was also her skating partner). In addition to these famous people, there are countless examples of equally courageous people all around us—maybe you (or the person next to you in an aerobics class) are just such a person. Well people tend to be hardy people; they see life as a challenge and have a positive attitude about change.

MAKING CHANGES

Establishing and maintaining a new lifestyle habit, like exercise, is not always easy. Researchers have been trying to figure out why some people successfully change and others do not. James Prochaska, John Norcross, and Carlo DiClemente and colleagues pioneered what is now known as the Transtheoretical Model of Change, sometimes known as the Stages of Change Model, and made us rethink what we know about how people change their behaviors. For years, behavior change programs assumed that everyone would benefit from the same action plan. Unfortunately, most of the people who attended programs (such as those for smoking cessation) failed to stay with the plan or failed to maintain the new behavior after the formal program ended. These types of programs can be effective, but only when you are ready. The Stages of Change Model originally described change as something that goes through five stages. A sixth stage has since been added. In the first stage, precontemplation, people are not even interested in change; in the second, contemplation, they are thinking about it; in the third, preparation, they are taking tentative steps toward making change (maybe experimenting a little); in the fourth, action, they are carrying out a plan; in the fifth, maintenance, they are sustaining the new behavior; and in the sixth,

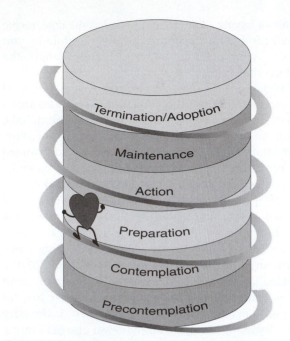

Figure 1.1 Stages of change.

termination/adoption, they have made the behavior a habit and maintained it for 5 or more years.

The Transtheoretical Model of Change proposes strategies for each of the stages. While there is overlap, the change strategies for one stage are different from the strategies for other stages. Precontemplators, for example, need strategies that help them see the value of changing, not action plans they haven't "bought into" yet. Programs that target change strategies to "where people are at" are more successful. As you can see in Figure 1.1, a person moves in an upward spiral through the stages. It is possible to skip a stage or slide backward, but in general the strategies help you move up the spiral toward permanent change.

Because you have signed up for an aerobics course, you have already taken a step from preparation into action. You may even be a maintainer or behavior adopter. The strategies in this text are aimed at helping you in your present stage. These strategies include the following:

- goal setting
- developing an individualized plan
- identifying and overcoming barriers to continued exercise (including how to restart in the event you stop exercising)
- finding and using sources of motivation
- measuring and evaluating your progress and goals

So in terms of exercise, you are already an action taker, a maintainer, or adopter—terrific! Even if this is the first regular exercise program you have attempted, you have made great progress just by signing up: You

have moved from preparation to action. By establishing a lifestyle that includes aerobic dance exercise, you are practicing preventive medicine and enhancing the quality of your life. The focus of this book is to help you do this in a safe, effective, and fun manner so that you will want to maintain and reap the many benefits of this wellness behavior all your life.

EXERCISE AND WELLNESS

Some people would have you believe that exercise is nothing but a sweaty, hair-messing, laundry-producing time-eater. But those of us who exercise regularly know that it is an energy-giving, life-prolonging, stress-reducing, socially fun thing to do—well worth a little sweat and laundry. Unfortunately, many of the people who start an exercise program don't stick with it long enough to feel the benefits that keep the veterans coming back. Aerobic dance exercise has obvious physical fitness benefits, which will be detailed in the next section. But it can also have a positive impact on mental, emotional, social, and spiritual wellness.

MENTAL BOOST

Exercise can lift your spirits. Aerobic exercise in particular can help lower anxiety and lift depression. The production of endorphins, hormones that act as natural painkillers and mood elevators, increases with regular aerobic exercise. Endorphins are believed to cause the euphoric feeling or "runner's high" that people feel after exercise. The runner's high is not limited to runners or to running; any aerobic activity can produce it. However, it usually takes 6 to 8 weeks of regular vigorous exercise training before you experience it; unfortunately, many people have dropped out of their program before this time. People who exercise enough to experience this feeling are motivated to continue exercising because of it. So while your initial motivation to exercise may be to look good, your motivation to continue may well become to feel good.

INCREASED PRODUCTIVITY

Businesses and insurance companies are now well aware that employees are more productive and absent less often when they exercise regularly. People who exercise will tell you that they feel refreshed and ready to tackle problems again after their workout. Solutions or creative ideas may even come to you while you are being physically active. When I was in college, during finals week a group of us would gather at 10:00 P.M. for a short, refreshing run. That may not be your preferred time or activity, but the point is that a little exercise, even during crunch times, can clear your mind and help you to be more productive.

GREATER SELF-ESTEEM

As people begin to look and feel better physically, they also tend to feel better about themselves. An improved self-image can make you more confident and self-assured, qualities that are nice to have when meeting people, dating, and making career decisions.

STRESS-BUSTER

Aerobic dance exercise also provides an opportunity to exercise out some of the worries and tensions of the day. It is a great release valve for stress. Some classes build in a few minutes of progressive relaxation at the end, a technique that can be used in a number of settings once you have learned it. A lot of people enjoy aerobic dance exercise because of the upbeat music that accompanies it. Music can be motivating, releasing, and energizing.

SOCIAL OPPORTUNITY

An aerobic dance exercise class is also a wonderful low-stress way to meet other active, energetic people. It can provide a social connection that might otherwise be lost in a busy day—something that may become more important when you graduate from college and have fewer opportunities to meet people. Having friends or family exercise with you is another way to build social time and fitness into your day.

MIND-BODY CONNECTION

More people are becoming attuned to the connection between the body and the mind. Exercising the body can have a positive effect on the mind, and tending the mind can have a positive effect on physical well-being. Yoga and pilates are two forms of exercise that help people focus on this connection. For some people, exercise can clear their minds of daily concerns and allow deeper thoughts and meanings to emerge. They leave the exercise feeling more centered and refocused. Although yoga is not a religion, it provides many people with a spiritual link to wellness.

HEALTH PROMOTION

Exercise results in numerous other benefits, including improved immune function, better sleep, injury prevention, and a more efficient metabolism. Teamed with a good diet, it helps control body fat, gives you energy, and helps you look and feel your best.

DISEASE PREVENTION

The number one killer of adults in the United States is heart disease. There are seven major risk factors for coronary heart disease (CHD) and stroke:

- smoking
- hypertension
- high blood cholesterol
- physical inactivity
- heredity
- gender
- increasing age

Exercise has long been considered good for your health. But when the American Heart Association added inactivity to the list of major heart disease risk factors, exercise became recognized as a serious member of the wellness team. In our high-tech world of remote controls and computers, it is important to get up and move. Individuals with poor fitness levels have an 8 times higher risk of death due to cardiovascular disease and a 5 times higher probability of dying from cancer (the second leading cause of death) than do persons who have good or excellent levels of fitness. Women who exercise regularly cut their risk of breast cancer in half.

Exercise also has a positive effect on some other major risk factors: smoking, elevated blood cholesterol, and hypertension (high blood pressure), and the contributory risk factors obesity and diabetes. As you will read in more detail shortly, regular aerobic exercise helps prevent plaque from adhering to the arteries and lowers blood pressure. In addition to reducing heart disease risk, this helps prevent strokes, the third leading cause of death. An active lifestyle also helps maintain a healthy body weight, which, in turn, lowers the risk of developing obesity and diabetes. Exercise may also help stop cancer by aiding people in their attempts to stop smoking (or never start). Because it is difficult to smoke and exercise at the same time, exercise is a good substitute activity during periods of craving. Exercise may also help prevent weight gain and/or offset some of the extra calories a smoker might eat after quitting. Exercise can also help offset or relieve stress. Although it isn't a panacea, exercise is one of the most positive things you can do for your health.

HOW MUCH EXERCISE IS ENOUGH?

A recurring question in exercise research is, How much is enough? The answer depends on your personal goals. Are you interested in improving health? Physical fitness? Both? And to what level? Moderate-intensity physical activities can enable you to achieve substantial health-related gains, and more vigorous exercise will allow you to achieve greater health benefits and higher levels of physical fitness. You may have heard several different guidelines for how much, and how hard, you should exercise. It is easy to be confused. Here is an abbreviated explanation of why there is more than one set of guidelines.

In the 1970s, the question was examined in terms of how much exercise or training would result in certain performance capabilities. For example, if I want to run fast (or far), what kind of training program should I use? The American College of Sports Medicine (ACSM) reviewed the research evidence and published its first set of exercise guidelines for healthy adults in 1975 and a position statement in 1978. For many, the ACSM guidelines have been the "gold standard." Their latest position stand revision was published in 1998. The ACSM periodically reviews new research evidence and publishes updates. These guidelines assume that you are willing to engage in physical activity that is vigorous enough to develop and maintain cardiorespiratory fitness, body composition, muscular strength and endurance, and flexibility. At this level of exercise, you will also achieve the many health-related benefits discussed later in this chapter. These guidelines are widely accepted and are the basis for the amount and intensity of exercise described in this book. The 1998 guidelines include workout intensity recommendations for low-fit individuals as well as moderate- and high-fit individuals.

As the wellness movement began in earnest, the research focus widened. The question was rephrased, How much exercise is necessary for health? The word "exercise" is often substituted with the phrase "physical activity" in discussions about health promotion. How much physical activity will result in health gains for individuals who are sedentary or active below the ACSM recommendations? The answer—for low-fit or sedentary individuals, even a small increase in physical activity starts to pay back in health benefits! It was discovered that many of the health benefits can be achieved at a moderate level of intensity, such as that used in a brisk walk, as long as it is done often. In 1995, the Centers for Disease Control and Prevention (CDC) and ACSM jointly made a new recommendation that every U.S. adult accumulate 30 minutes or more of moderate-intensity physical activity on most, preferably all, days of the week. In 1996 the Surgeon General Report, the American Heart Association, and a report from the National Institutes of Health all published similar guidelines. The news was out that you didn't have to run or engage in other strenuous, structured physical activity; by doing everyday physical chores, shoveling snow, walking the dog, or gardening, you could achieve health-enhancing fitness in 30 minutes. Even these 10-minute bouts can be effective.

Just as everyone was becoming familiar with this guideline, the Institute of Medicine (IOM) published a report in which they claimed that 30 minutes of moderate exercise was insufficient to maintain body weight in adults in a desired range. In 2002 they recommended that individuals complete 60 minutes of moderately intense physical activity each day. Suddenly the press was telling everyone to double their exercise minutes.

In 2004, Steven Blair, Michael LaMonte, and Milton Nichaman published an article tracing the evolution of physical activity recommendations. After an in-depth look at how each set of guidelines had been established, they suggested a careful blending of the recommendations for health-related physical activity. They recommended that individuals who were having trouble controlling their weight after meeting the 30 minutes per day of moderate-intensity physical activity and consuming an appropriate number of calories perform additional exercise or make additional caloric restrictions to reach energy balance and minimize the likelihood of further weight gain. They also recommended that individuals who were weight stable and meeting the physical activity guideline of 30 minutes a day consider building up to 60 minutes a day in order to receive additional health benefits.

Four years later a comprehensive review of the research was undertaken by an external committee appointed by the director of the U.S. Department of Health and Human Services (USDHHS). From the committee's report, along with input from government agencies and the public, the newest physical activity guidelines were born—welcome the 2008 *Physical Activity Guidelines for Americans*. These guidelines are not much different than the previous ones except that the emphasis is on total accumulation of minutes of activity a week versus a certain amount per day. As an example, scientific evidence does not allow researchers to say that the health benefits are any different for 5 days with 30 minutes of activity each day and 3 days with 50 minutes of activity each day. Thus you are free to accumulate the time in a variety of ways.

In brief, the *Physical Activity Guidelines for Americans* recommend that adults who want to attain substantial health benefits accumulate a minimum of 150 minutes of moderate-intensity or 75 minutes of vigorous-intensity aerobic physical activity every week; the guideline can also be met with a mixture of moderate and vigorous activity. Muscle-strengthening activities should be performed at least twice a week.

Separate guidelines are available for children and adolescents, older adults, and special populations. Visit the website at www.health.gov/paguidelines for a complete listing of the U.S. Department of Health and Human Services 2008 *Physical Activity Guidelines for Americans.*

More research needs to be done. There are still many questions, especially in regard to the connection between exercise and weight management. There is also a need for more information on exercise programming for special populations and different age groups. As we learn more, we can adjust and fine-tune individual workouts. Watch for new developments, but make sure they are being reported by credible sources.

How you use the guidelines and the level of physical activity you choose will depend on your goals. Goals can be health-related (weight management and disease prevention) or performance-related (for sport or competition). In Chapter 4, you will have the opportunity to use the guidelines (CDC/ACSM and USDHHS) to determine the proper intensity and duration of aerobic exercise to meet your goals. You should also keep in mind that although the USDHHS guidelines focused on activity for health enhancement, there are many other reasons to be physically active, including having fun with friends, engaging in the thrill of a game or sport, enjoying the outdoors, and improving your appearance.

THE PHYSIOLOGICAL BENEFITS OF EXERCISE

The remainder of this chapter is about how exercise, aerobic dance exercise in particular, promotes physical health. It is about how the body works and how exercise works on the body. Why do you need to know this? Because this information can help you take primary responsibility for your health. You can choose the benefits that are important to you and make sure that the exercises that result in those benefits are included in your exercise program. With a basic understanding of exercise physiology, you can talk with professionals on a more knowledgeable level, ask intelligent questions, and evaluate the quality of instruction you are receiving. Plus, if you understand how something works and believe that it is important, it is easier to stick with it. As you tangle up your feet on a new aerobic step or are challenged by a new overload, you will be able to fill your head with positive thoughts such as how your heart is getting stronger and healthier, fat is disappearing, and toned muscles are emerging.

The human body is intricately engineered and fantastically coordinated. At this very moment, inside you, millions of chemical reactions are occurring, brain signals are flying along nerve pathways, muscles are contracting and relaxing to maintain your posture against gravity, and food is being digested and converted to energy. All these things and many more are happening simultaneously, routinely, and without conscious thought. Each body system—cardiovascular, muscular, respiratory, and others (see the Benefits of Physical Activity box)—is influenced by exercise. Each system is affected in a manner specific to the kind of exercise performed. Aerobic dance exercise emphasizes improvement of the metabolic, cardiovascular, respiratory, and muscular systems.

At rest, the body is in a state of balance called **homeostasis,** in which energy is being produced at the same rate that it is being used. When you begin to exercise, your body uses energy faster than it is being produced. In an attempt to restore homeostasis, you breathe faster, your heart rate increases, your energy production increases, and you sweat more to dissipate heat. All these changes help you establish homeostasis at a higher level of energy production and utilization. When you stop exercising, the energy output decreases and your body adjusts once again. The changes involved in maintaining homeostasis are called short-term or acute adaptations.

Something that disturbs homeostasis and causes the body to make changes is called a stressor. Exercise is a stressor. When the body is stressed repeatedly over time, long-term or chronic adaptations take place. The right amount of stress causes healthy changes. Too much stress results in unhealthy changes. For example, taking an aerobic dance exercise class 3 to 5 times a week will increase your cardiorespiratory efficiency and tone your muscles. Taking two classes every day can lead to overuse injuries such as tendinitis and stress fractures. In the following chapters, you will learn how to set up a program with the amount of stress needed to maximize your long-term benefits. The following discussion examines the systems of the body most affected by participation in aerobic dance exercise and discusses the long-term benefits of exercise for each system.

THE METABOLIC SYSTEMS

The metabolic systems, often referred to as the energy systems, convert food into energy. The food you eat is broken down through various chemical pathways with the purpose of producing **adenosine triphosphate (ATP),** which is a high-energy phosphate molecule. When ATP is split apart, it releases energy that the cells in your body can use. Muscle cells use ATP to fuel contraction, and movement is possible as long as ATP is available. (Nonavailability of ATP results in rigor mortis.) It is extremely important, then, to have ways to resynthesize ATP when it has been broken down for energy.

BENEFITS OF PHYSICAL ACTIVITY

SKELETAL SYSTEM

- Increases bone density and strength
- Helps prevent osteoporosis (brittle bones)
- Helps maintain good bone alignment, which is especially important to the spine

CARDIOVASCULAR SYSTEM

- Decreases blood pressure
- Decreases blood cholesterol. Increases high-density lipoprotein (HDL)
- Decreases risk of cardiovascular disease
- Decreases resting heart rate (workload on the heart)
- Increases cardiac muscle strength
- Increases the number of capillaries
- Increases systemic and coronary circulation
- Increases blood/oxygen exchange to muscles
- Increases aerobic capacity
- Increases stroke volume (the amount of blood the heart ejects in one beat)
- Increases the functional capacity of asthmatics

RESPIRATORY SYSTEM

- Increases lung capacity
- Increases blood/oxygen exchange in the lungs
- Increases waste removal efficiency (carbon dioxide, or CO_2)
- Raises threshold for asthma-induced symptoms

MUSCULAR SYSTEM

- Increases muscular efficiency and coordination (neuromuscular benefit)
- Increases strength and/or endurance
- Increases muscle size (more so in men than women)
- Increases the ability of the muscles to use oxygen
- Increases fiber length (flexibility)

REPRODUCTIVE SYSTEM

- May enhance sexual pleasure because of increased muscular flexibility, endurance, and control
- May result in an improved ability to cope during delivery
- May result in a speedier recovery after giving birth

NERVOUS SYSTEM

- In combination with the muscular system, increases muscular efficiency and coordination
- Increases motor skill

OTHER

- Increases regular digestion and excretion
- Improves sleep quality
- Decreases risk of breast and colon cancer
- Decreases risk of non-insulin-dependent diabetes
- Improves the body's ability to use insulin
- Decreases body fat; improves body composition

PSYCHOLOGICAL BENEFITS

- Improves self-image, self-concept
- Decreases stress
- May decrease depression and anxiety
- Increases endorphins, sense of well-being
- May provide a means for increasing socialization

Source: J. G. Bishop and S. G. Aldana, *Step Up to Wellness: A Stage-Based Approach.* Copyright © 1999 by Allyn & Bacon. Reprinted by permission of Pearson Education, Inc.

There are two types of metabolic systems: aerobic and anaerobic. The type, intensity, and duration of activity you are engaged in determine how much energy is produced by each system. It is important to note that activities are not purely aerobic or anaerobic. When an activity is referred to as aerobic, that means the energy for movement is predominantly, but not exclusively, supplied by the aerobic system. When you perform exercises that emphasize the aerobic system, you get a different kind of conditioning than when you emphasize the anaerobic system. Familiarity with these systems can help you select activities that will lead toward your fitness goals.

ANAEROBIC METABOLISM

Anaerobic means "without oxygen."[2] During short, intense bursts of activity, such as running up a flight of stairs, the body cannot meet the muscles' demand for oxygen. For this situation, the body is equipped with two energy-producing systems that do not depend on oxygen: the phosphagen and lactic acid systems. These **anaerobic systems** are rapid sources of ATP for short periods of time. In a sense, the cells are making energy while they hold their breath.

PHOSPHAGEN SYSTEM   The most rapid anaerobic system is called the **phosphagen system.** This form of stored energy is used to get you going at the beginning of exercise, especially if you start quickly. It also allows you to leap out of your seat when someone yells "Free concert tickets!" Small amounts of high-energy phosphagens are stored directly in the muscle cell. As ATP is broken down, the high-energy phosphagens build it back up. The muscle can store only enough high-energy phosphagens to produce ATP for 1 to 6 seconds of activity. Training this system is important only if you want to participate in sports such as weight lifting or sprinting. The lactic acid and aerobic systems are much more important to lifetime fitness. As the phosphagen system is depleted, the lactic acid system takes over as the main energy producer.

LACTIC ACID SYSTEM   The **lactic acid system** (also known as **anaerobic glycolysis**) produces ATP by breaking down carbohydrate (glucose) without oxygen. Along with energy, **lactic acid** and heat are produced. If the anaerobic activity is intense enough, the lactic acid builds up and makes the muscle feel heavy and "burn." The buildup of lactic acid is associated with muscle exhaustion.

When you stop exercising or drop to a lower intensity, the concentration of lactic acid decreases. The excess heat is dissipated through sweat. You breathe hard after an anaerobic bout of exercise because your body requires oxygen to clear up the lactic acid and to return the cardiorespiratory system to homeostasis.

Activities that depend on the anaerobic metabolism for energy are usually short, intense, and powerful.

Predominantly anaerobic activities last for less than a minute. Sprints and strength-training exercises are examples of anaerobic exercises. Many exercises are partly anaerobic and partly aerobic. The lactic acid system also plays a major role in intense activities that last for 1 to 3 minutes. People like Bonnie Blair, an Olympic gold medalist in speed skating, who can perform well in a middle-distance event, must be in excellent condition both anaerobically and aerobically.

A number of exercise benefits are associated with anaerobic training. The most important are muscular strength and endurance and cardiorespiratory fitness. The latter is achieved using interval training, which involves a series of short intense bouts of exercise, such as sprints. Only short breaks are allowed between bouts. Since anaerobic training increases tolerance to lactic acid, someone in good anaerobic condition can sustain high-intensity activity longer than someone who is not.

AEROBIC METABOLISM

The **aerobic system** produces energy more slowly than the anaerobic systems, but it is capable of producing more energy per unit of food.[3] **Aerobic** means "with oxygen." The aerobic system breaks down carbohydrate **(aerobic glycolysis)** and fat **(fatty acid oxidation)** in the presence of oxygen to produce ATP (energy), carbon dioxide, water, and heat. Carbon dioxide is transported by the blood to the lungs, where it is exhaled from the body. Heat and water are released primarily through sweat.

It is easiest for the body to metabolize carbohydrate, so that is the primary source of fuel for the aerobic system. When the body is convinced that it will have to meet an elevated energy demand for a long period of time, it will conserve carbohydrate and use fat. It takes more energy to burn fat than carbohydrate, but fat is a much richer source of energy. The burning of fat is called fatty acid oxidation or beta oxidation.

Fatty acid oxidation must be coaxed into operation. To benefit from this process, you need to exercise for at least 20 minutes. If your goal is to burn fat, you would benefit more from exercising for a longer time at a moderate intensity than for a short time at a high intensity. High-intensity activities primarily burn carbohydrate, whereas low- to moderate-intensity activities burn both fat and carbohydrate. Low-intensity activities tend to burn a higher percentage of fat but also fewer calories per minute than moderate-intensity

---

2. Portions of this section also appear in J. G. Bishop and S. G. Aldana, *Step Up to Wellness: A Stage-Based Approach*, pp. 35–6. Copyright © 1999 by Allyn & Bacon. Reprinted by permission of Pearson Education, Inc.

3. Portions of this section also appear in J. G. Bishop and S. G. Aldana, *Step Up to Wellness: A Stage-Based Approach*, pp. 35–6. Copyright © 1999 by Allyn & Bacon. Reprinted by permission of Pearson Education, Inc.

activities. As a result, you must sustain a low-intensity activity for a longer period of time than a moderate one in order to burn the same amount of fat. For example, you would have to walk longer than jog to get the same fat-burning benefit.

Fat and carbohydrate are both being burned at rest and during exercise, but the percentages of each and the overall consumption of each vary with the intensity of activity. Although longer-duration activity is more apt to result in fat burning, any activity that burns calories will help prevent storage of fat. If you burn more calories than you take in, you will encourage fat loss and discourage fat storage. Exercise also increases your metabolism, which will stay elevated for a while burning some additional calories post-exercise.

Aerobic exercises are continuous, rhythmic activities using large-muscle groups. Swimming, cycling, brisk walking, cross-country skiing, and fast dancing are all aerobic activities.

THE CARDIOVASCULAR SYSTEM

To understand the cardiovascular system (heart, blood vessels, and blood) better, picture it as an elaborate grocery delivery and garbage removal system. The blood loads oxygen at the lungs, travels down the roadways of the arteries, and delivers it to the doorsteps of the cells. The cells take in the oxygen and other nutrients they need and unload waste products such as carbon dioxide into the blood. The blood then travels back toward the heart through the veins, unloading the waste products at the appropriate dump sites such as the lungs, liver, and kidneys. The heart is the pump that drives the whole system.

The speed of oxygen delivery and waste removal is controlled by the heart. When you start to exercise, your muscle cells call for more oxygen. Your heart picks up its pace so that oxygenated blood is moved to your cells more quickly. After exercise, your heart rate declines rapidly for 1 minute and then declines more slowly as your body reestablishes homeostasis (balance). During recovery, by-products such as lactic acid are removed or converted into other chemical forms. The more efficient your cardiovascular system, the more quickly the heart rate returns to a resting value.

The average healthy heart has a resting rate of 70 to 80 beats per minute (bpm). The amount of blood the heart ejects with one beat is called the **stroke volume.** The **cardiac output** is the amount of blood pumped out of the heart in 1 minute. Increasing either the heart rate or the stroke volume will increase the cardiac output. When you exercise, both the stroke volume and the heart rate increase, but the heart rate increases much more dramatically. Stroke volume increases to about 40% of maximum output; after that the increase in cardiac output is due to the heart rate. If the heart beats very fast, the stroke volume actually decreases because the chambers of the heart don't have enough time to completely fill.

Blood pressure is the pressure exerted by the blood against the walls of the arteries. When the heart is filling, the pressure in the arteries is fairly low. This is called the **diastolic pressure.** When the heart contracts, blood is forced out into the arteries, thus increasing the pressure of the blood against the arterial walls. This is called the **systolic pressure.** The body is infused with oxygen-rich blood during systole. Blood pressure is expressed as a fraction, with systolic pressure on top and diastolic pressure on the bottom. Resting blood pressure readings below 140/90 are considered normal.

When you exercise, your blood pressure rises because your heart contracts more often and pushes higher volumes of blood into your arteries. Healthy arteries stretch and can handle the extra blood flow without any problem. Blood pressure stays in a healthy range even with the added stress of exercise. To appreciate the ability of the arteries, imagine an airport or train station with hallways that can expand at prime time to accommodate the extra travelers. Diseases that harden the arteries (**arteriosclerosis**) or cause plaque buildup that narrows the arteries (**atherosclerosis**) cause the blood pressure to rise. Diseased arteries cannot withstand the same amount of stress as healthy arteries, so diseased arteries can severely limit your activity level.

Large arteries starting near the heart branch off into smaller and smaller arteries. The blood in the smallest arteries, called **capillaries,** delivers oxygen to the cells. The blood in the heart does not supply the heart with oxygen. Instead, small arteries that branch off the main artery near the heart take oxygen to the heart cells. These arteries are called **coronary arteries.** The heart is nourished with oxygen-rich blood during diastole through these coronary arteries.

Both aerobic and anaerobic exercise can improve cardiovascular fitness. However, to achieve cardiovascular fitness with anaerobic training, you must train at very high intensities. All-out efforts for short amounts of time are alternated with short rest periods. Many people find this kind of exercise difficult. In addition, it is too intense for beginners and older individuals. Aerobic dance exercise uses aerobic conditioning to achieve cardiovascular fitness. The more moderate intensity and continuous nature of aerobic conditioning seem to be more comfortable for most people. Because aerobic dance exercise uses aerobic conditioning to improve cardiovascular fitness, the benefits of cardiovascular training are discussed in terms of aerobic benefits.

BENEFITS OF EXERCISING THE CARDIOVASCULAR SYSTEM

The heart muscle becomes stronger with exercise. Like the skeletal muscles, the cardiac (heart) muscle can improve in strength. It increases a little in thickness and contracts with greater force. The stroke volume also increases, which means the heart can pump more blood with each beat or the same amount of blood with fewer beats. As a result, the resting heart rate (the rate at which the heart beats to sustain the body at rest) decreases. A few beats less per minute saves the heart a lot of beating over a lifetime.

The resting heart rate is influenced not only by the stroke volume, but also by other efficiency improvements in the circulatory system. People who are highly trained aerobically may have resting heart rates as low as 45 bpm. These are exceptional athletes. Among aerobic dance exercise veterans, it is not uncommon to hear about resting heart rates in the 60s, 50s, and even the 40s. Heredity also plays a role in establishing the resting heart rate. Some individuals who are not aerobically fit may have inherited a low resting heart rate. Similarly, some highly trained individuals have average (70 to 80 bpm) resting heart rates. But in general, as you train, your resting heart rate declines.

Exercise improves the ability of the cardiovascular system to deliver oxygen to the muscles. The ability of the blood to pick up and transport oxygen to the cells improves. The cells also improve in their ability to extract oxygen from the blood. The more oxygen you can supply to your cells and the more efficient your muscle cells become at using it, the longer you can exercise.

A trained individual can exercise longer and with less fatigue than an untrained individual. Think of two people in the same aerobics class working out at the same pace. The one in better shape is working out at a lower percentage of his or her maximum heart rate or aerobic capacity. In addition, the fit individual will enter into fatty acid oxidation more quickly than the unfit person.

Aerobic exercise also causes an increase in the number and size of mitochondria. Think of mitochondria as power plants located in the muscle cells. All aerobically generated energy is produced in the mitochondria. The mitochondria are more able to utilize fat as an energy source during exercise because the number of mitochondrial enzymes increases.

Imagine, for a moment, a city with only one main freeway. As rush hour hits, the freeway becomes congested. When an accident occurs, it stops traffic. Some cars head for the surface streets, but if these streets are inadequate, they too quickly get congested. However, if a city has a well-developed highway system and plenty of surface streets, traffic moves with ease even during peak hours.

Exercise increases the number of capillaries (surface streets) and, through cholesterol regulation, it helps keep the arteries (highways) clear. An increase in the number of capillaries means better oxygen/carbon dioxide exchange at the cellular level. It also means that when an artery becomes blocked, blood flow can be diverted to other healthy branches. This ability to divert blood flow is extremely important in the coronary network of arteries. Coronary circulation improves with endurance exercise: This helps prevent heart attacks.

Aerobic exercise increases the level of HDL (high-density lipoproteins) in your blood. HDL helps carry fat out of the bloodstream, which helps prevent it from forming plaque along the arterial walls. Plaque formation narrows arteries, thus restricting blood flow, raising blood pressure, and limiting stress-free activity. See the discussion on cholesterol in Chapter 12.

Evidence also indicates that exercise helps minimize the risk of having a heart attack and improves your chances of survival if you do have one. Improved cardiovascular fitness can also reduce stress-induced tension, alleviate depression for some individuals, and provide an overall sense of well-being.

THE RESPIRATORY SYSTEM

The respiratory system and the cardiovascular system work together to deliver oxygen to the cells. When you breathe in, you draw oxygen through the trachea and down the bronchial tubes into the lungs. The bronchi branch repeatedly and eventually become small alveolar ducts. At the ends of these ducts are numerous alveoli and alveolar sacs. It is between these alveoli and the tiny arteries and veins that oxygen and carbon dioxide are exchanged.

BENEFITS OF EXERCISING THE RESPIRATORY SYSTEM

Cardiorespiratory endurance exercises strengthen the respiratory muscles and increase the amount of air you can breathe into and out of your lungs (pulmonary ventilation). More surface area of the lung also becomes available for the exchange of oxygen and carbon dioxide. Each red blood cell has the capacity to carry one molecule of oxygen, yet blood is almost never 100% saturated. The blood moves by the lungs too quickly to load all the red blood cells with oxygen. Endurance training, however, can improve the blood's ability to load and unload oxygen.

THE SKELETAL SYSTEM

Each of the 206 bones in the human skeleton is a living entity. The bones you see when you look at a skeleton are dead. They give you a good idea of the shape and placement of living bones, but they do not represent live bone any more than the steak on your plate represents the living flesh of a cow. Living bones generate new bone tissue and repair and maintain healthy bone structure. Blood circulates through the bone tissue delivering nutrients.

BENEFITS OF EXERCISING THE SKELETAL SYSTEM

When you are active (walking, jumping, aerobic dancing, etc.), you stress your bones. The bones adapt by becoming stronger and more dense. Exercise helps prevent osteoporosis, a disease that causes bones to become porous and brittle. Osteoporosis is most common among postmenopausal women and is often the cause of broken hips or crushed vertebrae in elderly women. Proper nutritional care, particularly sufficient calcium intake, also plays an important role in preventing osteoporosis. As their life span increases, more men are developing osteoporosis. Men now represent one in every five cases. Exercise can help bone density increase during the young adult years and can help prevent bone loss in later years.

Although insufficient stress can cause bone weakening, too much stress can misshape, misalign, and even fracture a bone. The most common aerobic dance injury in this category is the lower leg stress fracture, which can be very painful and is so thin that it is difficult to observe on an X-ray image. Set reasonable levels of intensity, duration, and frequency, and buy good shoes to help prevent such an injury.

Good posture is vital for maintaining proper bone alignment. If you walk around with your shoulders forward, eventually your spine and shoulder girdle bones will adjust to that posture and make it impossible to stand straight. Poor posture also leads to muscular problems, aches, and pains. Think of posture and alignment throughout your aerobics class as well as during the day.

THE MUSCULAR SYSTEM

The three kinds of muscle are skeletal (striated), cardiac, and smooth. Skeletal muscles, attached to the bones by tendons, make it possible for us to move around; the heart is composed of cardiac muscle; and smooth muscle is found in internal organs. Both cardiac and smooth muscle are involuntary, which means they contract without conscious thought. You don't have to think about making your stomach wall contract during digestion, nor do you command your heart to beat. Skeletal muscles are voluntary: You make conscious decisions about how and when you want to move them. (Reflex movements of the skeletal muscles are the exception. During a reflex action, orders come from the spinal cord rather than the higher brain centers. The result is a very fast reaction that you don't consciously initiate.) Aerobic dance exercise develops both the cardiac and the skeletal muscles.

Muscles can only pull, not push; thus, they are paired together. One muscle pulls one way, the other muscle pulls the opposite way. When one is pulling, the other relaxes and stretches. The one doing the pulling is called the **agonist;** the one stretching is called the **antagonist.** When Popeye flexes his biceps, his lower arm is pulled closer to his upper arm. When he flexes his triceps (back of the upper arm), it pulls in the opposite direction, and his arm straightens out. When the biceps are working, the triceps are able to stretch and relax; when the triceps are working, the biceps are able to stretch and relax.

When you exercise muscles, it is important to work the muscle pairs equally. This way each stretches out the other, and strength balances are maintained. If you run on your toes throughout the aerobics section of a class, you have flexed (worked) your calf muscles the entire time. Stiffness will occur, and muscle imbalance may eventually lead to injury. Foot flexion exercises will work the muscles paired with the calf and allow the calf muscles to stretch. Because of this pairing, you can relieve a cramp in one muscle by flexing the opposite muscle: Relieve calf cramps by flexing the foot; relieve arch cramps by lifting up on the toes.

Don't confuse working a muscle with the pull of gravity or with the use of an eccentric (or negative) contraction. If you flex your arm using the biceps and then let it fall straight down, you are using gravity, not the triceps, to do the work. When you lower your arm slowly, the biceps are working in what is known as an eccentric contraction. An **eccentric contraction** is the controlled lengthening of a contracted muscle. You are using an eccentric contraction when you slowly lower a heavy box. Again, the triceps are not working. The opposite of an eccentric contraction is a concentric contraction. During a **concentric contraction,** the muscle is shortening. When you flex your arms, the biceps are doing a concentric contraction; they are shortening. Whether you are using concentric or eccentric contractions, you always want to move with control.

Muscles are composed of fibers. The power or strength of a contraction depends on how many muscle fibers are recruited by the nervous system. If you are doing something that takes all your strength, then most of the muscle fibers will contract at one time. If you are relaxing after class, only the fibers needed to maintain muscle tonus are used. Muscle tonus is the amount of tension needed in the muscle. During relaxation, only enough tension to maintain posture would be required.

Muscle spindles are specialized fibers that have stretch receptors. These spindles are responsible for the **stretch reflex.** When the muscle spindle's receptors are stretched suddenly, they send a signal to the spinal cord. The spinal cord sends back a message telling the surrounding muscle fibers to contract. The knee-jerk reflex is an example of this. When the doctor taps with a rubber hammer just below the knee, the patellar tendon, which attaches the thigh muscle to the bone, is suddenly stretched. The muscle spindles in the tendon react, the thigh muscle contracts, and the foot kicks.

Ballistic (bounce) **stretching** triggers the stretch reflex. Instead of relaxing and lengthening, the muscle gets the signal to contract. Proper **static stretching** does not excite the stretch receptors, so the muscle is able to relax and comfortably lengthen. Despite the stretch reflex, careful ballistic stretching can result in increased flexibility. However, it also carries a higher risk of tissue damage and muscle soreness than static stretching does.

Another kind of receptor, the Golgi tendon organ (GTO), sits among the muscle fibers. GTOs have high thresholds for tension, but if tension becomes too great during a muscle contraction, they alert the brain to send a back-off message to the muscles. The back-off or relax message actually stays in effect for a short while after the contraction is stopped. In **PNF** (proprioceptive neuromuscular facilitation) **stretching,** the response of the GTOs is purposefully elicited through an isometric contraction lasting 6 to 10 seconds. The muscle is stretched immediately after this contraction to take advantage of the relaxation phase induced by the GTO.

When the nervous system instructs a muscle to contract, it also alerts the antagonist (paired muscle) to relax. This is called reciprocal innervation. When you are trying to stretch a muscle, you can use reciprocal innervation by consciously contracting the opposing muscle. This is called **active** or **antagonist stretching.** For example, if you want to stretch your hamstring muscles, you can help them relax and lengthen by contracting your quadriceps muscles.

BENEFITS OF EXERCISING THE MUSCULAR SYSTEM
Muscles can improve in strength, endurance, and flexibility. The muscle-toning exercises used in aerobic dance exercise classes generally emphasize muscular endurance, but increases in strength can also occur, especially when exercise bands and weights are used. Flexibility is developed during the stretching segments of the class.

When muscles increase in strength, it may be the result of an increase in the size of the muscle fibers **(hypertrophy)** or improved neurological efficiency. For many years, it was believed that women's muscles did not hypertrophy like men's and that hormonal differences were the reason. Now, with better methods for measuring muscle tissue, we know that men's and women's muscles hypertrophy at the same rate. So why don't women get big muscles? The increase in muscle size is not as apparent in women's muscles because their muscle fibers are smaller than men's and therefore the percentage gain is less noticeable. To picture this, imagine doubling the size of both a needle and a pencil. The percentage gain (100%) is the same for both, but the size difference would be much more apparent for the pencil. Another factor is the higher quantity of fat women have stored between muscle fibers. If some of this fat, which is less dense than muscle, is lost at the same time that muscle size is gained, little or no difference in muscle circumference will occur. It is even possible to lose circumference and gain strength.

Gender hormonal differences may explain why women have smaller muscle fibers. It may also be that with prolonged training, women's bodies will tend toward strength gains through neuromuscular efficiency rather than by continued hypertrophy. More research is needed to answer these questions. One thing is clear: The vast majority of women do not build bulky muscles. A very small percentage of women may experience more hypertrophy than they desire. A change in training methods can resolve this problem. Men generally gain muscle size with strength training, but the amount of gain varies considerably between individuals and even between muscle groups in an individual. For example, a man may hypertrophy more in his shoulders than in his chest or vice versa even though he has trained both equally and has made similar strength gains in each.

You may experience a temporary increase in muscle size while you are exercising due to the increased amount of blood being pumped to the working muscle. Some refer to this as being "pumped." The size of the muscle will begin to decrease when you stop exercising and will return to normal when increased blood flow is no longer needed. Because most women's muscles are relatively small, this increase in size is not very apparent. However, if you are going to take body measurements, be sure to do so before or well after exercising.

Anabolic steroids are drugs that can be taken to enhance strength gains, but they have dangerous side effects. They are most often associated with strength training and/or sports competitions. Today, many competitions, including the Olympics, consider anabolic steroid use illegal. Clearly these drugs do not belong in a health-related program.

Muscle endurance improves with exercise because the muscle cells become more effective at extracting oxygen and other nutrients from the blood and using them in the production of cellular energy. The oxygen goes into a structure inside the cell called the mitochondrion. The mitochondrion is often called the powerhouse of the cell, since it is inside these little factories that simple sugars (carbohydrates after digestion) are converted into cellular energy (ATP). The muscle adapts to endurance exercise by increasing the number of mitochondria. More mitochondria mean more available ATP, which means more fuel for contractions. With more fuel available, movement (or exercise) can be sustained for a longer period of time. Think of all the ATP mitochondria must produce for an hour of aerobics. Or for a marathon run!

Improving strength, endurance, and flexibility results in greater work efficiency, an improved ability to meet emergencies, and a decreased chance of lower back pain and injury.

OTHER SYSTEMS

Other systems affected by exercise include the nervous and reproductive systems. The nervous system is a fantastic communications system. Electrical impulses speed along nerve pathways delivering messages from the brain and spinal column. Aerobic conditioning improves the coordination of these transmissions, which results in an ability to react with more speed, coordination, and strength. Skill and coordination improve as you learn which muscles to stimulate and which to inhibit. A clear example is the difference between a beginning and an advanced swimmer. Beginners use practically every muscle in their bodies to stay afloat. The advanced swimmer uses only the necessary muscles. Beginning aerobics students experience a similar effect. They may start out feeling clumsy, but they quickly improve.

The effect of exercise on the reproductive system is difficult to study. Some researchers believe that exercise enhances sexual pleasure because of increased muscular strength and control. Two more serious issues regarding the effect of exercise on the reproductive system include the temporary loss of menstruation that sometimes occurs during high-level aerobic training and the effects of exercise on pregnancy. This loss of menstruation seems to be reversible, and a training regimen of lower intensity is recommended for women trying to conceive.

Guidelines for pregnancy and exercise have been published by the American College of Obstetricians and Gynecologists (ACOG). Exercise is healthy before, during, and after pregnancy for most women. A pregnant woman should consult her physician concerning the amount and type of exercise she can perform. There is some evidence that babies born to exercising mothers have fewer birth defects and that the mother's recovery time is faster. Women interested in exercising through pregnancy should start exercising before they become pregnant. For more information concerning exercise and pregnancy, see Chapter 2.

OVERVIEW OF A WORKOUT

Exercise workouts are made up of several different components. This quick overview explains what you can expect as you begin your exercise class. Each of the components is discussed in much more detail in the chapters ahead. The workout begins with a 5- to 10-minute warm-up. During the warm-up, you will be doing easy, large-muscle activities to get your body warm and your heart beating a little faster. The warm-up also generally includes some stretches to ready your muscles to move through a good range of motion. The intensity of the warm-up should gradually increase until by the end you are just entering the intensity of exercise needed for the aerobic component.

The aerobic component consists of a variety of aerobic steps combined into a routine. Routines generally follow a 32–64 count pattern, which is taught in segments. Many styles and types of movements can be incorporated into these routines, making them a lot of fun to do. During the aerobic workout phase, you will be asked to monitor your intensity level using either heart rate, a talk test, or ratings of perceived exertion. You will receive instructions on how to do this early in the course, and worksheets are available at the back of your book. The aerobic workout (approximately 20–30 minutes long) is followed by a standing cool-down. During this component, your exercise intensity is slowly brought down. Resistance, or muscle-toning, exercises (15–20 minutes) are generally performed after the standing cool-down, although they can also be done after the warm-up and before the aerobics. These exercises are followed by some stretching (5–10 minutes) and, time permitting, some mind–body relaxation exercises. Music accompanies all of the class components. It is a great motivator for the workout portions and can be soothing and relaxing for the cool-down and stretch.

You only need a few things to be ready for class. Bring a positive attitude, some cool water to drink, a good pair of shoes, comfortable clothing that moves with you, and a towel if you sweat a lot or want one to put under you at times. Mats, ball, weights, steps, or other equipment is usually provided by the school unless otherwise specified.

SUMMARY

Wellness is both an attitude and a way of living. To be completely well, you must be in good physical, social, emotional, intellectual, and spiritual health. Individuals who practice healthy lifestyle habits will enjoy a higher quality of life and a reduced risk of disease and premature illness. Exercise, in addition to enhancing physical wellness, has a positive effect on the other four wellness components. For this reason, it is one of the most powerful lifestyle changes you can make. At the same time, it is recognized that change is not always easy and that people in different stages of readiness to change require different strategies. Behavior changes are most successful when you have "bought in," when you feel that the change is important for you. We are living in the information age; knowing how and why something works enables you to decide if it is important and relevant to you. Knowing how the body works and how exercise works on the body enhances your ability to make informed decisions. You can choose the benefits that are important to you and make sure that the exercises that result in those benefits are included in your exercise program. Staying active is the key to physical wellness, and aerobic dance exercise is a great way to do it.

KNOWLEDGE TIPS

1. Wellness is a way of life that involves taking responsibility for one's own well-being and practicing lifestyle habits that promote physical, social, emotional, mental, and spiritual health.

2. To lead a wellness lifestyle, you must be engaged in attitudes and behaviors that enhance quality of life and maximize personal potential.

3. Exercise is the remedy to inactivity, one of the heart disease risk factors. Exercise also helps to reduce the incidence of other risk factors, including obesity, hypertension, and high cholesterol.

4. Living a healthy lifestyle lowers your risk of premature death.

5. Exercise enhances all of the wellness components, albeit with a special emphasis on physical health.

6. Exercise causes short-term or acute responses, including an increased heart rate, increased systolic blood pressure, increased ventilation, and increased sweating.

7. Exercise causes long-term or chronic adaptations when it is done repeatedly over a period of time.

8. Aerobic exercises (continuous, rhythmic activities using large-muscle groups) use carbohydrate and fat for fuel.

9. Anaerobic exercises (intense activities of short duration) use carbohydrate for fuel.

10. The benefits of aerobically training the cardiovascular system include increased stroke volume, increased cardiac muscle strength, decreased resting heart rate, decreased blood pressure in individuals with hypertension, increased aerobic capacity, increased coronary circulation, decreased risk of heart disease, increased work capacity, increased level of HDL, increased oxygen delivery to the muscles, increased numbers of capillaries, and an increased number of mitochondria.

11. Two benefits of training the respiratory system are increased lung capacity and an increased ability to deliver oxygen to the blood.

12. The benefits of training the muscular system include increased strength, increased muscular endurance, increased flexibility, increased work capacity, decreased risk of lower back pain, and decreased risk of injury.

13. Some benefits of training the skeletal system are increased bone density, maintenance of good posture, and decreased risk of bone injury.

14. Other benefits of exercise include decreased mental tension, improved self-image, increased sense of well-being, regular digestion and excretion, improved sexual pleasure, and improved coordination and skill.

15. An aerobic dance exercise class consists of the following components: warm-up, aerobic workout, standing cool-down, muscle strength and endurance exercises, stretching, and relaxation.

THINK ABOUT IT

1. What does living a wellness lifestyle mean?

2. What are the benefits of being physically active?

3. How much exercise or physical activity is enough?

4. What is the difference between aerobic and anaerobic metabolism?

5. What type of activities draw predominantly on the aerobic system? the anaerobic system?

6. Why are people more successful at making behavior changes when they use the transtheoretical model for behavior change?

7. What strategies help you stick with a program when you are in the action phase?

8. What are the components of an aerobic dance exercise class?

REFERENCES

American Alliance for Health, Physical Education, Recreation, and Dance. *Health Related Physical Fitness: Test Manual.* Reston, VA: American Alliance for Health, Physical Education, Recreation, and Dance, 1980.

American College of Sports Medicine. *ACSM's Guidelines for Exercise Testing and Exercise Prescription.* 8th ed. Media, PA: Lippincott Williams & Wilkins, 2010.

American College of Sports Medicine. "The Recommended Quantity and Quality of Exercise for Developing and Maintaining Cardiorespiratory and Muscle Fitness in Healthy Adults." *Medicine and Science in Sports and Exercise* 30 (No. 6, 1998): 975–91.

Blair, S. N. "Physical Activity, Physical Fitness, and Health." *Research Quarterly for Exercise and Sport* 64 (December 1993): 365–76.

Boyer, J. L. "Effects of Chronic Exercise on Cardiovascular Function." *Physical Fitness Research Digest* 2 (1972): 1.

Cooper, K. H. *Aerobics.* New York: Bantam Books, 1968.

Corbin, C. B., G. Welk, W. R. Corbin, and K. A. Welk. *Concepts of Physical Fitness: Active Lifestyles for Wellness.* 14th ed. New York: McGraw-Hill Higher Education, 2006.

Editors of the University of California at Berkeley Wellness Letter, *The New Wellness Encyclopedia,* New York: Houghton Mifflin, 1995.

Estivill, M. "Therapeutic Aspects of Aerobic Dance Participation." *Health Care for Women International* 16 (No. 4, 1995): 341–50.

Fahey, T. D., P. M. Insel, and W. T. Roth. *Fit and Well: Core Concepts and Labs in Physical Fitness and Wellness.* 8th ed. New York: The McGraw-Hill Companies, 2009.

Hoeger, W. W. K., and S. A. Hoeger. *Lifetime Physical Fitness and Wellness: A Personalized Program.* 9th ed. Belmont, CA: Thompson Wadsworth, 2007.

Housh, T. J., D. J. Housh, and H. A. deVries. *Applied Exercise and Sport Physiology.* 2nd ed. Scottsdale, AZ: Holcomb Hathaway Publishers, 2006.

Imm, P. S. "Perceived Benefits of Participants in an Employees' Aerobic Fitness Program." *Perceptual and Motor Skills* 71 (December 1990): 753–4.

Jordan, P. *Fitness Theory and Practice.* Sherman Oaks, CA: Aerobics and Fitness Association of America, 1993.

Kannel, W. B., and P. Sorlie. "Some Health Benefits of Physical Activity: The Framingham Study." *Archives of Internal Medicine* 139 (1979): 857–61.

Kraus, H., and W. Raab. *Hypokinetic Disease.* Springfield, IL: C. C. Thomas, 1961.

Mathews, D. K., and E. L. Fox. *The Physiological Basis of Physical Education and Athletics.* Philadelphia: W. B. Saunders, 1976.

Paffenbarger, R. S., and R. T. Hyde. "Exercise as Protection Against Heart Attack." *New England Journal of Medicine* 302 (1980): 1026.

Paffenbarger, R. S., R. T. Hyde, A. L. Wing, and C. Hsieh. "Physical Activity, All-Cause Mortality, and Longevity of College Alumni." *New England Journal of Medicine* 314 (1986): 605–13.

Pate, R. R., et al. "Physical Activity and Public Health, a Recommendation from the Centers for Disease Control and Prevention and the American College of Sports Medicine." *Journal of the American Medical Association* 273 (No. 5, 1995): 402–7.

Pollock, M. L. "How Much Exercise Is Enough?" *The Physician and Sportsmedicine* 6 (No. 6, 1978): 50–6; 58–60; 63–4.

———. *Exercise in Health and Disease.* Philadelphia: W. B. Saunders, 1984.

Pollock, M. L., and S. N. Blair. "Analysis into Action: Exercise Prescription." *Journal of Physical Education and Recreation* 52 (No. 1, 1981): 30–5, 81.

Pollock, M. L., J. H. Wilmore, and S. M. Fox. *Health and Fitness Through Physical Activity.* New York: John Wiley & Sons, 1978.

Prochaska, J. O., and C. diClemente. "Toward a Comprehensive Behavior Change." In *Treating Addictive Behaviors,* W. Miller and N. Heather, eds. New York: Plenum, 1986.

Smith, E. L. "Exercise for Prevention of Osteoporosis: A Review." *The Physician and Sportsmedicine* (No. 3, 1982): 72–83.

Thomsen, D., and D. L. Ballor. "Physiological Responses During Aerobic Dance of Individuals Grouped by Aerobic Capacity and Dance Experience." *Research Quarterly for Exercise and Sport* 62 (March 1991): 68–72.

U.S. Department of Health and Human Services. *Physical Activity and Health: A Report of the Surgeon General.* Centers for Disease Control and Prevention, National Center for Chronic Disease Prevention and Health Promotion. Atlanta: The President's Council on Physical Fitness and Sports, 1996.

———. 2008 *Physical Activity Guidelines for Americans.* U.S. Department of Health and Human Services, 2008.

Watterson, V. V. "The Effects of Aerobic Dance on Cardiovascular Fitness." *The Physician and Sportsmedicine* 12 (No. 10, 1984): 138–45.

White, T. P., and Editors of the University of California at Berkeley Wellness Letter. *The Wellness Guide to Lifelong Fitness.* Rebus, NY: Random House, 1993.

Williford, H. N., M. Scharff-Olson, and D. L. Blessing. "The Physiological Effects of Aerobic Dance: A Review." *Sports Medicine* 8 (No. 6, December 1989): 335–45.

Wilmore, J. H. and Costill, D. L. *Physiology of Sport and Exercise.* 3rd ed. Champaign, IL: Human Kinetics, 2004.

2

Individual Differences: Let's Talk About You

"I never looked at asthma, my condition, as being a handicap. My attitude was to beat asthma. I wasn't going to allow asthma to get the best of me."

JACKIE JOYNER-KERSEE

- Is there such a thing as a one-size-fits-all exercise program?
- Should I exercise if I have a health condition such as asthma or diabetes?
- What should I do if an exercise doesn't feel good or is hard for me?

EVEN though the information in this text is based on research and on strategies and techniques practiced by numerous professionals, exercise programs can and should be adjusted to accommodate each individual's needs. Research works with statistical measures such as the "mean" or "average" score, but people are not statistics; they can be average, above or below average, or above in one way and below in another. Sometimes, what is good for the "average" participant or for the "majority of" participants requires adjustments to meet individual needs. You, your instructor, and a health care professional (as needed) can work together to custom design the optimal program for you. Here is an example of this type of teamwork.

A student confided in her instructor that for years she had tried to do a proper curl-up but still couldn't get her back to round sufficiently. Partway through the curl-up, most of her back would lift off the floor as a unit. This put considerable stress on her lower back and resulted in back pain. The problem appeared to be more than weak abdominal muscles. A consultation with her physician revealed that two bones in her lower spine were fused. Armed with this information, her instructor modified the curl-up. When performing on a mat, the student was instructed to pull lightly with her hands underneath her thighs at the point where she felt her lower back engage. The instructor also used a pilates approach to help the student gain as much rounding (mobility) of the spine as possible. Finally, the instructor suggested that the student perform curl-ups on a stability ball so that her back was supported on a comfortable surface throughout the movement. These adaptations allowed the student to reduce the stress on her lower back and to strengthen her abdominal muscles safely and effectively.

If you experience a problem with part of your exercise program, talk with your instructor or physician and as a team develop a safe and effective program.

Blindly following someone else's exercise program or technique is usually not a good idea. Aerobic dance exercise students often fall into the habit of imitating every movement the instructor makes. Instructors joke about how a whole class will follow their movements to wipe hair out of their eyes or scratch an itch. One day, as a test, I instructed my class in the hazards of exercises such as deep knee bends and then proceeded to put a series of these "bad" exercises into the routines. To my dismay, most of my class followed along.

Here is another story, with a twist, to illustrate the importance of paying attention to individual differences: A track coach once told me that for years the many high-jump coaches and athletes who carefully studied and copied the exact form of 1968 Olympic high-jump champion Dick Fosbury, the creator of the "Fosbury Flop," cheated themselves of jumping height by unwittingly imitating poor head positioning. He explained that Fosbury had hurt his neck high jumping into sawdust before the days of foam pits and, as a result, kept his neck in a protective rather than optimal position. I have had the opportunity to talk with Dick Fosbury, and guess what? Chuckling, he informed me that the story isn't true at all, but he quickly added that the point of the story is very true. According to Fosbury, he was not successful at imitating other great high jumpers of his day. He was able to achieve his gold medal height only by accommodating his body type and abilities and inventing (evolving) a new way to jump. Fosbury added that he believes strongly in studying and learning from other successful people; he does not believe that we can imitate perfectly what someone else does, nor should we try. Instead, real success comes when we take into account our individual differences and make the appropriate adjustments. On rare occasions, an individual's "adjustments," like Dick Fosbury's, revolutionize how something is done; in most cases, only slight variations or adjustments are needed.

In aerobic dance exercise, there are a number of situations that require individuals to make adjustments in order to optimize their workouts. Here are just a few examples.

- A student's fitness level may differ from the level of workout being presented. In this case, intensity can be increased or decreased by techniques described in Chapters 8 to 10, such as increasing or decreasing arm work or amplitude (i.e., "largeness" of movements) during aerobics, or increasing or decreasing the amount of weight used during resistance training.

- A student with an injury or physical disability may require modification of an exercise or exercise position. For instance, a person with a sore shoulder may need to eliminate overhead arm movements. A person with a hearing impairment may need louder music, preferential positioning near the instructor, and hand cues as well as verbal cues from the instructor.

- An overweight student may discover that the jumping in high-impact aerobics is too hard on his or her joints. In most cases, moderate- or low-impact movements can be easily substituted for high-impact movements. Additional options would be to switch to water aerobics or to use a cardiorespiratory endurance machine like an elliptical trainer or a rower.

- As a woman's pregnancy advances, she needs to make adjustments in her workout to ensure the safety of the fetus and to provide personal comfort.

- A person on medications that affect heart rate will need to substitute ratings of perceived exertion (see Chapter 4) for pulse monitoring to estimate exercise intensity.

Good aerobic dance instructors will demonstrate how to perform exercises at several levels of intensity to accommodate students who range from less fit beginners to highly fit advanced students. It is important for individuals to learn which of the demonstrated levels of intensity is appropriate for them and to be aware that the correct level of intensity will vary according to the type of exercise being performed. Although instructors present many modifications and levels, some individual modifications may not be demonstrated to the whole class. Instructors have to be careful of demonstrating advanced moves and positions in a class of mixed abilities because too often students, regardless of fitness level, follow every movement of the instructor. If you require modifications not presented by the instructor, be sure to ask for help. An instructor will happily share ways with you, one on one, to increase (or decrease) the intensity of your program.

Your experience with aerobic dance exercise and your age can both influence the type of program you want and need. Veterans are more apt to want variety and challenging step combinations, whereas beginners are happy when instructors stay with simple combinations and lots of repetition. People who have taken classes for a while with one instructor become accustomed to that person's patterns and sequences and may find it difficult, at least initially, to follow a new instructor. Age differences can involve everything from goals to music tastes. College students in their twenties want different things out of their exercise programs than do students in their forties or sixties. As your goals change, so too should your program.

Gender raises a number of exercise programming issues. Women need special considerations for exercising during pregnancy or the discomfort of menstruation. The average man has more strength than a woman, especially in the upper body, and may need different exercises or more resistance during exercises to improve strength. Different movements may make men and women feel uncomfortable exercising. Men, for example, may feel self-conscious handling dance steps, whereas women may be embarrassed when they can't perform a full set of a muscle endurance exercise. As with all gender issues, there is a certain amount of crossover—women who feel they have two left feet and men who can't do a push-up yet, for example.

Music preference also plays a role in how much an individual enjoys an aerobics class. Some instructors use a wide variety of music; others concentrate on one type of music. Many use music sets that are specially produced for aerobics classes, with a mix of songs set to a steady beat. The music and class style can range from salsa to funk to rock and roll to swing to country-western to boxing jabs and kicks. Most instructors are open to music suggestions, but don't expect an instructor to use your music immediately; it takes some time to put together an effective routine. When choice is available, look for an instructor who uses a style and type of music that makes *you* want to get up and move.

Injury or disabilities may limit you from performing certain exercises. Many times there are simple substitutions, alternative positions, or even alternative activities that you can perform while the class performs the original action. Some conditions, such as hearing loss, may require bringing in resources such as an interpreter, or having the instructor wear a microphone. Most college campuses are equipped to handle these situations; sometimes you just have to ask the question.

Some things in this text are necessarily based on the "average" person. For example, research tells us that the fastest our heart can beat can be estimated by plugging our age into a formula. The newest formula (see Chapter 4) estimates a 20-year-old's maximum heart rate to be 206 beats per minute. Some 20-year-olds, however, have maximum heart rates greater than 230 bpm, whereas others cannot exceed 170 bpm. This does not mean that the formula should be thrown out—it provides a good estimate for most people—but it does mean that for a few people some fine-tuning will be required.

The remainder of this chapter describes some of the special conditions for which modifications can and should be made to a standard aerobic dance exercise class.

EXERCISE AND BACK CARE

An alarmingly high number of people experience lower back pain at some time in their lives. Strong, flexible muscles, good posture, and good exercise techniques can all help prevent lower back pain. If you already suffer from chronic back pain, it is important to start with a medical examination to determine the underlying cause(s). When appropriate, the doctor or physical therapist will provide you with exercises to alleviate pain and correct muscular weakness and inflexibility. It is also important to know which exercises you should avoid. Inform your instructor, and establish a time during class when you can do your prescribed exercises.

When the hamstring (back of thigh) muscles are too tight, they pull the pelvis down, thus rounding your lower back. When the hip flexor (front of thigh) muscles are inflexible, they pull the pelvis forward, thus causing a swayback. Both of these positions cause lower back pain. A good stretching program can alleviate these problems. Weak abdominal muscles and poor posture are the other two biggest culprits in back pain—both of which can be corrected with proper exercise, attention and awareness, and correction of your posture during daily tasks. There are tips throughout the text on how to properly care for your back, including a set of guidelines for back care in Chapter 6, but here is a summary of some of the most important points.

1. When standing for any length of time, stand with your knees slightly bent.
2. When standing or sitting, keep your pelvis in a neutral position that allows normal (not exaggerated) curvatures of the spine.
3. Stabilize your back during exercises by contracting your abdominal muscles.
4. Avoid leaning forward or backward with a straight back and without support.
5. Strengthen your abdominal and back muscles.
6. Develop good flexibility in both the hamstrings and hip flexors (quadriceps and iliopsoas).
7. Use your legs when lifting heavy objects.
8. Turn with your feet, not your waist, when putting down heavy objects.
9. Carry heavy objects close to your body.
10. And finally, here is one exercise you can—and should!—perform anywhere, anytime: Tuck your chin in and pull your shoulders back slightly. You will feel immediate relief in your upper back and neck.

EXERCISE AND ASTHMA

Asthma is a condition in which the muscles surrounding the airways constrict, thus causing shortness of breath, wheezing, and coughing. Allergies, infections, emotion, air temperature, and exercise can trigger an attack. When exercise is the trigger, it is called exercise-induced asthma (EIA). The labored breathing caused by bronchial constriction may discourage people with asthma from exercising. However, people with controlled asthma can—and should—exercise. Here are some of the benefits of exercising with controlled asthma.

- Tolerance to exercise increases. Research has shown that for most people with asthma, aerobic exercise improves their cardiorespiratory system, which, in turn, raises the exertion level at which symptoms begin to occur. This means that a person with asthma can be more physically active while experiencing fewer difficulties.

- Boosts self-esteem and self-confidence. Being able to do something good for your body and being able to perform as well (or better) than others boosts self-esteem. Individuals with asthma often get trapped into a downward cycle of reducing activity each time symptoms appear. This ultimately results in an inactive lifestyle. As individuals successfully work out, self-confidence grows. Amy Van Dyken, four-time Olympic gold medalist in swimming; Jackie Joyner-Kersee, triple Olympic track and field gold medalist; Bill Koch, America's Cup champion in cross-country skiing; Mary Jo Fernandez, two-time Olympic gold medalist and pro in tennis; and Jerome "The Bus" Bettis, all-pro running back for the Pittsburgh Steelers, all have asthma. These people are inspiring, but remember that anyone, not just world champions, can enjoy the benefits of exercise and feel good about themselves.
- Allows the person to gain all the wellness benefits of regular exercise.

If you have asthma, consult with your physician before beginning an exercise program, then share pertinent information with your instructor. If you experience EIA, try to recognize early symptoms and then lower your intensity or take a break as needed. If you use bronchodilator medication, bring your inhaler to class, let your instructor know where it is prior to each session, and use it at the first sign of wheezing. Taking medications prior to vigorous exercise may help prevent EIA. Check with your physician concerning your medications.

Here are some additional tips for exercising with controlled asthma.

1. Use a long warm-up. Symptoms often occur in the first 15 minutes. A longer warm-up allows you to ease into the activity and to handle any symptoms that might occur. Try to schedule your exercise classes/activities so that you can arrive early and begin to warm up ahead of time as needed. A good warm-up, even if you have symptoms, often leads to a period of time when more intense exercise can be performed with fewer problems.
2. If the continuous nature of an aerobic dance exercise doesn't work for you, as it doesn't for some people with asthma, try doing an interval approach. Do a series of 5 minutes of workout alternated with rest or walking in place. Discuss this with your instructor and physician.
3. Be particularly careful on days when environmental conditions are more likely to trigger an attack, such as days when it is hot or cold, or when there is a high pollen count or smog alert. Avoid exercising in an environment that triggers your asthma.
4. Drink plenty of fluids.
5. Increase the length of the cool-down as needed. EIA attacks can occur after exercise as well as during it. A good cool-down helps. Try to schedule your exercise classes/activities so that you have ample time to cool down.
6. Be prepared in the event of an asthmatic attack, and educate those around you so that they can get you assistance, if needed.
7. Do not exercise if you are experiencing symptoms such as wheezing prior to class.
8. Consider water aerobics. Most people with asthma have fewer symptoms in the moist, warm air of an indoor pool.
9. Set an appropriate exercise intensity and duration in consultation with your physician and instructor, and then work to gradually increase your symptom-free exercise time.

EXERCISE AND OBESITY

We know that one of the greatest health concerns in the United States is obesity, and we know that exercise along with good nutrition can help reduce it. Yet, many exercise programs do not make overweight individuals feel comfortable. Here are some guidelines that can help you if you are overweight and in an aerobic dance exercise class. Also see the box, Do I Belong Here?

1. Feel no compulsion to keep up. It is critical that you work at an intensity that will allow you to keep going rather than start hurting and want to quit. Use low-intensity versions of movements. Walk in place if the steps are too hard. Take rests as needed. You may only be able to do a few minutes of activity in a row—that's okay. Endurance will come.
2. Enjoy the music, and use little movements to feel connected to the workout when you are resting. Keep time with your head and shoulders. Tap your toe.
3. Lower the workout intensity by eliminating or decreasing the size of arm movements as needed—especially those above shoulder height.
4. Avoid movements that create joint pain. Work toward smooth fluid movements rather than bouncy ones. Ask the instructor for alternative exercises if one is uncomfortable.
5. Consider using some of the cardio machines that are easy on the joints for cross-training

DO I BELONG HERE?

One overweight student confessed that when she went on vacation, she visited a club to take a step class. She had been enjoying an intermediate step class at home, but when she walked into this class, she felt as though everyone questioned whether she could handle the class. She assured them she could. At the end of the class, some well-meaning members congratulated her on doing so well but said it in such a way that it had the "you did a great job considering how heavy you are" feeling to it. She just wanted to enjoy an hour of exercise.

How about this guy on his first day of class? He's concerned he'll be expected to wear form-fitting clothes, and he's not sure his form is something he's ready to share. He wonders whether others will question why he signed up. He can't do the basic steps without getting confused, and what if everyone is watching when he only completes 3 out of 10 push-ups? Maybe, he thinks . . . I'll drop this class.

Everyone belongs!! Here are a few ideas that might make you feel more comfortable.

- Sign up for class with a supportive friend.

- Look around at others, and smile. You'll find when you look up that "the whole class" isn't looking right at you and that the ones you smile at will either become new friends or stare less.

- Position yourself to one side so that you can see the instructor and most of your classmates well. This way you are watching them instead of the reverse.

- Proclaim improvements and make positive comments about getting through the class. Others will likely start to agree and cheer you on.

- Modify exercises so that you can complete them. Or do one move for every two or three that the instructor does. This will let you keep going and finish with the group.

- If you tire easily, walk in place, tap your toe, or move your arms to the music.

- Don't want to wear the form-fitting attire? How about a t-shirt that says something like, "I'm here for my health, what are you here for?" Or "Are you looking at me?" Or, "Wow, look at me!" or something even better you think up.

- Socialize. You'll find others will enjoy a word of encouragement, too.

on days you don't have aerobics class. The elliptical trainer, stationary bike, and recumbent stepper (performed in a sitting position) are all good choices.

6. Water activities are also excellent cross-training activities that reduce joint strain and prevent overheating. If you are self-conscious in a bathing suit, wear a big t-shirt and exercise shorts in the water.

7. Perform resistance training exercises to increase strength and stamina so that daily tasks such as climbing stairs become easier. Again, avoid exercises or weight loads that aggravate your joints.

8. Find a supportive exercise partner. It helps when you have someone to go to class with or meet there who is looking forward to seeing you.

9. Remind yourself that research shows that overweight and fit individuals have less health risk than the lean and unfit.

10. Know that you can look good exercising. Queen Latifah is a big woman, and her moves are smooth!

If you don't feel well exercising, check with your physician. Obese and overweight individuals are at risk for other health problems such as diabetes and arthritis. Exercise is still usually recommended, but additional adjustments may be needed. (Obesity, weight management, and nutrition are further discussed and defined in Chapter 12.)

EXERCISE AND DIABETES

Diabetes mellitus is a group of metabolic diseases in which the pancreas fails to produce sufficient insulin (Type I) or the body is unable to effectively use the insulin it does produce (Type II). Insulin's role is to regulate the amount of sugar **(glucose)** in the blood and move the sugar into cells when it is needed. Muscle cells, for example, use the glucose to produce energy for movement.

If diabetes is untreated, the blood sugar can reach dangerously low, or high, concentrations. If blood sugar drops too low, a person becomes hypoglycemic. This can be caused by taking too much diabetic medicine, delaying or missing a meal, exercising more than normal, or drinking alcoholic beverages. When hypoglycemic, a

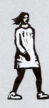

WORKOUT TIPS FOR PEOPLE WITH DIABETES

If you have diabetes, make sure to do the following when you exercise.

- Get a thorough medical exam before you start a new exercise plan.

- Watch for low blood glucose levels. If you take insulin or oral diabetes medicine, you may have low blood sugar during, immediately after, or up to 12 hours following exercise. Medications can be adjusted to prevent this. Careful monitoring of blood glucose may be required before, during, and after exercise.

  Update your exercise plan regularly with your doctor. Regular exercise may result in a need for less insulin or lower doses of diabetes pills. Your doctor can also teach you how to adjust your medicine for the days when you perform a different exercise plan.

BEFORE EXERCISE

- Ask your health care team whether you should check your blood glucose level before exercising.

- If you take diabetes medicines that can cause low blood glucose, ask your health care team whether you should
  - change the amount you take before you exercise
  - have a snack if your blood glucose level is below 100

DURING EXERCISE

- Wear your medical identification (ID) bracelet or necklace or carry your ID in your pocket.

- Always carry food or glucose tablets so you'll be ready to treat low blood glucose.

- If you'll be exercising for more than an hour, check your blood glucose at regular intervals. You may need snacks before you finish.

AFTER EXERCISE

- Check to see how exercise affected your blood glucose level.

Source: http://www.diabetes.niddk.nih.gov/dm/pubs/physical_ez/index.htm.

person should eat an easily digested carbohydrate or glucose tablets and get the blood sugar up before exercising.

If blood sugar is too high, the person becomes hyperglycemic and needs insulin. Hyperglycemia can happen if a person with diabetes misses a dose of diabetes medicine, eats too much, or doesn't get enough medicine. Infection, illness, and stress can also raise blood sugar. When blood sugar is not controlled, a person has a higher risk of serious diseases such as kidney failure, nerve disorders, eye problems, and heart disease.

People with Type I (insulin-dependent) diabetes control their glucose levels through diet, exercise, and insulin injections or an insulin pump. The vast majority of people with diabetes have Type II (non–insulin-dependent) diabetes. Some people with Type II diabetes can control their blood sugar using a good exercise and diet regimen. These individuals seldom have a low blood glucose problem. Other people with Type II diabetes need to augment their body's production of insulin with either oral medication or injections.

People with diabetes should exercise for several important reasons.

- Aerobic exercise helps make muscle cells more permeable to glucose. This means that glucose can more easily leave the bloodstream and enter the muscle cell where it can be used for energy.

- Aerobic exercise seems to allow the body to be more effective at using available insulin.
- Exercise helps control body weight and composition. Most people with Type II diabetes are overweight.
- Exercise helps reduce the amount of cholesterol and other fats circulating in the blood, thus effectively lowering an otherwise elevated risk for heart disease.
- Regular, moderate exercise helps a person with diabetes maintain normal blood glucose levels and, in some cases, may reduce the amount of insulin a person needs to take. Any changes should, of course, be made under the guidance of a physician.

If you have diabetes and are starting an exercise program, get a thorough medical examination and discuss your exercise plan with your health care team. You will probably be able to take part in both aerobic and light resistance training (weight training) exercise. In some cases, the bouncing nature of aerobic dance exercise is not recommended. When you are cleared for exercise, you will need to make ongoing adjustments to your exercise, meals, and medicines as you get in shape. You will want to follow all of the normal exercise procedures of warming up and working at an appropriate intensity, but you will also need to add some additional safety steps that take your diabetes into account. You should stay well hydrated and take extra good care of your feet. Wear good aerobic or cross-trainer shoes, wear good smooth socks that wick away moisture, keep your feet dry and free of athlete's foot, and inspect them frequently. See the Workout Tips for People with Diabetes box for some safety tips concerning blood sugar monitoring. Report any problems to a doctor immediately. And finally, keep your instructor informed so that you can work together to provide you with the best exercise experience.

EXERCISE AND PREGNANCY

Exercise is a positive health habit that, in most cases, can be continued through pregnancy. It is important, however, to recognize the demands pregnancy places on a woman's body and to make adjustments accordingly. It is better to start an exercise program before pregnancy, but it is certainly possible to begin with light exercising during pregnancy. Women who have been exercising regularly prior to conception may be able to continue in a regular aerobic dance exercise class, as long as they make appropriate adjustments to their intensity and avoid contraindicated exercises. As pregnancy advances, many women prefer to take a class specifically designed for pregnant women or continue with a non-weight-bearing activity such as cycling or swimming. If you are pregnant or considering pregnancy, discuss an exercise plan with your physician.

Exercising during pregnancy has many physical and mental benefits. It can:

- increase your energy
- improve your mood
- help reduce and prevent backaches
- improve muscle tone, strength, and endurance
- help you sleep better
- help reduce constipation, bloating, and swelling
- (may) help prevent or treat gestational diabetes
- (may) help you cope with the mental and physical demands of giving birth

The American College of Obstetricians and Gynecologists (ACOG) publishes exercise guidelines for healthy pregnant women. For a complete and free set of guidelines, contact ACOG directly.[1] The following guidelines are consistent with those published by ACOG.

1. Exercise intensity should be regulated according to a pregnant woman's symptoms. It is important to recognize that oxygen availability for aerobic exercise is decreased during pregnancy. In light of this, some women find they need to make substantial modifications, whereas others find they can exercise at near pre-pregnancy intensities. All pregnant women should stop exercising when they feel fatigued and should not exercise to exhaustion. The old intensity guideline of 140 bpm has been replaced with this new, more individualized guideline.

2. Regular exercise, at least 3 times a week, is preferred to intermittent activity. Even mild to moderate regular exercise will result in substantial health benefits.

3. After the first trimester, avoid exercises that involve lying on the back. This position is associated with a decrease in cardiac output, which means that less oxygen is circulated into the blood. Because vigorous exercise preferentially distributes blood to the muscles and away from places such as the uterus, avoiding exercises that involve lying on the back and watching your intensity will ensure that the uterus receives an adequate supply of oxygen. Standing motionless for long periods of time allows blood to pool in the legs and should also be avoided.

4. Pregnant women should pay special attention to staying well hydrated and to avoiding overheating. Drink plenty of water, layer comfortable clothing, and remove layers as you warm up. Attend to heat dissipation throughout the pregnancy, but pay special attention to it in the first trimester. Avoid or modify overly hot or moderately hot but humid environments. If you live in a hot climate and want to exercise outdoors, consider taking a water aerobics course.

5. Consume enough calories to sustain a healthy pregnancy. A woman must eat about 300 more calories per day when she is pregnant. Exercise also requires additional calories, so an exercising pregnant woman must be sure to consume enough food.

6. As the pregnancy advances, some women may be able to continue with weight-bearing activities, but others will find that non-weight-bearing activities such as swimming or cycling are more comfortable and minimize risk of injury.

7. Avoid any activity that risks even mild trauma to the abdomen. This includes activities in which a loss of balance can result in a fall. As the fetus develops and a woman's abdomen increases, her center of gravity shifts. Especially late in the pregnancy (third trimester), this can result in clumsiness and

---

1. American College of Obstetricians and Gynecologists, *Exercise During Pregnancy and the Postpartum Period* (ACOG Technical Bulletin 189) (Washington, DC: ACOG, 1994).

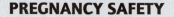

PREGNANCY SAFETY

Stop exercising and call your doctor if you develop any of these symptoms:

- vaginal bleeding
- dizziness or feeling faint
- increased shortness of breath
- chest pain

- headache
- muscle weakness
- calf pain or swelling
- uterine contractions
- decreased fetal movement
- fluid leaking from the vagina

easier loss of balance. Activities that could hurt either the fetus or the mother should be avoided, especially in the third trimester.

8. Many of the bodily changes that occur during pregnancy persist for 4 to 6 weeks following childbirth. For this reason, postpartum exercise should be started gradually and be based on the individual's physical capacity.

These recommendations are intended for healthy women with normal pregnancies. Discuss pregnancy and exercise with your physician to determine how these guidelines apply to you. In some cases, exercise is not recommended, but usually with the right precautions, exercise can enhance pregnancy. See the Pregnancy Safety box for a few situations in which a pregnant woman should stop exercising and contact her doctor.

If your doctor agrees that exercise is healthy for you, discuss frequency, intensity, and duration. During flexibility work, be careful not to overstretch, because your ligaments will tend to be looser and more relaxed. If you feel clumsy or uncoordinated, try not to let it frustrate you. Instead, simplify the steps or walk in place and enjoy the music. Finally, make sure your instructor is aware of your pregnancy (or recent childbirth), and provide him or her with the names and phone numbers of your physician, the hospital, and the relative you want contacted in case of an emergency. If you will enter into your second or third trimester during a semester-long course, talk with the instructor ahead of time concerning alternatives in the event that weight-bearing aerobic dance becomes uncomfortable for you. You might, for example, be able to leave the floor after the warm-up, cycle during the aerobic portion of class, and then return to class for muscle toning and stretching. This kind of solution is preferable to dropping the course.

Some women are able to begin exercising within days of giving birth, but most need 4 to 6 weeks to recover and manage the new responsibilities of taking care of a newborn. When cleared to exercise by their physicians, women find that exercise helps them regain their shape, rebuild their fitness, and enjoy a greater sense of well-being.

EXERCISE AND JOINT PAIN

Joint pain can be the result of disease or injury. Because there are many causes, some of which can be serious, a person with joint pain should consult a physician prior to beginning an exercise program. There are some things that you can do to prevent joint pain and/or to keep from aggravating pain with which you are allowed to exercise.

1. Do not perform an exercise that hurts. Ask for a modification or second exercise that may attain the same benefit. For example, a stretch that requires a kneeling position is contraindicated for someone with knee pain. A similar exercise in a lying down position can usually be substituted.

2. Wear good shoes. Most of the complaints in aerobic dance exercise have to do with the feet, shins, and knees. Supportive, well-cushioned shoes can help prevent many of these problems. See Appendix 2 for more details.

3. Exercise using good alignment and technique. If you start to tire and break form, take a break and begin again when you can do the exercise correctly. You want joints to move in their proper direction (planes) and not experience unnecessary torque or shearing forces. Information on exercise technique is provided throughout this book. You can also ask your instructor to check your technique.

4. When adding resistance such as weights, do it gradually, and never add resistance when joint soreness exists. If a joint does become painful, rest, ice it, and seek a physician's advice.

5. Develop flexibility to allow a healthy range of motion around the joint, and develop strength in the muscles to help support joints.

EXERCISE AND HYPERTENSION

Blood pressure that is higher than normal results in a condition called **hypertension**. Hypertension affects more than 30% of people in the United States; as many as half of these people are unaware that they have high blood pressure. For this reason, it is often referred to as the silent killer. People with hypertension have a higher risk of developing heart disease or suffering a stroke. Hypertension places an increased strain on the heart, so the additional strain of exercise must be carefully applied and monitored. Exercise can, however, be therapeutic because it helps improve the efficiency of the cardiovascular system. Before exercising, individuals with high blood pressure need to obtain both medical clearance and guidelines about how much and how intense the exercise should be.

If you have hypertension, be sure to tell your instructor and make sure that he or she is prepared in the event of an emergency. Your instructor should also be informed of any medications you are taking and any changes in medication that occur during the course. Some medications influence heart rate; in this event, your instructor will teach you how to use ratings of perceived exertion (RPE; see Chapter 4) to monitor your exercise intensity. Also be sure to let the instructor know of any symptoms you experience.

Certain exercises tend to raise blood pressure more sharply than others. These should be avoided unless otherwise approved by your physician. Isometric exercises (in which you push against an immovable object) may spike blood pressure and should be avoided. Resistance training (such as lifting weights) can be a healthy part of an overall fitness program for some people with hypertension, but it should not be considered the best kind of stand-alone program because it does not help reduce blood pressure the way aerobic exercise does. If you have hypertension, or are at risk for hypertension, check with your physician to see whether you should use resistance exercises and, if so, at what intensity.

Individuals with hypertension should begin exercising with an extra-long warm-up. As with all exercisers, they should start at a low intensity and gradually build up to a moderate intensity. Low-impact aerobics may be a better choice than high-impact or step aerobics. A longer cool-down is also recommended. Individuals with hypertension may also experience more orthostatic hypotension—the dizziness and light-headedness that accompany standing up too quickly. Therefore, they should be careful as they move from floor exercises to standing exercises and avoid exercises that involve dropping the head below the knees.

EXERCISE AND LOW-RISK CORONARY ARTERY DISEASE

Building fitness, especially cardiorespiratory fitness, is very important in both the prevention and rehabilitation of **coronary artery disease (CAD)**. It is one of the keys to maintaining a good quality of life. Individuals with moderate- to high-risk CAD should begin exercising in a rehabilitation program under a physician's care. After being thoroughly evaluated by a physician, people with low-risk CAD may be recommended to a regular exercise program. If you have low-risk CAD, be sure to obtain an exercise prescription from your physician, and then share this with your instructor. The instructor may want to talk directly to your physician. Start with low-intensity exercise; gradually work on duration first, and then intensity. Monitor your intensity frequently using heart rate (if you are not on heart-rate-altering medications) or ratings of perceived exertion. If resistance equipment such as weights or exercise bands are used in class, clear this with your physician. When performing resistance exercises with or without weights, be sure to breathe. Holding your breath, overzealously gripping weights, and performing isometric exercises may unnecessarily drive up your blood pressure. Be sure to tell the instructor of any abnormal symptoms you experience before, during, or after exercise. Finally, check to make sure an emergency protocol is in place in case you need help.

EXERCISE AND AGING

There is no age limit on who can enjoy the benefits of exercise. Through exercise, older adults can:

- improve their muscular strength and endurance, flexibility, and aerobic capacity
- take off or prevent unwanted fat and increase muscle mass
- help control the swelling and pain of arthritic joints
- enjoy the company of others during group exercise (such as low-impact or aquatic aerobics classes), including other active seniors
- boost metabolism (metabolism slows as you age), which helps combat weight gains that are common among the sedentary elderly

The Surgeon General states that muscle-strengthening exercises can reduce the risk of falls and fractures in older adults and can improve their ability to live independently.

If you are an older adult in a college aerobic dance exercise class, you will probably need to make some modifications. Most high-impact aerobic steps can be modified into low-impact steps. Ask your instructor to demonstrate this. At times you may want to simply walk in place. If having your arms overhead is tiring or makes you light-headed, use lower arm positions or leave them by your sides. If you are on any medications that alter heart rate (ask your physician), you may want to use RPE (see Chapter 4) to monitor your exercise intensity. If you don't have any joint problems and are adding weights for the first time, start with small amounts of weight and gradually work up. If you have arthritis, high blood pressure, or heart disease, ask your physician about using weights or exercise bands. If you are on any medications, also check with your physician for any exercise implications. For example, nitroglycerine taken right before exercise can cause hypoglycemia (low blood sugar). Wear layers of clothing so that you don't become too hot or overcooled in class, or en route to or from class. A longer cool-down may be needed. If you find this to be true, lower your intensity sooner in the standing aerobics portion of class, or spend additional time walking after class. Finally, if you have difficulty with some exercise positions, speak to your instructor about alternatives or using equipment such as a mat that will make you more comfortable. Older individuals in college courses are often inspirations to their younger counterparts—real "wellness" role models!

SUMMARY

You are an individual—unique. An exercise program can be adjusted to meet your special needs. Programs are designed around the "average person" but are not intended to be limited to this. Good instructors try to provide and demonstrate alternative exercises, positions, and intensity levels. Being able to take advantage of this information and working with the instructor concerning individual needs will provide you with the very best program. Individual differences may be due to age, gender, ethnicity, pregnancy, aging, disability, injury, disease, or personal preferences.

KNOWLEDGE TIPS

1. An aerobic dance exercise program can be adjusted to accommodate people's individual differences.

2. Individual differences arise for numerous reasons, including experience, age, gender, ethnicity, pregnancy, aging, disability, injury, disease, and personal preferences.

3. Any exercise modifications due to pregnancy, illness, disease, disability, or injury should be made in conjunction with a physician.

4. Flexibility and strength work can prevent and in some cases relieve back pain.

5. People with asthma who exercise aerobically can raise the exertion level at which symptoms occur. This allows them to enjoy more symptom-free activity.

6. Aerobic exercise can be modified to accommodate the comfort and abilities of obese individuals.

7. Exercise can help people with diabetes control blood sugar, lose weight, and improve the body's use of insulin.

8. Aerobic exercise can help lower blood pressure.

9. Aerobic exercise can reduce the risk of cardiovascular disease and is therapeutic for those who already have it.

10. People of all ages can enjoy exercise. For older adults, exercise helps improve coordination, strengthen muscles, sustain bones, decrease falls, and increase the ability to live independently.

THINK ABOUT IT

1. Why is it important to adjust an exercise or exercise plan to meet the needs of an individual?

2. Think about a friend in the class and identify ways that you are the same and different and how these characteristics might influence your individual exercise plans.

3. Is it possible to exercise safely if you are asthmatic? diabetic? overweight? hypertensive?

4. What are some things you can do to prevent low back pain?

5. Who should make the decisions about exercising while pregnant?

6. Can you think of one way you would individualize your aerobic exercise to better meet your needs?

REFERENCES

American College of Obstetricians and Gynecologists. *Getting in Shape After Your Baby Is Born.* (AP131). Washington, DC: American College of Obstetricians and Gynecologists, 2000.

——. *Exercise During Pregnancy.* (AP119). Washington, DC: American College of Obstetricians and Gynecologists, 2003.

——. *Easing Back Pain During Pregnancy.* (AP115) Washington, DC: American College of Obstetricians and Gynecologists, 1997.

American Council on Exercise. *Aerobics Instructor Manual: ACE's Guide for Fitness Professionals.* San Diego, CA: American Council on Exercise, 2000.

Estivill, M. "Therapeutic Aspects of Aerobic Dance Participation." *Health Care for Women International* 16 (No. 4, 1995): 341–50.

Lokey, E. A., Z. V. Tran, C. L. Wells, B. C. Myers, and A. C. Tran. "Effects of Physical Exercise on Pregnancy Outcomes: A Meta-analytic Review." *Medicine and Science in Sports & Exercise* 23 (No. 11, 1991): 1234–9.

Wells, C. L. *Women, Sport, and Performance.* Champaign, IL: Human Kinetics, 1985.

3

Fitness Components and Exercise Principles

"Failure comes only when we forget our ideals and objectives and principles."

JAWAHARLAL NEHRU

- Do I have to play sports to get fit?
- What types of exercises do I need to do to be healthy?
- Are there some basic rules or guidelines to follow for exercise?

COMPONENTS OF FITNESS

Exercising for health is different from training for competition. To fine-tune your performance for competition, you have to train long hours at high intensities. You may also have to place your body in mechanically difficult positions. For example, volleyball players and weight lifters drop into deep knee positions that place stress on their knee ligaments. Gymnasts constantly hyperextend their backs, thus placing pressure on their vertebral discs, and pitchers risk injuring their elbows when they throw curve balls. The motivation for such intense practice and performance comes from a deep-seated drive to excel and a desire to win recognition and awards.

Many positive outcomes are associated with competition—health can be one of them. However, a higher risk of injury is associated with high-intensity training. It may also surprise you to learn that not all highly skilled competitors are physically fit. For example, some excellent golfers and baseball players carry extra pounds of fat and lack good cardiorespiratory conditioning.

To exercise for health, you can train at a moderate intensity, enjoy the physiological and psychological benefits of exercise, and at the same time limit the risk of injury. It's time to discard the myth that it is good to exercise until you drop. Lifetime fitness is built on activities that are enjoyable and, when done correctly, free from pain. There are five health-related components of physical fitness:

1. cardiorespiratory endurance
2. body composition
3. flexibility
4. muscular strength
5. muscular endurance

Sometimes muscular strength and endurance are considered one component (muscular fitness), thus making the total number of health-related components four. Any improvement in these five areas will improve your health (see the box, Can You..., on page 28). There are also skill-related components of fitness:

1. agility
2. balance
3. coordination
4. power
5. reaction time
6. speed

Strength is often included as a seventh component because it plays an important role in skilled performance. Kinesthetic awareness (awareness of where your body is in space) may also be included as a skill-related component. Because aerobic dance exercise is primarily concerned with developing and maintaining physical health, exercises that concentrate on the five health-related components are emphasized. This emphasis does not exclude the possibility of improving some of the skill-related components, especially coordination, agility, and balance.

Regular physical activity is one of the key ingredients to health. Therefore, skill-related components can have a positive effect on your health because when you are good at something (skilled), you tend to do it more often. Standard aerobics classes don't require a lot of

CAN YOU . . .

. . . identify exercises or activities that will result in positive changes in each of the following health-related fitness components?

- cardiorespiratory endurance

- body composition
- flexibility
- muscular strength
- muscular endurance

---

skill. The routines usually consist of lots of repetitions of basic steps. You might feel a little clumsy at first, but this feeling will disappear with a few lessons. More advanced classes may use more intricate movement patterns and power steps that challenge not only fitness but also agility and coordination.

CARDIORESPIRATORY ENDURANCE

Cardiorespiratory endurance is the ability to perform large-muscle movements over a sustained period of time. Defined another way, it is the ability of the circulatory (heart, blood, blood vessels) and respiratory (lungs) systems to deliver fuel, especially oxygen, to the muscles during continuous exercise. Fit individuals have a heart–lung capacity that allows them to persist in physical activity for relatively long periods of time without undue fatigue. (The terms "cardiovascular endurance" and "cardiorespiratory endurance" are often used interchangeably. The latter will be used in this text because it reflects the important relationship between the respiratory and circulatory systems.)

Cardiorespiratory endurance is improved during the aerobic portion of the exercise class. Some of the health benefits associated with cardiorespiratory endurance include a stronger heart, improved circulation to the heart, increased oxygen transportation by the blood, an increased level of high-density lipoproteins (HDL), a lower risk of coronary heart disease, a better chance of surviving a heart attack, a decreased level of blood fat (cholesterol), a lowered resting heart rate, lower blood pressure, improved body composition, and a better chance of living a longer, healthier life.

BODY COMPOSITION

Body composition refers to the relative amounts of lean body mass and fat in your body. **Lean body mass (LBM)** includes bones, muscles, and connective tissue. **Fat** includes subcutaneous fat (the fat deposits stored *between* the muscles and the skin) and intramuscular fat (the fat

stored *within* the muscles). The percentage of fat you have can be measured several ways, including the skin-fold technique and underwater weighing (see Chapter 12). A certain amount of fat is essential for health. Too high or too low of a percentage of fat is unhealthy.

Body composition can be changed by decreasing the body's amount of fat, increasing the body's amount of lean body mass, or both. You can change your body composition through a sound diet and exercise program. Fat (along with carbohydrate) is metabolized during aerobic exercise, whereas muscle (lean body mass) can be added through strength training exercises. Increasing muscle mass has the added benefit of increasing your resting metabolic rate, which means your body is burning more calories while at rest. This can help you maintain a healthy weight after a weight-loss diet.

Maintaining a healthy body composition reduces the risk of heart disease, stroke, some cancers, diabetes, hypertension, high blood cholesterol, and arthritis. In addition, it makes you look and feel better, and increases your body's work capacity.

FLEXIBILITY

Flexibility is the ability to move a joint or a combination of joints through a full range of motion. Muscles, tendons, ligaments, and bone structures all limit a joint to a normal range of motion. When muscles and tendons tighten and shorten, the range of motion in the joint is restricted. Simple tasks such as turning in a car seat to check traffic or picking something up off the floor can become difficult. When ligaments and tendons are overstretched or damaged, the joint becomes loose and dislocates easily. Strengthening the muscles around a joint may help stabilize a loose joint, or surgery may be required. (A physician should be consulted to provide advice on which exercises are appropriate for rehabilitating a loose or injured joint.)

Working on flexibility by stretching during the warm-up and cool-down periods of an aerobics class helps maintain and improve range of motion. The warm-up involves a type of stretching called dynamic stretching. This is an active stretch of the muscles achieved through easy rhythmic movements. Following this, or intermixed with it, may be some static or held stretching. This stretching regimen prepares the body for more vigorous movement. The best way to develop or improve flexibility is to perform static stretches after a good workout, when the muscles are really warm and pliable. Health benefits associated with good flexibility include freedom of movement (which represents independence for older individuals), improved postural alignment and physical appearance, greater work efficiency, less risk of muscle or joint injury, and decreased chance of developing lower back pain. Flexibility can also enhance sport skill performance, decrease muscle tension, and promote relaxation.

MUSCULAR ENDURANCE

Muscular endurance is the ability of a muscle, or group of muscles, to apply a submaximal force repeatedly or to sustain a muscular contraction for a period of time. Leg lifts are an example of repeatedly applied force. Holding the leg in a raised position for 10 seconds is an example of a sustained contraction. During leg lifts, the muscles go through a range of motion while applying force. This is an example of a **dynamic contraction.** During a dynamic contraction, muscle fibers contract and shorten. When the leg is held in one position, the muscles are in a **static** or **isometric contraction.** During a sustained isometric contraction, muscle fibers contract but don't shorten.

Most muscle-toning exercises are done using dynamic contractions, because they strengthen the muscle through its entire range of motion. Muscular endurance is usually developed by performing a high number of repetitions (approximately 8–15) with light to medium resistance. Isometric contractions strengthen a muscle in a particular position, which can be particularly useful for therapeutic purposes and improving posture. The wall sit is a good example. People with high blood pressure should check with their physician before doing isometric contractions, which can cause a rapid rise in peripheral resistance (blood pressure). The benefits of improving muscular endurance include less fatigue during regular activity, an increased ability to do work, and a reduced risk of injury.

MUSCULAR STRENGTH

Muscular strength is the ability of a muscle, or group of muscles, to exert force against a resistance. The number of pounds you can lift one time with your arms is a measure of maximal muscular strength. You can improve your muscular strength by lifting relatively heavy weights in a small number of repetitions. Aerobic dance exercise classes have traditionally placed more emphasis on endurance than on strength, but the use of exercise bands, weights, weighted balls, bars, stability balls, and step aerobics has enabled participants to improve both muscular endurance and strength. A well-designed weight training program is the best way to further increase strength. Strength training, like endurance training, usually emphasizes dynamic contractions. The health benefits related to muscular strength include an increased ability to do physical work, a decreased risk of injury, and a decreased risk of back pain.

PRINCIPLES OF EXERCISE

As you work to improve or maintain your fitness level in each of the five health-related components of fitness, use the following principles of exercise to guide you.

THE PRINCIPLE OF OVERLOAD

When the human body is stressed repeatedly over a period of time, it responds by adapting to the stress. Regular exercise stresses the body, which adapts by becoming stronger and more efficient. Another word for "stress" is "overload." When the muscles, including the heart muscle, are overloaded or stressed more than normal amounts, fitness gains occur. This is the **principle of overload.** When you overload, you are temporarily increasing the amount or intensity of an exercise. As your body adapts, you experience a training effect and the exercise becomes easier. To continue to improve your physical fitness, you have to continue to overload. For example, if you can normally do 10 push-ups, create an overload to the arm and chest muscles by doing 11 or 12. When 12 becomes easy, overload again by doing 13 or 14, and so on. Overload can also be achieved by doing a harder version of the push-up rather than more push-ups. See the Overload box on page 30 to begin applying the principle of overload. When you reach your desired level of fitness, you can stop overloading. To maintain your fitness level, continue to perform your new "normal" amount. Doing less than normal will result in deconditioning.

A minimum amount and intensity of exercise must be performed before fitness improvement begins. This minimum level of exercise is called the **threshold of training.** To improve your physical fitness, you must engage in activities at an intensity above your

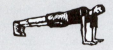

OVERLOAD: FOR ONCE IT'S A GOOD THING!

Remember, overloading in exercise is a good thing as long as you do it gradually. Here are some examples of how you can create progressive overloads. Can you apply these ideas to specific exercises?

- **Flexibility:** Stretch the muscle just longer than its normal length.

- **Strength:** Increase the amount of resistance against which the muscle normally moves, OR increase the number of repetitions and/or sets of an exercise you perform.

- **Muscular endurance:** Increase the number of repetitions (or sets of repetitions) you normally perform, OR increase the resistance against which the muscle is moving while maintaining a moderate to high number of repetitions, OR hold an isometric contraction for a longer time than normal.

- **Cardiorespiratory endurance:** Place a demand that is greater than normal on the heart and lungs by sustaining a longer bout of aerobic exercise, OR increase the intensity of the exercise by working at a higher level (higher heart rate), OR perform aerobic exercise on more days of the week.

threshold of training. The threshold of training for a beginner is relatively low. As you become more fit, your threshold of training will increase.

THE PRINCIPLE OF PROGRESSION

The **principle of progression** is an extension of the principle of overload. Basically, this principle means that you should gradually increase your overload over a period of time. Too rapid of an overload can make you really stiff and sore or even result in injury. Overload and progression are so interrelated that fitness professionals usually speak in terms of doing appropriate progressive overloads. Beginners will want to progressively overload by increasing the duration and frequency with which they perform activities before adding intensity. For example, a beginning aerobics student who can only do 10 minutes of continuous low-intensity aerobics will want to slowly extend that to about 20 minutes of aerobic activity for 3 to 5 days before thinking about increasing to a moderate intensity workout. Similarly, with push-ups, beginners would want to improve from 5 modified (on knees) push-ups to 10 to 15 before attempting push-ups performed on the toes. More advanced participants can gradually add intensity. People who fail to progress may be exercising too infrequently or not overloading enough to stimulate change.

THE FIT (OR FITT) PRINCIPLE

The FIT (or FITT) principle describes exercise and provides guidance about the appropriate amounts and intensity of exercise needed to attain health and performance benefits. The optimal range of exercise for health-related physical fitness is called the **fitness target zone.** The lower limit of the zone is the threshold of training; the upper limit is the maximum amount and intensity of exercise recommended for health. The best-known target zone is the one for cardiorespiratory endurance. However, target zones exist for each of the health-related components of fitness.

Three variables are involved in locating and exercising within your target zones: the frequency with which you train (number of times per week), the intensity at which you train, and the amount of time you train per session. These three variables are often remembered by the acronym **FIT**—the *F* stands for **frequency,** the *I* for **intensity,** and the *T* for **time** (or **duration**). Each of the health-related fitness components has optimal ranges (fitness target zones) for these three variables.

The FIT principle sometimes is called the **FITT principle;** here, the extra *T* stands for "type of exercise." Therefore, to describe your exercise using the FITT principle, you would specify the Frequency, Intensity, and Time you perform a certain Type of activity.

The target zone for aerobic endurance is described in more detail in Chapter 4. The target zones for flexibility and muscular strength and endurance are described in Chapters 7 and 8. Each of these chapters will discuss how to adjust the frequency, intensity, and duration of your exercise so that you get the most out of your aerobic dance exercise.

THE PRINCIPLE OF INDIVIDUALITY

Everyone is unique, and this includes people's responses to exercise. The **principle of individuality** holds that no two people react exactly the same way to exercise. Two men with the ability to lift the same amount of weight can have significantly different muscle circumferences. Two women eating the same diet, attending the same exercise class, and working out at the same intensity may lose inches or pounds in different places at different rates. This means that the only person you can really compare yourself to is you. Your rate of progress and the way you progress are unique to you.

Many fitness tests provide norms, averages, or percentiles for you to compare your scores against. These are helpful guidelines, but they should not be considered the gold standard. Norms simply state what a tested group of people were able to do. The norms for a push-up test performed by athletes would be considerably higher than the norms for a push-up test performed by senior citizens. The best fitness test norms are age adjusted and based on scores from large populations. The fitness tests in the worksheets section at the back of this book were selected with these criteria in mind. Compare yourself to these norms, but most importantly, compare yourself to yourself.

THE PRINCIPLE OF SPECIFICITY

Would you ever practice stretching your shoulders so that you could touch your toes or do a set of abdominal curls to tone your legs? Of course not. You would select exercises that would accomplish your goal. When you make these selections, you are using the **principle of specificity,** which states that placing a specific demand on the body results in a specific adaptation.

If you create a demand on the body by doing strength exercises, the body adapts by building stronger muscles. If you create a demand by doing aerobic exercises, the body adapts by improving the cardiorespiratory system. Note that the adaptation is specific to the demand—strength exercises result in strength, not in cardiorespiratory endurance.

Different occupations place different demands on the body. As a result, pianists have strong fingers, construction workers have well-developed shoulder and arm muscles, ice cream scoopers have one strong arm, and aerobic dance instructors have toned muscles and healthy hearts. (If an occupation does create muscle imbalances, as in the ice cream scooper with only one strong arm, an exercise program can often correct the imbalance.)

THE PRINCIPLE OF REGULARITY

Sometimes referred to as the **principle of reversibility,** the **use/disuse principle** is succinctly defined by the well-known phrase "use it or lose it." Within 2 weeks

of the time you stop exercising, your body begins to adapt to the lack of activity. The loss of competitive edge can be even faster. Cardiorespiratory and flexibility losses occur more rapidly than strength and endurance losses. Nobody is protected from these negative adaptations. The only way to be fit is to be active on a regular basis. (Worksheet 2 will help you track your progress and stay motivated.) Varsity college athletes who stop exercising when they graduate are ultimately no better off than people who never exercised. So—keep moving!

THE PRINCIPLE OF OVERUSE

Overuse results from violating the principle of overload. When you overdo (which is the essence of the **principle of overuse**), you create problems. Injuries, especially chronic injuries such as shinsplints and tendinitis, start to appear. Some people actually become addicted to exercise, a sign of which is the refusal to exercise fewer than 7 days a week. Addiction leads to overtraining. Signs of overtraining are the previously mentioned chronic injuries and an elevated resting heart rate. Overuse may also be the result of a violation of the principle of individuality. A person trying to keep up with another person may overload too quickly. Three sets of 10 push-ups may be an appropriate load for one individual but may be overuse for another.

SUMMARY

Your instructor has probably incorporated exercises for all five health-related fitness components into your aerobic dance exercise. Think through the class and see if you can identify at least one exercise for each fitness component.

Even though you may not know it, you are probably an expert at using the principles of exercise. For example, have you ever increased the frequency, intensity, or duration of your workout to make it more challenging (overload)? Have you ever asked someone for a better exercise to achieve a goal like a flatter abdomen or thinner thighs (specificity)? Have you ever wondered why your friend is adapting more quickly or more slowly than you are to certain parts of the class (individuality)? Have you ever noticed how you have more energy when you are on an exercise program than when you stop your program (reversibility)? Now you can consciously put these principles to work for you by creating a positive exercise plan that best fits your needs.

KNOWLEDGE TIPS

1. The five health-related fitness components are cardiorespiratory endurance, body composition, flexibility, muscular strength, and muscular endurance.

2. The six skill-related components of fitness are agility, balance, coordination, power, reaction time, and speed; strength is often included as a skill-related component as well.

3. Aerobic dance exercise is designed to improve all of the health-related components of fitness and some of the skill-related components of fitness.

4. To overload, you must go just beyond the point of comfort by increasing frequency, intensity, or time.

5. A progressive overload is one that occurs gradually over time.

6. The FIT principle uses the variables of frequency, intensity, and time to describe beneficial fitness target zones for the health-related components of physical fitness.

7. Individuals respond to exercise differently.

8. The body makes specific adaptations in accord with the demands placed on it.

9. Deconditioning occurs with disuse.

10. Overuse results in undue fatigue, chronic injury, and other problems.

THINK ABOUT IT

1. What is the difference between health-related and skill-related fitness? Can you name the components for each?

2. How is exercising for health different from exercising for sport and competition?

3. Which components of physical fitness are targeted in an aerobic dance exercise class?

4. Identify one or more health benefits for each health-related component of fitness.

5. Describe a progressive overload for both cardiorespiratory endurance and muscular fitness.

6. Explain why varsity athletes are no better off than anyone else if they stop being physically active. Which principle of exercise speaks to this?

7. Is it healthy to perform both aerobic and muscular resistance training in the same day? Explain why or why not.

8. Does an individual have to be skilled in order to be fit? Explain your answer.

9. Explain the FITT principle.

10. What are some signs that a person is overdoing his or her fitness program?

REFERENCES

American College of Sports Medicine. *ACSM's Guidelines for Exercise Testing and Exercise Prescription.* 8th ed. Media, PA: Lippincott Williams & Wilkins, 2010.

Corbin, C. B., G. Welk, W. R. Corbin, and K. A. Welk. *Concepts of Physical Fitness: Active Lifestyles for Wellness.* 14th ed. New York: McGraw-Hill Higher Education, 2006.

Physical Best and NASPE. *Physical Education for Lifelong Fitness: The Physical Best Teacher's Guide.* 2nd ed. Champaign, IL: Human Kinetics, 2005.

4

The Aerobic Target Zone

"Life begets life. Energy creates energy. It is by spending oneself that one becomes rich."

SARAH BERNHARDT

- How much aerobic exercise do I need to do?
- How will I know if I'm exercising hard enough?
- Why do I see people taking their pulse or looking at their heart-rate monitors during aerobic exercise?

AEROBIC exercise has a lot of benefits; the amount and type of benefits you will experience depend on the intensity with which you perform. In Chapter 1 you learned that you can get substantial health benefits by doing a minimum of 150 minutes per week of moderate-intensity aerobic physical activity *or* 75 minutes per week of vigorous-intensity aerobic activity *or* an equivalent combination of moderate and vigorous activity. Research tells us that moderate-level activity (brisk walk) is the minimum level one must reach in order to gain benefits. But greater gains in health and fitness occur when a person performs exercise at a higher level, one which substantially increases heart rate and breathing. The aerobic target zone described in this chapter ranges between moderately vigorous to vigorous intensity to promote optimal benefits but with the allowance that levels below the zone can benefit those in class who are just getting started and need to build endurance. If you perform the aerobic portion of class at a level similar to a brisk walk, you may need to supplement class with additional exercise. If you jog and jump your way through class, you will probably achieve or come close to your 75-minute minimum of vigorous activity for the week. Additional minutes can result in even greater health and fitness and additional performance benefits, but the amount and intensity of your workouts should be in line with your goals. Compared to health-oriented goals, high-end performance goals come at a price, such as demanding time commitments and potential injuries.

Like all target zones, the **aerobic target zone** is composed of three variables: frequency, intensity, and time (duration). In this chapter, you will learn how often, how hard, and how long you must perform aerobic exercise to improve your cardiorespiratory endurance and to enjoy the associated health benefits.

Please note that this chapter is only about the target zone for aerobic exercise. The target zones for flexibility, muscular strength, and muscular endurance are described in Chapters 7 and 9.

FREQUENCY

According to the American College of Sports Medicine (ACSM), optimal aerobic training occurs when you exercise 3 to 5 times a week at the intensities discussed in the next section. The exceptions to this are deconditioned or unfit individuals who may be able to improve their cardiorespiratory fitness by exercising just twice a week. Exercise benefits start to plateau at a frequency of 5 times a week. Exercising more than this seems to result in minimal benefits, whereas risk of injury, especially to the extremities, increases abruptly.

People who exercise at low-end intensities (see next section) may need to exercise more than 3 days a week to burn enough calories to meet weight-loss goals. If weight loss is a primary goal, frequency can range from 3 to 7 days a week, depending on intensity, duration, and mode of exercise. Workouts of moderate intensity with longer duration and less impact are generally recommended for weight loss. For more information on weight loss and exercise, see Chapter 12.

High-frequency exercisers (e.g., those working toward weight loss, instructors, and individuals training

33

for competition) can minimize impact stress by using low-impact, nonimpact, or non-weight-bearing activities as well as high-impact aerobics. Low-impact exercises include step, low-impact, and aqua (water) aerobics as well as brisk walking; nonimpact exercises include slide aerobics, some special forms of aerobic dance, and non-weight-bearing exercises such as swimming, rowing, cycling, and deep-water running. Activities and their impact stress will be discussed in more detail later in Chapter 8.

Exercise addicts are people who feel compelled to work out every single day. Addicts are more prone to overuse injuries such as shinsplints and tendinitis and may develop such an obsession for exercise that they begin to value it above everything else. Like any addiction, this leads to an unhealthy lifestyle. Physical fitness must always be balanced with the other wellness components: social, emotional, intellectual, and spiritual health.

INTENSITY

This section contains a number of abbreviated terms. To make your reading of the text easier, a quick reference list of abbreviations is provided.

HR	= heart rate
EHR	= exercise heart rate
RHR	= resting heart rate
THR	= training heart rate range (target zone)
MHR	= maximum heart rate
PreHR	= pre-exercise heart rate
RecHR	= recovery heart rate
HRR	= heart rate reserve (MHR − RHR)
VO_2max	= maximum volume of oxygen consumed

There are a number of ways to monitor the intensity of your aerobic workout. You may have heard of several different intensity ranges and wonder which range is the right one for you. This decision will be clear when you know where the ranges come from and how they are related. To fully understand intensity monitoring, you first need to understand oxygen's role in aerobic exercise and how it relates to heart rate and ratings of perceived exertion.

The word "aerobic" actually means "with oxygen." It is only when a steady supply of oxygen is available to the muscles that aerobic exercise can be performed. The oxygen you breathe into your lungs is picked up by red blood cells and delivered to your muscles. Inside the muscle cells, oxygen is used in the chemical processes that convert food (carbohydrates, fats, and proteins)

into energy for muscular contraction. The more intensely you exercise, the more oxygen your muscles need. The more oxygen you are able to supply, the more exercise you will be able to do. As you increase your exercise intensity, your breathing becomes faster and deeper to bring in more oxygen, your heart beats faster to speed up the delivery of the oxygen, and your muscles use more food and oxygen to produce movement. As exercise becomes more and more intense, the rate and volume of oxygen entering the body continues to increase until finally the body is consuming oxygen as rapidly as it can. This maximum volume of **oxygen consumption** (measured in liters per minute or milliliters per minute per kilogram of body weight) is called **VO_2max;** you may also see it referred to as "maximum oxygen uptake (MOU)." If exercise intensity is increased any further, the muscles' demand for oxygen cannot be met. You can exercise at these very high intensities for only a short time before total exhaustion makes you stop.

Exercising near or at VO_2max is not fun. In fact, it's agonizingly difficult. The good news is that you can improve your aerobic fitness by exercising at an intensity well below maximum. The ACSM periodically reviews the available research on exercise and recommends guidelines for exercise testing and prescription. In 2000, the ACSM revised their recommendations. They now recommend exercising between 40 and 50% (40/50) to 85% of oxygen uptake reserve. (Oxygen uptake reserve is the difference between your maximum oxygen uptake—VO_2max—and your resting oxygen uptake.) The lower range of 40 to 50% is for deconditioned or unfit participants, who can improve their aerobic capacity by exercising at low levels of intensity. As endurance improves, participants can begin to work at higher levels. The goal for an average healthy person is to exercise in the middle of the range. The upper part of the range is for advanced participants and those interested in competition.

This is all fine and good if you have a way to measure how much oxygen you are using, but who can count oxygen molecules while exercising? You can't, but exercise scientists can. The only way to directly measure your oxygen consumption is to take part in a supervised laboratory test during which you exercise on a stationary bicycle or treadmill (or other ergometric device) while hooked up to machines that monitor your oxygen consumption and **heart rate.** These kinds of tests are wonderful tools for research and for working with special populations, but they are too elaborate and individualized to be of any practical benefit to the average group exercise participant.

This brings us to an important discovery that was made by Martti Karvonen in the 1960s. He discovered that there is a near linear relationship between oxygen consumption and heart rate during cardiorespiratory exercise. When one goes up, the other goes up at about the same rate. This means that you can substitute heart-rate measures for oxygen measures. Your intensity range for aerobic exercise can be based on how fast your heart beats versus how much oxygen you consume. In summary, you can use heart rate to monitor the intensity of aerobic exercise because it is an indirect measure of oxygen consumption.

Scientists have developed two heart-rate formulas to determine an exercise intensity range. The heart-rate formulas calculate a range of acceptable heart rates—something that you can easily count by taking your pulse, which is the wave of pressure felt in the arteries when the heart beats. There are two heart-rate formulas instead of one for the same reason that we measure apples in both bushels and pounds: Both are effective measures, depending on the circumstances.

The **maximum heart-rate formula** is fairly conservative and can be calculated as long as the age of the participant is known. The ACSM recommends an intensity of exercise corresponding to between 55 and 65% (55/65) to 90% of maximum heart rate. The lower range is reserved for less fit individuals and the high end for very highly fit individuals. For healthy active adults, the range is usually calculated using 70 to 85% of maximum heart rate.

The heart-rate reserve, or **Karvonen formula,** is more individualized, using both age and resting heart rate in its calculations. The ACSM recommendation for this formula is identical to the one for oxygen uptake reserve: exercise between 50 and 60% (50/60) to 85% of heart-rate reserve. For active healthy adults, this formula is usually calculated using 60 to 80% of heart-rate reserve. If you are unfit or deconditioned, you will want to use the lower portion of the range. Again, the very high intensities are significant only for competitors. As the intensity rises, so do the risks of injury and the amount of discomfort felt during the exercise. Competitive athletes have to exercise at these intensities to maintain the winning edge, but the fitness gains are not significant in relation to the risk of injury for the person interested in achieving health-related cardiorespiratory fitness.

MONITORING INTENSITY BY HEART RATE

When the intensity range is measured by heart rate, it is called the **training heart-rate range** (or target heart rate zone), usually abbreviated **THR.** To achieve aerobic conditioning, you must exercise hard enough to keep your heart rate within your THR. To calculate your THR, you can use either the maximum heart-rate formula or the Karvonen formula. The Karvonen formula is more accurate, but to use it you must know your true **resting heart rate (RHR),** which is the rate at which the heart beats when the body is at rest. Although that is not difficult, it takes several days to measure. In the meantime, you may want to get started by using the quick, easy, and conservative maximum heart-rate formula. Individuals whose heart rates are influenced by disease or medications should not use heart rate to monitor intensity. Turn instead to page 40 for alternative methods of monitoring exercise intensity.

In both formulas, you will calculate a lower and an upper limit for your THR. To do this, you will need to know your **maximum heart rate (MHR).** MHR is the fastest rate your heart can beat. The most accurate way to determine your MHR is to exercise to absolute exhaustion while your heart rate is monitored by an EKG (electrocardiograph) machine. Fortunately for you, there is a faster and easier way to estimate your MHR. Researchers discovered that the MHR drops an average of one beat each year of an individual's life. Through statistical extrapolation, researchers determined that a newborn's MHR is about 220 beats per minute (bpm). A one-year-old would have an MHR of 219 bpm, a two-year-old 218 bpm, and so on. So, until recently, to calculate your MHR all you had to do was subtract your age from 220. For a 20-year-old, this would mean a MHR of 200 bpm. More recent research has found that this formula generally overpredicted maximum heart rates in people aged 20–40 and underpredicted them for individuals over 40. A new formula has been developed, and it is this newer version that will be used in the examples in this book. (Please note, however, that at this time, both formulas are still being used by professionals in the exercise field.) The new formula is as follows:

$$207 - (0.7 \times age) = MHR$$

By this formula, a 20-year-old will have a MHR of 193 bpm.

$$207 - (0.7 \times 20) = 207 - 14 = 193 \text{ bpm}$$

MAXIMUM HEART RATE FORMULA (ZERO TO PEAK FORMULA)

THR is a range with an upper and a lower limit. To calculate the lower limit (threshold) of your THR, multiply your MHR by 70%. To calculate the upper limit, multiply your MHR by 85%. Remember that when you multiply by a percentage, you are multiplying by a fraction. For example, $70\% = 70/100 = 0.70$

$$MHR \times 0.70 = \text{lower limit of THR}$$

$$MHR \times 0.85 = \text{upper limit of THR}$$

The THR for a 20-year-old person is calculated below. A space for figuring your THR is provided at the back of the book on Worksheet 3.

STEP ONE	STEP TWO	STEP THREE
207	193	193
− (0.7 × 20)	× .70	× .85
193	135.1	164.1
(MHR)	(lower limit of THR)	(upper limit of THR)

Thus, the THR for this individual is 135 to 164 bpm.

Your **exercise heart rate (EHR)** is the speed at which your heart is beating during exercise. Your EHR should fall within your THR. If your EHR is higher than your THR, you are exercising too intensely. If it is lower, you aren't exercising hard enough. To find your EHR, either take your pulse while you are exercising or complete your count within 15 seconds of the time you stop. When you stop exercising, your heart rate stays at a level close to your EHR for about 15 seconds, then drops off quickly as your body recovers. During the first 15 seconds, you have time to locate your pulse (most people require 2 to 4 seconds) and take a 10-second pulse count. Multiply the number of beats you count in 10 seconds by 6 to determine your pulse in beats per minute. For example:

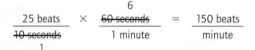

Exercisers often take a 6-second count, because mentally multiplying by 10 is easy. The problem with this method is that if you miscount your heart rate, you are multiplying your error by 10. When your heart is beating very fast, it is easy to miscount by 1, even 2 beats. A 2-beat miscount becomes an error of 20 beats. If instead you use the 10-second count, a 2-beat miscount represents only a 12-beat error. Almost all fitness experts recommend the 10-second count.

To eliminate the problem of mentally multiplying by 6, convert your THR from beats per minute to beats per 10 seconds by dividing the top and bottom of the range by 6 and rounding off to the nearest whole number. The range of 135 to 164 bpm, which was calculated in steps one, two, and three, is converted below in steps four and five.

STEP FOUR	STEP FIVE
$\frac{135}{6}$ = 22.5	$\frac{164}{6}$ = 27.3

THR = 23–27 beats/10 sec.

Looking at this example, you can see that a 20-year-old who counts an EHR of 26 beats during a 10-second count is well within the recommended THR.

KARVONEN METHOD (HEART-RATE RESERVE FORMULA)

In this formula, percentages of the **heart–rate reserve (HRR)** are calculated. The HRR is the MHR minus the resting heart rate (RHR) in beats per minute. The RHR is added back in after a percentage of the HRR has been calculated. The formula looks like this:

(MHR − RHR) X 0.60 + RHR = lower limit THR
(MHR − RHR) X 0.80 + RHR = upper limit THR

Before using this formula, you need an accurate count of your RHR. Take your RHR first thing in the morning while you are still lying in bed. (Relax for a few minutes if your alarm clock has jolted you into consciousness.) Count your pulse for 1 minute to get the rate in beats per minute. Take this RHR on two or three different mornings to determine the average rate.

Provided below is an example of the THR for a 20-year-old individual with an RHR of 75 bpm. To calculate your THR using the Karvonen method, use Worksheet 4 at the back of the book.

STEP ONE	STEP TWO
207	193
− (0.7 × 20)	− 75
193 (MHR)	118 (HRR)

STEP THREE	STEP FOUR
118	70.8
× .60	+ 75
70.8	145.8 (lower limit THR in bpm)

STEP FIVE	STEP SIX
118	94.4
× .80	+ 75
94.4	169.4 (upper limit THR in bpm)

The range is 145 to 169 bpm (Figure 4.1). Divided by 6 and rounded to the nearest whole number, the

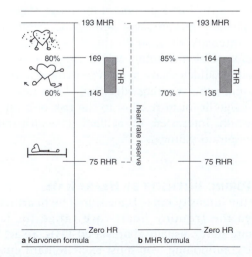

Figure 4.1 (a) THR calculated using the Karvonen formula for a 20-year-old with 75 bpm for RHR. (b) THR calculated using the maximum heart-rate formula for a 20-year-old.

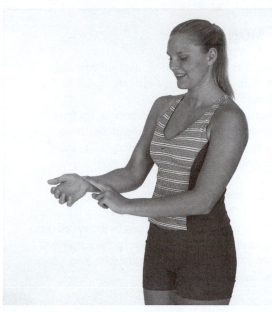

Figure 4.2 Radial artery.

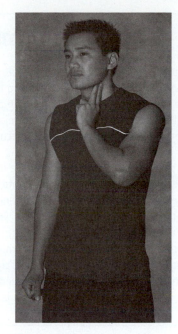

Figure 4.3 Carotid artery.

range is 24 to 28 beats per 10 seconds. One advantage of using the Karvonen formula is that you can adjust your THR as your RHR declines with training.

TAKING YOUR PULSE

When you press gently on an **artery,** you can feel the pulsing of the blood as it is pushed through the arteries by the heart. The arteries most commonly used for taking the pulse during exercise are the radial and carotid arteries.

The **radial artery** is located on the inside of your wrist. You can feel it beside your forearm tendons on the thumb side (Figure 4.2). The **carotid artery** is just to the side (either side) of your voice box (larynx). You can feel it in the valley between your Adam's apple and your neck muscles (Figure 4.3).

To feel your pulse, use two fingers to press gently but firmly on the artery. Do not use your thumb; it also has a pulse and will cause you to miscount. If you can't feel your pulse, you may be pressing too lightly or too hard. Pressing too hard on an artery squeezes it shut so that you can no longer feel any pulsing. Try different pressures while sitting quietly until you can feel and count your pulse easily. Then practice taking it while you move around the room. If you have a lot of trouble counting your pulse, place your hand over your heart and count beats.

Although most people can use the carotid site without experiencing any problems, a word of caution is in order. Special receptors located in the walls of the carotid artery are responsible for detecting changes in pressure. If you put pressure on these baroreceptors

while taking your pulse (or massage them while looking for your pulse), they send a message to the heart to slow down. This slowing heart rate can cause dizziness or faintness in some people. If your heart rate does slow down, your pulse count will not be accurate. Try taking your pulse at both your carotid and radial sites. If you find the carotid gives you a slower count, use the radial site.

When taking your pulse, count complete cardiac cycles. A pulse throb constitutes the end of a cardiac cycle. If the instructor says "go" and you immediately feel a throb, don't count it (or, call it zero). If the instructor says "go" and there is a pause and then a beat, go ahead and count it as number 1. Continue to count until the instructor stops you.

OTHER HEART RATES

Other heart rates in addition to the EHR are useful to monitor and compare. For example, the RHR is a useful indicator of cardiorespiratory fitness. As your fitness improves, your heart becomes stronger and your circulatory system more efficient. This means that your heart can beat fewer times per minute and still accomplish the same amount of work. Think of how many times you have to work the handle on an inefficient pump to get a gallon of water compared to the number of times you have to work the handle on an efficient pump. Your heart acts like a pump. As your heart and circulatory system improve, you will be able to see a decline in your RHR. Remember the principle of individuality; some people's RHRs will decline quickly and dramatically, while those of others

SELECTING A HEART-RATE MONITOR

Heart-rate monitors have improved significantly and the cost of good ones has dropped, thus making them a more affordable tool for individuals embarking on an aerobics program. They generally consist of a lightweight wireless transmitter that is worn comfortably and securely around the chest (below the bustline) that picks up the heartbeat and sends a signal to a watchlike receiver worn on the wrist where it displays heart rate in beats per minute. Other versions make use of technology that measures heart rate by finger touch on the wrist receiver, but these are generally less accurate. A good monitor will track total exercise time, time in your training zone, and average heart rate. It will also have an alarm that lets you know when you drop below or exceed your training zone. More expensive models include more options, such as a calorie counter, data storage, and an improved ability to screen out heart-rate signals from other nearby monitors.

A heart-rate monitor is only as good as the formulas and information in its memory. A monitor that allows you to input information such as your resting heart rate, height, weight, gender, and age will be more accurate than one that does not. Although these devices are great training tools that offer immediate feedback and reinforcement, they are by no means necessary equipment for an aerobic workout. Heart rate can be monitored accurately and easily just by counting your pulse. Finger and earlobe monitors that you may encounter on older fitness equipment are not reliable.

will hardly decline at all. An average RHR is 70 to 80 bpm. Highly trained athletes often have RHRs as low as 45, but some elite runners have RHRs in the 60s and 70s. (These athletes are highly efficient in some other physiological way.) Take your RHR periodically to see if it is declining.

Besides heredity and exercise, a number of other factors influence the RHR. Medication, illness, stress, overtraining, temperature, caffeine, and smoking are a few of the major influences. Because many of these influences are transient, you probably won't pick them up in a morning RHR reading. They will, however, often show up in a heart rate taken right before class. For example, your **pre-exercise heart rate (PreHR)** can be elevated if you are still digesting a meal, just drank a cup of caffeinated coffee or a can of soda, ran to class, or are anxious about a test in the next class. Take your PreHR before you begin exercising, plot it on the chart provided in Worksheet 5, and see whether you can identify reasons for any fluctuations you discover.

Another useful heart rate to monitor is your **recovery heart rate (RecHR),** which reflects the speed with which your cardiorespiratory system can return to its pre-exercise state after you stop exercising. It is often used as an indicator of fitness because a physically fit person with an efficient cardiorespiratory system recovers from exercise more quickly than an unfit person exercising at the same intensity. The heart rate drops rapidly during the first minute of recovery,

then more slowly, and gradually drops to normal. A good guideline is to be able to return to a heart rate below 120 bpm within 2 minutes. If you are not below 120 bpm in 5 minutes, your THR is probably too high for your fitness level. (You may also have performed too active a cool-down.) Continue to cool down until your pulse is below 120 bpm.

To monitor your RecHR, take your pulse immediately after the aerobic portion of class and again 1 minute later. Record your RecHR on the chart provided in Worksheet 5. Your instructor may want to use a 2-, 3-, or 5-minute recovery time instead of a 1-minute time. Any recovery time will work as long as you are consistent, although more fit people may want to use the shorter times because most of their recovery will occur in the first 2 minutes. You should see an improved recovery rate after about 6 to 12 weeks of aerobic conditioning.

Keeping track of these heart rates can make you more aware of the kinds of things (exercise, stress, caffeine, and others) that affect your body. Figure 4.4 is an example of a heart rate chart in progress for a 20-year-old individual. The THR is drawn in bold lines. The PreHR, EHR, and RecHR have been recorded for each exercise session. Lines connecting the same types of heart rates have been drawn to make it easier to see the trends. Some trends to look for include a more consistent EHR with practice, a lower RecHR over time, and an increased ability to work in the upper portion of the THR.

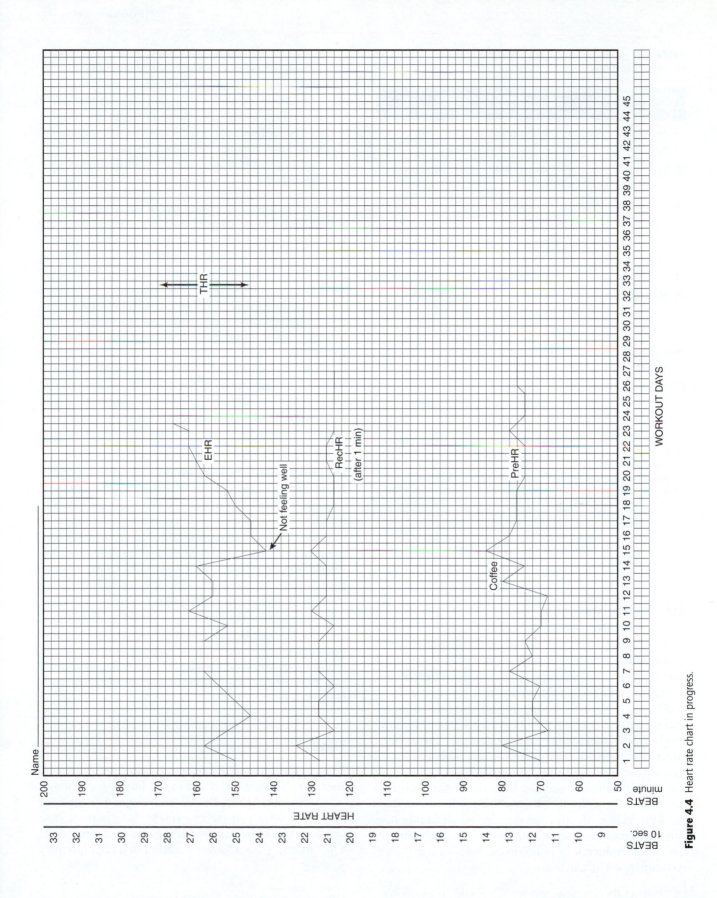

Figure 4.4 Heart rate chart in progress.

Table 4.1 Category and Category-Ratio Scales for Ratings of Perceived Exertions

BORG–RPE SCALE* (CATEGORY SCALE)		BORG CR 10 SCALE (CATEGORY RATIO SCALE)	
6	No exertion at all	0	Nothing at all	
7	Extremely light	0.3		
8		0.5	Extremely weak	Just noticeable
9	Very light	0.7		
10		1	Very weak	
11	Light	1.5		
12		2	Weak	Light
13	Somewhat hard	2.5		
14		3	Moderate	
15	Hard (heavy)	4		
16		5	Strong	Heavy
17	Very hard	6		
18		7	Very strong	
19	Extremely hard	8		
20	Maximal exertion	9		
		10	Extremely strong	"Maximal"
		11		
		•	Absolute maximum	Highest possible

*Copyright Gunnar Borg.
Detailed information about the Borg Scales is given in the book by Borg, G., *Borg's Perceived Exertion and Pain Scales.* Champaign, IL, Human Kinetics, 1998. For correct usage it is necessary to follow the instructions given in the folders: (1) Borg, G., 1994, 2002, the BORG–RPE-SCALE, A method for measuring perceived exertion, and (2) Borg, G., 1998, 2002, the BORG CR 10 SCALE, A method for measuring intensity of experience, e.g., perceived exertion and pain. Order from Borg Products USA, Inc. Att: Joseph V. Myers III, 1579 F. Monroe Drive, #416 Atlanta, GA 30324, USA.

ALTERNATIVE METHODS OF MONITORING INTENSITY

A Swedish physiologist named Gunnar Borg discovered a relationship between the perception of exercise intensity and heart rate. He developed the **ratings of perceived exertion (RPE)** scales shown in Table 4.1. To use these scales, you look at the numbers and word descriptions and select the number that best represents how hard you feel (perceive) you are exercising. An aerobic training effect is associated with perceived exertion ratings of "somewhat hard" to "hard," approximately 12 to 16 on the original category scale and ratings of 4 to 5 on the category-ratio scale. Research evidence indicates that the RPE scale is an effective way for adults to monitor aerobic intensity as long as standardized instructions are used to introduce it. The following are Gunnar Borg's recommended instructions:

> During the exercise test we want you to pay close attention to how hard you feel the exercise

work rate is. This feeling should reflect your total amount of exertion and fatigue, combining all sensations and feelings of physical stress, effort, and fatigue. Don't concern yourself with any one factor such as leg pain, shortness of breath or exercise intensity, but try to concentrate on your total, inner feeling of exertion. Try not to underestimate or overestimate your feelings of exertion; be as accurate as you can.[1]

One big advantage of ratings of perceived exertion is that they can be used to monitor exercise intensity when heart rate is not reliable. If, for example, you are on a medication that affects heart rate, or if you aren't good at taking a pulse count, RPE can be a good method for estimating workout intensity. If your heart rate is a valid way to estimate intensity, you may want to compare heart rates with ratings of perceived exertion to see where your training range falls on the RPE scales.

Another quick, easy (and less scientific) method for estimating intensity is the talk test. You should be able to talk comfortably while working out. If you can't, your workout intensity is too high. If you can sing comfortably, your intensity is probably too low.

WHEN TO MONITOR INTENSITY

Using the pulse check, the RPE scale, or the talk test, you can monitor your level of exertion periodically during your workout. It is a good idea to check your intensity level 5 to 10 minutes into the aerobic workout to make sure you have reached your training intensity. Check again at the peak of the aerobic section to make sure you aren't too high. Check once again toward the end of the aerobic section to see whether you were able to maintain the training intensity to the end. If you check your intensity only at the end of class and find that you are too high or too low, it is too late to modify your workout. In addition, your finishing heart rate may not be indicative of the intensity of your entire workout.

TIME

Time, or the duration of exercise, is linked with intensity. Together they need to result in the burning of enough calories to meet health, fitness, and weight management goals. The total volume of exercise is important. You can burn the same number of calories by exercising at a low intensity for a longer duration or a high intensity

---

1. Borg, G., *Borg's Perceived Exertion and Pain Scales*, Champaign, IL: Human Kinetics, 1998

for a short duration. To accommodate differences in intensity, the ACSM recommends 20 to 60 minutes of continuous or intermittent (10-minute bouts) exercise accumulated through the day, and advises that 20 to 30 minutes of exercise (not including warm-up and cool-down) at intensities equal to 70 to 85% of MHR or 60 to 80% of HRR will allow most individuals to reach their health, fitness, and weight management goals. In addition, Dr. Kenneth Cooper, director of the Institute for Aerobics Research in Dallas, Texas, recommends limiting running to 80 to 90 minutes a week at 3 times a week for 30 minutes or 4 times a week for 20 minutes. He believes that the additional benefits gained by running more (other than additional weight loss) do not outweigh the increased risk of bone, joint, and muscle injury.

Because the impact stress in high-impact aerobic dance exercise is equal to or greater than that of running, it makes sense to limit a high-impact aerobic segment to 20 to 30 minutes per session. If you want to exercise aerobically for a longer duration, you can supplement your aerobic dance exercise with a nonimpact, low-impact, or non-weight-bearing activity. Activities such as a brisk walk can be done for up to an hour with little worry of overuse injury. Individuals, such as competitors and instructors, who choose to perform moderate- to high-intensity aerobics for more than 30 minutes, do so for reasons other than health.

EXERCISE LEVELS

Individuals who have not been exercising regularly, who are returning to exercise after childbirth or an injury, or who are substantially overweight (overfat) should start exercising at the low end of the target zones. For some beginners, even threshold amounts of exercise may be too much of an overload. In this event, start with small, manageable workout segments, 3 to 10 minutes long. Start with walking, cycling, swimming, or easy dance steps, and work up to more formal aerobic dance exercises. To overload, first increase the frequency of the short bouts, and then start to increase duration by putting short bouts together. When you can exercise for 20 to 30 minutes, overload by increasing intensity. If burning fat is your goal, use longer durations up to 30 to 60 minutes (depending on the activity), at low to moderate intensities. As you become more fit, you will find that you have to use more arm work and larger ranges of motion to challenge your aerobic system. Big movements are recommended, but avoid the use of momentum and do not overextend the limits of your flexibility.

Research has shown that aerobic dance activity results in cardiorespiratory training similar to that of jogging and cycling. However, physiologists have not yet determined whether regular aerobic dance activity can train and maintain very high fitness levels. If you are interested in a competitive level of aerobic conditioning, you may have to combine aerobic dance training with other forms of aerobic exercise. I have had a few highly fit runners in my classes who, even with vigorous movement, were unable to reach the upper ranges of their THR. These individuals used aerobic dance exercise for light workout days and change of pace, while everyone else worked up a heavy sweat! Step aerobics, particularly with power moves, can probably challenge even the most fit. Advanced participants, give it a try!

COMMONLY ASKED QUESTIONS

Is it safe for a fit person's heart rate to exceed the age-related training heart rate zone?

Remember that the THR is calculated based on averages. It is possible that an individual has a higher maximum heart rate than the estimate derived from the formula. If this is true, then it would make sense to raise the THR. Perceived exertion can be considered in this case. As long as the person is healthy and it "feels" right, the zone can be adjusted upward. Recovery rates can also be used to help reestablish a zone.

Can I achieve aerobic conditioning if I am not in the zone?

If you are a low-fit individual, you can achieve aerobic conditioning at the lower intensities, as discussed in the text. Too low a level will not result in aerobic fitness changes but may still provide some health-related benefits. Moderately vigorous physical activity, such as brisk walking, results in health benefits.

I have trouble finding my pulse. What should I do?

Try locating your pulse at the wrist, neck, and temple. Practice this outside class for a couple of days. If you are still unsuccessful, try putting your hand on your chest and counting beats. If you are still unsuccessful, try the talk test and/or ratings of perceived exertion. A heart-rate monitor would also solve the problem.

I am highly fit and can't get my heart rate high in my zone. What can I do?

Use propulsion steps, travel more, raise and lower your center of gravity as much as possible, and use arm movements with every step. Ask your instructor for specific modifications. Also, remember you can achieve a good workout in the middle of the zone.

Other questions pertaining to fat burning can be found in Chapter 8.

SUMMARY

To improve aerobic fitness, exercise above your aerobic threshold and within your aerobic target zone. For less fit individuals, threshold intensities will be lower than for fit individuals. The target zone is described by the FIT variables: frequency, intensity, and time. Optimum cardiorespiratory fitness occurs when you exercise 3 to 5 times a week, at 50–60% to 85% of heart rate reserve, for 20 to 60 minutes. When aerobic dance exercise is the mode of training, the duration of high-impact aerobic routines should be shortened to 20 to 30 minutes and, for most active individuals, performed at an intensity of 60 to 80% of heart rate reserve. This level of exercise will promote health and minimize overuse injuries. Longer aerobic workouts can be safely performed if low-impact or nonimpact activities are used. Beginners should start out near their low end or threshold levels of frequency, intensity, and time. This usually means exercising 3 times a week for 20 minutes at an intensity equal to 50 to 60% of HRR. When beginners need to start out below threshold, they should first gradually increase time and frequency and then intensity. Advanced participants can, of course, work out at the higher end of their ranges.

A final note: Remember that heart rate formulas are based on averages; although they provide good estimates for most people, there are individuals for whom the range may need to be adjusted. If your training range seems too high or too low, speak with your instructor.

KNOWLEDGE TIPS

1. Participants can monitor the intensity of an aerobic workout using heart rate (pulse) counts, ratings of perceived exertion, or the talk test.

2. To obtain an EHR, the pulse should be counted for 10 seconds using the radial or carotid site within 15 seconds of stopping. If a heart-rate monitor is being used, heart rate can be checked while exercising.

3. Participants should monitor their intensity several times during the workout to make sure they are working in their aerobic target zone.

4. The best measures of oxygen consumption and MHR are obtained through direct measurement during a graded exercise stress test (on a treadmill, stationary bicycle, or other ergonomic device).

5. Heart rate and oxygen consumption have a nearly linear relationship.

6. The Karvonen formula (heart-rate reserve formula) estimates THR using age and resting heart rate. The intensity range is usually calculated as 60 to 80% of HRR. However, less fit individuals can use 50 to 60% of HRR.

7. The MHR formula estimates THR by taking a direct percentage of the MHR. The intensity range is usually calculated as 70 to 85% of the MHR. However, less fit individuals can use 60 to 70% of MHR.

8. Ratings of perceived exertion can be used to monitor intensity and are particularly useful when heart rate is not a reliable or valid indicator of intensity.

9. The RHR and RecHR are also useful indicators of fitness.

10. Optimal exercise frequency is 3 to 5 times a week with an exception of additional frequency for weight-loss purposes.

11. Optimal duration for the aerobic segment of a high-impact aerobic dance exercise class is 20 to 30 minutes.

THINK ABOUT IT

1. What is the FITT principle for aerobic exercise? Explain how it is adjusted based on fitness level.

2. Identify and explain three methods of estimating (monitoring) intensity during aerobic activity. What is the target zone using each method?

3. Why are there two different heart-rate formulas for estimating the aerobic target zone?

4. Explain how to properly count one's pulse.

5. When should you monitor the intensity of your workout? How often?

6. If weight loss is the primary goal, how does this influence the FITT principle?

7. Explain how a person performing movements at a low level (low amplitude, smaller ranges of motion, low impact) and a person performing movements at a high level (propulsion moves, jumping, etc.) can both be working within their target heart-rate zones.

8. How can two people be performing the same exercise at the same tempo (jumping jacks on a beat) and one person have a higher heart rate than the other person?

9. If a person is over his or her target zone, what kinds of adjustment can be made to get into zone? (*Hint:* There are ways to stay on the beat and still make adjustments.)

10. What are the implications of being below, in, and above your aerobic target zone?

REFERENCES

American College of Sports Medicine. "The Recommended Quantity and Quality of Exercise for Developing and Maintaining Cardiorespiratory and Muscle Fitness in Healthy Adults." *Medicine and Science in Sports and Exercise* 30 (No. 6, 1998): 975–91.

Åstrand, P. O., and K. Rodahl. *Textbook of Work Physiology.* 2nd ed. New York: McGraw-Hill, 1977.

Bell, J. M., and E. J. Bassey. "A Comparison of the Relation Between Oxygen Uptake and Heart Rate During Different Styles of Aerobic Dance and a Traditional Step Test in Women." *European Journal of Applied Physiology* 68 (No. 1, 1994): 20–4.

Borg, G. *Borg's Perceived Exertion and Pain Scales.* Champaign, IL: Human Kinetics, 1998.

——. "Psychophysical Bases of Perceived Exertion." *Medicine and Science in Sports and Exercise* 14 (No. 5, 1982): 377–81.

Cearly, M., R. Moffatt, and K. Knutzen. "The Effects of Two- and Three-Day-per-Week Aerobic Dance Programs on Maximal Oxygen Uptake." *Research Quarterly for Exercise and Sport* 55 (1984):172–4.

Cooper, K. H. *Aerobics.* New York: Bantam Books, 1968.

Couldry, W., C. B. Corbin, and A. Wilcox. "Carotid vs. Radial Pulse Counts." *The Physician and Sportsmedicine* 10 (No. 12, 1982): 67–72.

Foster, C. "Physiological Requirements of Aerobic Dancing." *Research Quarterly* 46 (1975):120–2.

Garber, C. E., J. S. McKinney, and R. A. Carleton. "Is Aerobic Dance an Effective Alternative to Walk-Jog Exercise Training?" *Journal of Sports Medicine and Physical Fitness* 32 (No. 2, 1992): 136–41.

Gellish, R. L., B. R. Goslin, R. E. Olson, A. McDonald, G. D. Russi, and V. K. Moudgil. "Longitudinal Modeling of the Relationship Between Age and Maximal Heart Rate." *Medicine and Science in Sports and Exercise* 39 (No. 5, 2007): 822–9.

Hooper, P. L., and B. J. Noland. "Aerobic Dance Program Improves Cardiovascular Fitness in Men." *The Physician and Sportsmedicine* 12 (No. 5, 1984): 132–5.

Igbanugo, V. and B. Gutin. "The Energy Cost of Aerobic Dancing." *Research Quarterly* 49 (1978): 308–15.

Jackson, A. S. "Estimating Maximum Heart Rate from Age: Is It a Linear Relationship?" *Medicine and Science in Sports and Exercise* 39 (No. 5, 2007): 821.

Karvonen, M., E. Kentala, and O. Mustalof. "The Effects of Training on Heart Rate: A Longitudinal Study." *Annales de Medicinae Experimentalis et Biologiae Fenniae* 35 (1957): 307–15.

Koltyn, K. F., and W. P. Morgan. "Efficacy of Perceptual Versus Heart Rate Monitoring in the Development of Endurance." *British Journal of Sports Medicine* 26 (No. 2, June 1992): 132–4.

Lind, A. R., and G. W. McNichol. "Cardiovascular Responses to Holding and Carrying Weights by Hand and by Shoulder Harness." *Journal of Applied Physiology* 25 (1968): 261–7.

Mahurin, J., and T. P. Martin. "Anaerobic Threshold: A Trainable Component of Cardiovascular Fitness." *Motor Skills: Theory Into Practice* 6 (1982): 41.

McArdle, W., L. Zwiren, and J. R. Magel. "Validity of the Postexercise Heart Rate as a Means of Estimating Heart Rate During Work of Varying Intensities." *Research Quarterly* 40 (1969): 523–8.

Parker, S. B., B. F. Hurley, D. P. Hanlon, and P. Vaccaro. "Failure of Target Heart Rate to Accurately Monitor Intensity During Aerobic Dance." *Medicine and Science in Sports and Exercise* 21 (1989): 230–4.

Pollock, M. L. "How Much Exercise Is Enough?" *The Physician and Sportsmedicine* 6 (No. 6, 1978): 50–6; 58–60; 63–4.

Reeves., B. D., and L. A. Darby. "Physiological Responses of Female Experienced and Novice Aerobic Dancers During Graded Exercise Tests: Treadmill vs. Dance Exercise." (Abstract). *Medicine and Science in Sports and Exercise* 24 (1992, Suppl.): S97.

Reeves, B. D., L. A. Darby, C. L. Moss, and C. Armstrong. "Energy Costs and Vertical Forces of High-Impact and Low-Impact Aerobic Dance Sequences." (Abstract). *Research Quarterly for Exercise and Sport* 63 (1992, Suppl.): A28.

Schaeffer, S. A., L. A. Darby, K. D. Browder, and B. D. Reeves. "Perceived Exertion and Metabolic Responses of Women During Aerobic Dance Exercise." *Perceptual Motor Skills* 81 (No. 2, 1995): 691–700.

Scharff-Olson, M., H. N. Williford, and F. H. Smith. "The Heart Rate VO$_2$ Relationship of Aerobic Dance: A Comparison of Target Heart Rate Methods." *Journal of Sports Medicine and Physical Fitness* 32 (No. 4, 1992): 372–7.

Skinner, J. S., R. Hursler, V. Bergsteinova, and E. R. Buskirk. "The Validity and Reliability of a Rating Scale of Perceived Exertion." *Medicine and Science in Sports* 5 (No. 2, 1973): 94–6.

Tanaka, H., K. D. Monahan, and D. R. Seals. "Age-Predicted Maximal Heart Rate Revisited." *Journal of American College of Cardiology* 37 (2001): 153–6.

U.S. Department of Health and Human Services. *2008 Physical Activity Guidelines for Americans.* U.S. Department of Health and Human Services, 2008.

5

Setting Goals and Reaching Your Dream

"Habit is a cable; we weave a thread of it each day, and at last we cannot break it."

HORACE MANN

- I set goals but don't seem to reach them. What should I do differently?
- How can I track and measure my progress?
- What will keep me motivated?

Do you dream of looking svelte, sporting beautifully toned muscles, living longer, and feeling radiantly full of energy? Millions of people do, and they enroll in exercise classes, buy fancy outfits and expensive equipment, and talk enthusiastically about the fun and benefits. Then, within 6 months, 30 to 70% of these people drop out of their program. Even many former varsity athletes and coaches who have spent most of their lives promoting fitness are overweight (overfat) and out of shape. The irony is that while more than 60% of adults don't exercise regularly (25% don't exercise at all), most have a good attitude about exercise and think it would be a good thing for them to do.

Why, then, do so many people quit exercising or never get started? Physical educators, fitness specialists, and exercise scientists have been trying to answer that question. While there is still much to learn, there is substantial information we can put to work. The reasons that people don't start are usually different from the reasons people quit. You have already conquered all the barriers that keep people from starting (congratulations!), so this chapter will focus on how to keep your commitment to exercise going—for a lifetime.

Now, let's back up for a moment. If you have dreams, the first thing you need to do to turn those dreams into realities is establish some very specific, realistic goals. Many times people have an idea of what they want but don't take the time to nail it down. And sometimes what we want is media driven rather than realistic. There is not one beautiful body type; there are

many. Therefore, individualize your goals to bring your body type to its full potential and to attain personal health. Writing goals will be the first step in reaching your dream. Step two is to find and use sources of motivation. Third, select an activity (or activities), such as aerobic dance exercise, that will help you reach your goals. Because you are already in an aerobic dance exercise course, let's hope it is the right vehicle for reaching at least some of your goals. Fourth, establish a method for measuring your progress. Fifth, set up a periodic review of your goals and program to make sure they still reflect what you wish to accomplish. And finally, identify barriers, supports, and strategies to prevent relapses and to help you restart if you do temporarily stop exercising.

As you take these steps, you will be using the behavior change strategies introduced in Chapter 1. Reaching a goal usually involves change, and behavior change doesn't happen easily or by sheer willpower alone. These strategies will support your efforts and make success a little easier to reach.

STEP ONE: ESTABLISHING YOUR FITNESS GOALS

THE BASIS FOR YOUR GOALS

A goal is a statement of what you want to happen. Base your fitness goals on what you would like to accomplish through an exercise program. Write down any ideas that come to mind. In addition to basing your goals on personal desire, you can use the five health-related fitness components—cardiorespiratory endurance, muscular strength and endurance, flexibility, and body composition—as guidelines.

Set your goals using personal interest (desire); fitness test results; and knowledge of what is realistic, feasible, and healthy. Guidelines in this chapter, information in other parts of this book, fitness test scores, and guidance from your instructor will help you to refine the goals you identify and to select goals you may not have considered.

This chapter focuses on physical fitness goals. Some very valuable goals cannot be measured by fitness tests or, in some cases, cannot be adequately tested for at all. Your list might also include some of these goals, such as increased social involvement, improvement of self-concept, improvement of self-confidence, achievement of relaxation, and having fun. You can often measure progress toward goals such as these by keeping a journal. For example, if your goal is to have more energy and be more productive, then keeping a journal that tracks your accomplishments and how you feel at the end of a day will give you an idea of how you are progressing.

SPECIFIC GOALS

When asked to write down their goals for the semester, the majority of college students write things such as:

- lose weight
- lose inches
- last longer in the class
- look better
- become more fit
- firm up my body

The ideas expressed provide a good starting point, but they are ambiguous; there are no concrete ways to measure success. For example, does the loss of one pound constitute success? Does looking better mean an attractive appearance or how you look doing the exercises? Does lasting longer mean during the muscle-toning exercises, aerobic exercises, or both? At what point is the body firm?

These goals can be rewritten to be more specific. They might read like this:

- lose 10 pounds (lbs) in the next 10 weeks (a safe 1-lb loss per week)
- lose 1 inch from each thigh, my waist, and my hips by the end of the semester
- complete 20 minutes of standing aerobics at 60 to 80% of my maximum heart rate by the end of 6 weeks

- tone and firm my legs, as represented by losing 1 inch from my thighs and being able to do 15 leg lifts in a row with a medium-weight exercise band by the end of the semester
- complete all 3 minutes of the step test by the end of 6 weeks
- improve my curl-up score from a poor rating to an average rating in 8 weeks

These very specific goals can be measured, full or partial success can be noted and celebrated, and new goals can be set. Information throughout this book will help you identify specific goals.

REALISTIC GOALS

Beginners and overzealous participants have a tendency to choose unrealistic goals. When you set goals that are too difficult, you set yourself up for failure. Yet, goals that are too easy aren't very motivating. Three guidelines for writing challenging and yet attainable goals are (1) allow enough time to reach the goal, (2) set safe goals, and (3) base goals on correct information.

1. Positive adaptations do not occur overnight. It usually takes 6 to 8 weeks to make significant cardiorespiratory and muscular gains. It can take longer to strengthen ligaments, bones, and tendons. Be patient, and write your goals with time expectations of at least 6 to 8 weeks. People who expect quick results often quit the program before it has had a chance to work. Start with conservative goals so you have success early in the program.

2. To set safe goals, consider your medical history, your present condition, your age, and the amount of time that has passed since you last exercised. Set up a pace and program that are comfortable for you. There is no need to start out too fast and get stiff, sore, or injured. The idea is to have fun and feel good about exercising.

   Many unsafe goals arise from the desire to obtain quick results. For example, people who want very rapid weight loss starve themselves and, at the same time, attempt to attend an exercise class. Without a sufficient intake of carbohydrates, they don't have enough energy to exercise. They may feel listless, tired, dizzy, or even faint during class. Starvation diets result in significant loss of muscle and water, not just fat. The body may even start conserving and storing fat as an energy source because the caloric intake is so low.

3. Misconceptions can wreak havoc on goals. For example, a person with a goal of losing

abdominal fat might embark on an intense program of curl-ups. When he or she can do 100 curl-ups a day yet finds the fat still there, discouragement is sure to set in. The problem is that fat is lost through aerobic exercise, not through anaerobic exercise such as curl-ups. The result of doing curl-ups will be strong abdominal muscles hiding under a layer of fat. In addition, fat cannot be taken off in one specific spot (spot reduction); it comes off in a general way from all over the body.

Faulty reasoning can also be dangerous. There have been cases of pregnant women whose reason for exercising during pregnancy was to keep their figures. These women were trying to prevent normal weight gains; if allowed to continue, they would endanger the health of their babies. Pregnant women can benefit from exercise as long as it is done correctly and with the supervision of a doctor.

The best way to avoid making these kinds of mistakes is to read about fitness from reliable sources (books and articles written by professionals and materials published by recognized associations such as the American College of Sports Medicine, the National Academy of Sportsmedicine, the American College of Obstetricians and Gynecologists, the American Alliance for Health, Physical Education, Recreation, and Dance, and the National Strength and Conditioning Association) and to talk with professionals like your instructor.

It is also important to remember the principle of individuality as you try to set realistic goals. Two people on an identical exercise program will respond differently. It can be motivating to compare yourself against norms or averages or even classmates, but remember, the comparison that counts is you against you.

SHORT- AND LONG-RANGE GOALS

Take your dream, your long-range goal, and break it down into short-range goals. If your dream is to lose 3 inches off your waist, make short-term goals of ½ inch every 8 weeks. Reaching the short-term goal will give you the confidence and motivation to keep going. One step at a time will take you to your dream.

When you don't establish short-term goals, you set yourself up for total success or total failure: There is nothing in between. If reaching your goal takes a while and you have no intermediate steps of success to celebrate, it is easy to get discouraged and quit. Think of the people who climb Mt. Everest: They are pleased when they establish base camp, and they cheer as they establish each successive camp up the mountain. Their goal is the summit, but they recognize that success comes in stages.

Fitness professionals can help you set realistic, specific goals, tell you what a realistic rate of achievement is, provide encouragement, and evaluate and adjust your program. These people are service oriented and want to help you. They are your instructor, physical fitness educators in your public and private schools, directors, exercise physiologists, trainers in fitness clubs, owners and directors of private fitness businesses, personal trainers, professors and instructors of fitness and wellness at colleges and universities, health promotions instructors and directors in the workplace, and instructors and coordinators at recreation centers, YMCAs/YWCAs, and corporate programs. Seek them out.

STEPS TO GOAL WRITING
1. In general terms, decide what you want to do.
2. Assess where you are right now.
3. Make your general goal more specific, using information from your assessment (Step 2).
4. Decide how you are going to accomplish your goal.
5. Add a time frame.
6. Write a very specific goal incorporating all the information from the first five steps.
7. Decide how you will evaluate/monitor your progress.

EXAMPLE

General Statement: I want to lose weight.

Assessment: Measure (or have a professional measure) my percentage of body fat.

More Specific Goal: I want to move from 30% body fat to 24% body fat.

Plan (Mode): I will combine three days of walking and three days of low-impact aerobics with my present weight-loss diet.

Time Frame: I will lower my body fat by 6% in the next 6 weeks. (For a woman weighing 100 to 200 lbs, this represents a 6- to 12-lb loss, a 1- to 2-lb loss per week.)

Very Specific Goal: I will lose 6% body fat in the next 6 weeks using 30 minutes of brisk walking on Tuesday, Thursday, and Saturday, and attending a low-impact aerobics class on Monday, Wednesday, and Friday. I will combine this with my present 1,500-calorie balanced diet.

Evaluation of Progress: I will have my body fat measured again in 6 weeks.

STEP TWO: FINDING MOTIVATION

People usually start exercising to look good, but the main reason habitual exercisers give for continuing is that exercise feels good. Endorphins, hormonelike substances, are released during aerobic exercise; scientists believe that in addition to masking pain, endorphins are responsible for the uplifting feeling that follows a good workout. Unfortunately, many people just starting out have never felt this exercise "high" and can't identify with it. And since it takes 6 to 8 weeks to work into the exercise high, many quit before they experience this wonderful benefit.

In the beginning, you may feel a little stiff, sore, and awkward. The trick is to get past this discomfort so that you can experience the good feelings that come from exercise. When you do experience the exercise high, often accompanied by an increased sense of energy, you'll find it motivates you to keep on exercising.

There are two forms of motivation: intrinsic and extrinsic. **Intrinsic motivation** comes from inside you. If you exercise because you want to look and feel better, then you are intrinsically motivated. When you personally believe in something, you will be more motivated to do it than if someone else is telling you to do it. Find an exercise program that is taught in a style that you like, at a place you enjoy, and at a time and in a location that is convenient for you—aspects that support your intrinsic motivation. If you do this, you will be more likely to stick with your program. Positive talk is also a very powerful tool. Check into the conversation going on inside your head. Is it negative? Are you thinking of bad experiences with exercise? Or previous failures? Try to turn that around and get the little voice inside you to tell you that you can do it, that you are going to enjoy the new feelings that the program will generate. Also, try to picture yourself (visualize) doing the exercise well. During a quiet time, close your eyes and watch yourself (or feel yourself) go through the steps and exercises you've learned. Mental practice can actually make you better at physical activities. Many times, when people begin a new activity, they think that others are watching them and judging them. Get outside of yourself and look around—you will probably be relieved to see that other participants are busy trying to do the exercise and aren't looking at you at all. Be sure to give yourself some positive talk right after the workout. Reaffirm your goals, and congratulate yourself on taking one more step toward them. You can be your own best motivator.

You may already be one of those rare and wonderful people who has the internal desire and discipline to exercise all of your life. If so, fantastic! But if you are like most of us, you need the occasional proverbial "kick in the pants" to keep motivated. Motivation that comes from outside you is called **extrinsic motivation**. Here are a few sources of extrinsic motivation you can tap.

1. Find another person who also wants to exercise, and make a pact to meet at a designated place on workout days. Knowing the other person is waiting for you will get you there. Carpools with rotating drivers also provide an extra incentive to show up, especially if you are the driver.

2. Get the people around you—friends, family, and fellow employees—to support or join you in your exercise endeavors. Plan family outings that involve hiking, swimming, cycling, and other forms of exercise. Organize a college or worksite team to participate in a local road race or aerobithon.

3. Find sources of feedback and reinforcement. Get to know your instructor, and find out if you are doing things correctly. A good instructor will be positive and upbeat, will provide feedback periodically, and will miss you when you are not there. It is much more difficult to miss a class when the instructor or participants are going to give you a hard time for not being there.

4. Write down your goals, and look at them periodically. Some people like to post their goals on their bathroom mirror or refrigerator door so they will see them often. Perhaps it will help you to tell someone about your goals, especially if that person is in a position to help you attain them. For example, your instructor may be able to introduce you to someone else with the same goal.

5. Set aside a specific time for your exercise, and let others know so that you won't be interrupted.

6. Do something nice for yourself and others when you reach a short-term goal.

7. Finally, accept that you will have lapses. We are all human. Illness, emergencies, vacation, or even boredom can take you temporarily off your program. It doesn't mean that you are a miserable failure. Just pick a date to begin again, and go forth with new resolve.

STEP THREE: CHOOSING THE ACTIVITY

If your goal is to be aerobically fit, you have a wide variety of activities from which to choose: aerobic dancing, walking, swimming, cycling, rowing, cross-country skiing, stair stepping, jumping rope, and many others. Select an activity you enjoy. For the sake of this book, let's assume you've decided on aerobic dance exercise.

You can select one or more new activities. Using two or more activities in your exercise program is called cross-training. A lot of people find this prevents boredom. Doing things you enjoy will help you stick with exercise and make it a lifetime habit.

STEP FOUR: TRACKING YOUR PROGRESS

To measure progress, you must have a starting point; a good one is your present fitness level. You can measure it using one of the many fitness tests that have been developed over the years. Or if physical activity is your goal, you can use a pedometer to determine your baseline number of steps per day. (See the box Using a Pedometer on the following page.) The tests contained in this text were selected because of their relationship to the health-related fitness components. Table 5.1 is a list of these tests under their appropriate fitness component heading. Each test is described in detail on the designated worksheet provided at the back of the book or in the appropriate chapter. The norms provided with these tests should give you a general idea of how well you scored. Don't be too concerned with the norms; it is more important to compare your scores at the beginning of a program to your scores later in the program.

Some fitness tests can be taken right at the beginning of a program. Other, more difficult tests, such as the 12-minute walk/run test and the 1.5-mile timed run test, should be taken only after you've been exercising for about 6 weeks. Retake the tests after about 8 to 12 weeks to see how you are progressing. It is very motivating to see tangible evidence of improvement. (You may even see improvement in 6 weeks, but don't be discouraged if it takes a little longer. Changes in cardiorespiratory endurance can take longer than improvements in muscular strength and endurance.) You may discover that you are very fit in one component and not so fit in another. Follow a program that lets you maintain your strengths and improve your weaknesses.

To track your progress, several worksheets have been provided with this text (in the worksheets section). Worksheet 2 provides a place to record your fitness and healthy weight scores over several test periods. Worksheet 5 lets you plot your heart rates over time, including resting heart rate (RHR), so that you

Table 5.1 Fitness Tests

FITNESS TESTS	
CARDIORESPIRATORY ENDURANCE TESTS	
Step Test	Worksheet 9
12-Minute Walk/Run	Worksheet 10
1.5-Mile Timed Run	Worksheet 11
FLEXIBILITY TESTS	
Trunk Forward Flexion Test	Worksheet 12
Quick-Check Flexibility Tests	Worksheet 13
MUSCULAR STRENGTH AND ENDURANCE TESTS	
Partial Curl-Up Test	Worksheet 14
Push-Up Test	Worksheet 15
BODY COMPOSITION TESTS	
Body Fat Assessments	Chapter 12
Healthy Weight Assessments	Worksheet 16

can look for trends such as a lowering in RHR over time. Worksheet 7 is a fitness log on which you can track all of your physical activity and make comments about how you are feeling during or about the exercise/activity. The latter helps you to evaluate nonfitness but related goals like gaining self-confidence, finding new friends, and so on. Worksheet 8 helps you establish a baseline, set a goal, and track your steps using a pedometer. Keeping track of your progress can be both insightful and motivating.

STEP FIVE: EVALUATING THE PROGRAM AND YOUR GOALS

After you have been exercising for 8 to 12 weeks, it is important to take an objective look at your program to see if it is accomplishing what you intended. Look at your goals and at your most recent fitness test scores. If your goals also included things such as meeting new people, ask yourself how many new friends you have made or read back over your journal to look for patterns of improvement. If the results of your program don't indicate achievement toward your goals, something is wrong; change the goals, or change the program.

Sometimes goals change. For example, teenagers often base their goals on a desire to have an attractive body, while adults place more emphasis on weight control and a healthy body. As retirement approaches, people tend to shift their goals again, this time toward sociability and maintaining physical independence.

USING A PEDOMETER

Pedometers are fun, inexpensive devices that help you track your physical activity by counting the number of steps you take. A popular goal for pedometer stepping is 10,000 steps a day for adults. Although having a 10,000-step goal can be fun to strive for, the best thing to do is find out how many steps you typically take and then challenge yourself to gradually take more. The following baseline and goal-setting approach is recommended:[1]

- A baseline count is determined by wearing the pedometer for 8 days (adults and adolescents) and determining the average number of steps/day.

- When the baseline average is determined, a 10% increase of steps is calculated and added to the baseline number every two weeks with an overall goal of achieving about 4,000 to 6,000 steps above the baseline.

- If your baseline is already 10,000 or more, you can set a higher step goal or simply maintain your baseline amount.

- Use Worksheet 8 on pages 231–232 to calculate your baseline and your goals and chart your steps.

TESTING YOUR PEDOMETER

When you get your new pedometer home, give it a test run to make sure it is reasonably accurate.

- Walk or jog 100 steps and then look at the step count; a count within 2–3 steps is acceptable. (This is not an expensive piece of equipment, so it will likely not be "exact.")

- Most pedometer research is done using models with up to 2% error. Some models will have more error, and you can decide what is acceptable to you.

POSITIONING YOUR PEDOMETER

Position your pedometer on your waistline directly above (inline with) the right knee; the pedometer should sit vertically to react to the up and down motion of a step.

- Tilting of the pedometer can interfere with the counting mechanism. Tilt may be the result of a loose waistband or abdominal fat pushing down on the top of the pedometer.

- If the accuracy of your pedometer is more than a few steps off, try wearing it more to the right (slightly in front of, or over the hip); as a last resort, try placing it in the center of your back.

- Fasten the leash, if present, as this will save it from hitting the floor (or falling in the toilet—more common than you'd think!) if it comes off your waistband.

FEATURES

Newer pedometers can count steps, convert steps to distance using stride length, calculate calories burned, estimate intensity using steps per minute (spm), and keep track of bouts of exercise at designated levels of exertion.

1. R. P. Pangrazi, A. Beighle, and C. L. Sidman. *Pedometer Power: Using Pedometers in School and Community.* Champaign, IL: Human Kinetics, 2003.

Keep your goals up to date, and adjust your program whenever your goals change.

Sometimes you don't follow your own exercise plan. Here are some examples of how this can happen:

- The instructor and class may have a plan (priorities) different from yours.
- You get injured and have to modify your plan.
- You don't like part of the plan and decide not to do it, or you don't have enough time to work at your whole plan. When these things happen, reassess your priorities and try to create a new exercise plan.

If the class you are in is different from what you expected and you cannot change classes, see if the instructor will let you individualize your workout enough to satisfy you both. For example, if you really want to develop strong abdominal muscles and the class emphasis is on leg work, see if you can do some abdominal exercises while the class continues with leg work.

When you aren't doing something because you dislike it, see if another exercise can accomplish the same thing. For instance, some people don't like or can't do push-ups. An arm-pushing exercise using an exercise band can be substituted. If no substitutes are practical, decide whether an exercise is important enough to you or your health to do it anyway.

In the event of injury, extend the time period on your goal and be patient. If you don't have enough time to work on your entire plan, determine your highest priorities and put time where you need it most.

Sometimes your personal exercise program isn't working. You may be using insufficient overloads or the wrong exercises. Check with your instructor or other fitness professionals for ideas.

In other cases, the program is working, but it is not reflected in the goals. Take, for example, a person whose goal is to lose weight. Eight weeks of aerobics later, she is discouraged because she has gained weight. Upon closer examination, however, she discovers that she has lost inches and has a lower percentage of body fat; she actually lost fat and gained muscle. Because muscle weighs more than fat, she gained weight. The program worked, but the evaluation tool she used (weighing herself versus a body fat measurement) did not reflect the improvement.

Sometimes, a new and better exercise program comes along. If you hear of a new program, find out if it is based on solid information and backed by people with good credentials. Exercise research generates new information, which results in new and sometimes better program ideas. For example, 40 years ago it was thought that weight training would inhibit strength. Football players were not allowed to lift weights! Today we know that weight training is a good way to improve muscular strength, and it is being incorporated into aerobic dance exercise through the use of dumbbells, bars, weighted balls, exercise bands, and stability balls. Be open-minded when it comes to new ideas, but beware of promises of instant success.

STEP SIX: PROTECTING YOUR COMMITMENT

Starting an exercise program takes initiative; sticking to one requires motivation and a good game plan—one that includes contingency plans. Even the most committed people can find themselves suddenly sidelined by an injury or illness. Other things that can disrupt your normal routine and interfere with an exercise program include vacations, business travel, pregnancy, emergencies, or helping others. Think for a minute and identify the things that could cause you to stop exercising—even for a day. These are called barriers, in this case, barriers toward continued exercise. Now decide how you can break through these barriers. Think about how you can prevent these situations, continue to exercise during certain conditions, or get started again once the disruptive situation has been resolved.

Some examples may make this clearer. When your college or university breaks for a holiday, do you stop exercising until after the break? If yes, how can you prevent this relapse? You could make arrangements to attend an exercise class with a parent at home, use a videotape, or get together with friends to play a sport like tennis. If you travel on business, try taking a brisk walk after checking in or before a meal, or bringing an exercise band and jump rope, or check to see whether the hotel has an exercise room. Some hotels have arrangements with nearby health clubs; you might even be able to take an aerobics class. There are a lot of exciting options for exercise on a vacation, everything from a jog on the beach to a brisk walk down Fifth Avenue. The key is to plan it into the vacation and, if others are involved, plan things you can do together. Try to include two to three fitness activities per week. If you find yourself talking with relatives all day, see if someone would like to walk and talk. If you are planning a pregnancy, look into special exercise programs now for later in the pregnancy, because you will probably be less motivated to do so later. Also, set up a plan for returning to exercise following childbirth. Share these ideas with your physician.

When the flu season catches up with you, you will need to take some time off. Exercise is a stressor; while you are sick or injured, you need to let your body use its resources to make you well. Sometimes, caring for someone else through an illness or crisis can throw you off your exercise routine. In cases like these, you need some strategies for getting started again. When an instructor is marking you absent, that always provides motivation. But when you are no longer enrolled in a course, the motivation must come from within. Some people find that writing down a start date helps them. Others make a pact with someone else, and they start together. Or maybe setting out your exercise clothes is enough to get you going. Decide *now* what you will do if you stop or have to take a break.

Sustaining a wellness behavior like exercise can be difficult at times. Identifying strategies and people who will support you in your efforts gives you somewhere to turn when you feel your commitment wavering. A number of supports have already been discussed under the section on motivation. Positive reinforcement, feeling good about yourself, and having social support for what you are doing go a long way in staying motivated. When you are doing well, look around and see whether someone else needs a word of encouragement!

SUMMARY

Adhering to exercise can be a problem. You can protect your commitment to exercise by taking the time to identify goals, barriers, and supports. With the help of your instructor, determine your fitness goals and set up a plan of action. Make the plan specific and realistic, then stick with it. Check your progress, and celebrate improvement. Update your fitness plan throughout your life, and it will continue to bring you satisfaction and joy.

KNOWLEDGE TIPS

1. The dropout rate in exercise programs is between 30 and 70% within 6 months of beginning the program. Certain strategies may improve adherence.

2. Goals can be based on personal desires, fitness test scores, information from knowledgeable sources, and advice from professional educators.

3. Establish clear, specific, and (whenever possible) measurable goals.

4. For motivational purposes, break long-range goals into a series of short-range goals.

5. Intrinsic motivation comes from within yourself and is the most powerful form of motivation. Extrinsic motivation comes from outside sources. Use both.

6. Select exercise activities that will help you reach your goals. Vary these activities as needed.

7. Use fitness tests to measure your current fitness levels, and continue to check your progress using the same tests. Use journals to track your progress in nonfitness goals such as building self-confidence and making new friends.

8. Periodically evaluate your exercise goals and programs to make sure that they are up to date and complement each other.

9. Identify barriers and strategies to break through them. Plan how you will exercise during special situations such as vacations, business travel, and pregnancy.

10. Plan now what you will do to get yourself started again if you stop exercising in the future.

THINK ABOUT IT

1. Why is it so hard for people to attain their exercise goals?

2. Why is it helpful to set goals?

3. What are the qualities of good goals?

4. Give examples of intrinsic and extrinsic motivation. Which kind has the most lasting effect? Why?

5. Why is it important to have baseline information?

6. What are some common barriers to achieving fitness goals and what are some strategies for overcoming these barriers?

7. What are some ways that you can track your progress?

8. If you stop exercising for a period of time, how will you get yourself to start again?

REFERENCES

Crouter, S. E., P. L. Schneider, M. Karabulut, and D. R. Bassett, Jr. "Validity of 10 Electronic Pedometers for Measuring Steps, Distance, and Energy Cost." *Medicine & Science in Sports & Exercise* 35 (No. 8, 2003):1455–60.

Cuddihy, T. F., R. P. Pangrazi, and L. M. Tomson. "Pedometers: Answers to FAQs from Teachers." *JOPERD* 76 (No. 2, 2005): 36–40, 55.

Dishman, R. K. "Exercise Compliance: A New View for Public Health." *The Physician and Sportsmedicine* 14 (No. 5, 1986): 127–43.

Graser, S. V., R. P. Pangrazi, and W. J. Vincent. "Step It Up: Activity Intensity Using Pedometers; If You Think Pedometers Can't Measure MVPA, Think Again." *JOPHERD* 22 (No. 3, 2009): 22–4.

Hatano, Y. "Use of the Pedometer for Promoting Daily Walking Exercise." *International Council for Health, Physical Education and Recreation* 29 (1993): 4–8.

Kravitz, L., and D. Furst. "Influence of Reward and Social Support on Exercise Adherence in Aerobic Dance Classes." *Psychological Reports* 69 (No. 2, 1991): 423–6.

Marcus, B. H., and A. L. Stanton. "Evaluation of Relapse Prevention and Reinforcement Interventions to Promote Exercise Adherence in Sedentary Females." *Research Quarterly for Exercise and Sport* 64 (No. 4, 1993): 447–52.

Marshall, S. J., S. S. Levy, C. E. Tudor-Locke, F. W. Kolkhorst, K. M. Wooten, J. MingMing, C. A. Macera, and B. E. Ainsworth. "Translating Physical Activity Recommendations into a Pedometer-Based Step Goal: 3000 Steps in 30 Minutes." *American Journal of Preventive Medicine* 36 (No. 5, 2009): 410–5.

Martin, J. E., and P. M. Dubbert. "Adherence to Exercise." In *Exercise and Sports Sciences Review*, R. J. Terjung, ed. New York: Macmillan, 1985.

Physical Best and NASPE. *Physical Education for Lifelong Fitness: The Physical Best Teacher's Guide.* 2nd ed. Champaign, IL: Human Kinetics, 2005.

Schneider, P. L., S. E. Crouter, O. Lukajic, and D. R. Bassett. "Accuracy and Reliability of 10 Pedometers for Measuring Steps Over a 400-m Walk." *Medicine & Science in Sports & Exercise* 35 (No. 10, 2003): 1779–84.

Schneider, P. L., S. E. Crouter, and D. R. Bassett, Jr. "Pedometer Measures of Free-Living Physical Activity: Comparison of 13 Models." *Medicine & Science in Sports & Exercise* 36 (No. 2, 2004): 331–5.

Shephard, R. J. "Motivation: The Key to Fitness Compliance." *The Physician and Sportsmedicine* 13 (No. 6, 1985): 88–98.

Tudor-Locke, C., Y. Hatano, R. P. Pangrazi, and M. Kang. "Revisiting 'How Many Steps are Enough?'" *Medicine & Science in Sports & Exercise* 40 (No. 7 Suppl., 2008): 537–43.

Welk, G. J., J. A. Differding, R. W. Thompson, S. N. Blair, J. Dziura, and P. Hart. "The Utility of the Digi-Walker Step Counter to Assess Daily Physical Activity Patterns." *Medicine & Science in Sports & Exercise* 32 (No. 9 Suppl., 2000), S481–88.

6

Posture: A Dynamic Concept

Stand up tall every time you walk through a doorframe; if nothing else, you will always make a grand entrance.

- How can I achieve good posture and body alignment during exercise?
- What should I do to take care of my back?
- What is core training?

BODY position can make a big difference in how you feel during and after an activity. For example, good sitting posture during computer use can save neck, shoulder, and back strain. Correct body alignment during exercise ensures the full benefit of the exercise and helps prevent injuries. Correct bending and lifting postures also save your back and let you do more with less fatigue. Good posture and alignment are not just about standing up straight; they are about a dynamic process of repositioning your body segments to produce the best possible mechanical (and sometimes aesthetic) advantage at all times.

The position of your body in space when sitting, standing, and lying down is called **body posture. Body alignment** has to do with how the different segments of your body are positioned in relation to each other. Within each posture, different alignments are possible. Sitting posture, for example, can be with a straight or a rounded back. Different alignments are appropriate at different times. An intentional sway back in the cat stretch (sagging the back before arching it upward) gives a healthy stretch of the back muscles. That same sway back while running in place is a liability that can result in low back pain. This text is packed with descriptions and photographs identifying correct postures and alignments for specific exercises. Careful attention to these and helpful feedback from your instructor can help you attain good exercise alignment.

It should also be noted that yoga, pilates, and formal dance training have a strong focus on body alignment during a wide variety of body postures. The exercises included in these programs will develop the

flexibility and strength necessary to hold well-aligned positions. The result—excellent body postures.

FLEXIBILITY AND POSTURE

Poor flexibility can actually pull you out of good alignment. When the hip flexors (muscles that cross the hip joint and attach to the top of the pelvis) are shortened due to muscle tightness, they pull the pelvis forward. This causes excessive curvature of the lumbar (lower) spine, a condition known as lordosis (see the Your Back and How to Care for It box on pages 55–57). If the hamstrings (the muscles on the back of the legs that attach to the bottom of the pelvis) are tight, they pull the pelvis down and back. This flattens the lumbar curve and rounds the low back. Either condition can cause low back pain and referred leg pain. Good flexibility in both of these sets of muscles allows the pelvis to stay in a neutral position. This becomes even more important during movements like kicks to the front and back, which require hip flexibility in order to prevent low back strain.

MUSCLE STRENGTH AND BODY ALIGNMENT

Strong and long are what you want. Strong muscles provide support and stabilization in addition to performing specific movements. Strong abdominal and spinal muscles are vital to protecting and stabilizing the back. When the body is in proper alignment during muscular strength and endurance exercises, the intended muscles get the proper workout. When the alignment is incorrect, muscles other than the target muscle(s) get recruited. Allowing other muscles to take part of the load defeats the original purpose: strengthening the target muscle(s). It can even lead to unnecessary soreness or injury. For example, a straight-leg sit-up allows the hip flexor muscles to assist the abdominal muscles in lifting the torso. This means that the abdominal muscles do not get as heavy a load as intended. And worse, the iliopsoas (a hip flexor that attaches in the low back), if not countered by strong abdominal muscles, will pull and arch the lower back off the floor—an unhealthy strain on the back. Good alignment becomes even more important when weights or bands are added to an exercise.

Muscular strength imbalances can also compromise posture. Developing the chest muscles without doing corresponding exercises for the upper back can result in rounded shoulders. The stronger chest muscles pull the shoulders forward. Opposing muscles should be exercised equally. Improving the strength and endurance of muscles also helps you maintain good body posture during prolonged exercise or activity. Injuries are most likely to occur when you become fatigued and start to lose exercise technique.

CORE TRAINING

Core training is the use of a variety of resistance exercises to develop the muscles that support and stabilize the middle of the body, especially the spine. The "core" includes the abdominals, back, chest, buttocks, and shoulder girdle muscles. Traditional exercises such as curl-ups, push-ups, and pelvic tilts can be used to accomplish core strength, but optimum effectiveness depends on being able to "access" deep spinal and pelvic muscles when you perform these movements. Pilates is a special technique that teaches you how to use these deeper muscles with an emphasis on the connection between the "core" or "power-house" and the rest of the body. It accomplishes this using both mat exercises and specialized equipment. Yoga also works the core muscles through special postures called asanas. (See Chapter 11 for more on pilates and yoga.) Core training has a number of benefits, including improved posture, greater functional strength, better balance, a lower risk of injury, and improved sports performance.

When the core (center) is strong and stable, we can more easily transfer force and movement out to the extremities, which allows us to move more easily, with less stress and strain. To illustrate how core strength translates into limb strength and stability, try the following: (1) While seated, extend your arm out to the side. Have a partner push it back while you

Figure 6.1 Stability exercise using a partner and a stability ball. One partner pushes the ball in a variety of directions while the other partner uses core muscles to maintain body alignment.

remain relatively passive. (2) As your partner pushes for a second time, react by resisting the movement with your arm and shoulder muscles. (3) This time as your partner pushes, react by resisting the movement using your arm, shoulder, and *abdominal* muscles—contract them as you resist. Using the core (especially if it is strong) can help you maintain good posture and apply force or resistance as needed.

Reactive movement is the idea of a movement response to a stimulus. You do this when you slip on something; you react by quickly employing movements that help you regain your balance. There are some very effective ways to use this idea in core training. Situations that produce an unstable environment force the body to use muscles—core muscles—to react to maintain the body's position. Stability balls offer one such unique way to train. To balance or stabilize yourself on the ball during an exercise, you call into action the core muscles. Stability resistance training can also be done on a Bosu ball or core board. The Bosu ball looks like a stability ball cut in half. You can put the flat or rounded side down and perform exercises while balancing on top. The board is designed to tilt, twist, torque, and recoil as you perform exercises on it. When the board or ball moves, you have to react to that movement by stabilizing your body. Each time you react, you get a little bit stronger! Figure 6.1 demonstrates a fun stability exercise you can perform with a partner. *(text continues on page 58)*

YOUR BACK AND HOW TO CARE FOR IT

Whatever the cause of low back pain, part of its treatment is the correction of faulty posture. But good posture is not simply a matter of "standing tall." It refers to correct use of the body at all times. In fact, for the body to function in the best of health, it must be so used that no strain is put on muscles, joints, bones, and ligaments. To prevent low back pain, avoiding strain must become a way of life, practiced while lying, sitting, standing, walking, working, and exercising. When body position is correct, internal organs have enough room to function normally, and blood circulates more freely.

With the help of this guide, you can begin to correct the positions and movements that bring on or aggravate backache. You should pay particular attention to the positions recommended for resting, because it is possible to strain the muscles of the back and neck even while lying in bed. By learning to live with good posture, under all circumstances, you will gradually develop the proper carriage and stronger muscles needed to protect and support your hard-working back.

How to Stay on Your Feet Without Tiring Your Back

To prevent strain and pain in everyday activities, it is restful to change from one task to another before fatigue sets in. Some people can lie down between chores; others should check body position frequently, drawing in the abdomen, flattening the back, bending the knees slightly.

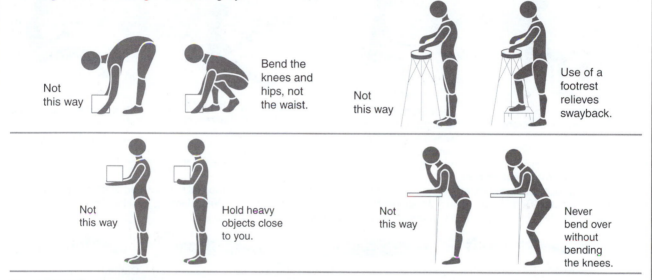

Not this way — Bend the knees and hips, not the waist.

Not this way — Use of a footrest relieves swayback.

Not this way — Hold heavy objects close to you.

Not this way — Never bend over without bending the knees.

Check Your Carriage Here

In correct, fully erect posture, a line dropped from the ear will go through the tip of the shoulder, middle of hip, back of kneecaps, and front of anklebone.

Incorrect: Lower back is arched or hollow.

Incorrect: Upper back is stooped, lower back is arched, abdomen sags.

Incorrect: Note how, in strained position, pelvis tilts forward, chin is out, and ribs are down, crowding internal organs.

Correct: In correct position, chin is in, head up, back flattened, pelvis held straight.

To Find the Correct Standing Position

Stand one foot away from wall. Now sit against wall, bending knees slightly. Tighten abdominal and buttock muscles. This will tilt the pelvis back and flatten the lower spine. Holding this position, inch up the wall to standing position by straightening the legs. Now walk around the room, maintaining the same posture. Place back against wall again to see whether you have held the position.

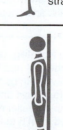
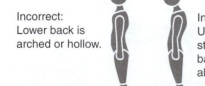
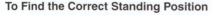

(continued)

How to Sit Correctly

A back's best friend is a straight, hard chair. If you can't get the chair you prefer, learn to sit properly on whatever chair you get. To correct sitting position from forward slump: Throw head well back, then bend it forward to pull in the chin. This will straighten the back. Now tighten abdominal muscles to raise the chest. Check position frequently.

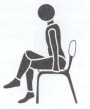

Relieve strain by sitting well forward, flatten back by tightening abdominal muscles, and cross knees.

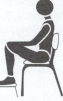

Use of footrest relieves swayback. Aim is to have knees higher than hips.

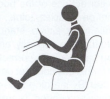

Correct way to sit while driving, close to pedals. Use seat belt or hard backrest, available commercially.

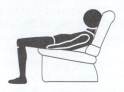

TV slump leads to "dowager's hump," strains neck and shoulders.

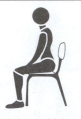

If chair is too high, swayback is increased.

Keep neck and back in as straight of a line as possible with the spine. Bend forward from the hips.

Driver's seat too far from pedals emphasizes curve in lower back.

Strained reading position. Forward thrusting strains muscles of neck and head.

How to Put Your Back to Bed

For proper bed posture, a firm mattress is essential. Bedboards, sold commercially or devised at home, may be used with soft mattresses. Bedboards, preferably, should be made of 3/4-inch plywood. Faulty sleeping positions intensify swayback and result not only in backache but in numbness, tingling, and pain in arms and legs.

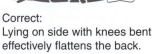
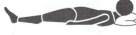
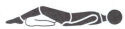
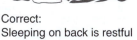

Incorrect:
Lying flat on back makes swayback worse.

Correct:
Lying on side with knees bent effectively flattens the back. Flat pillow may be used to support neck, especially when shoulders are broad.

Incorrect:
Use of high pillow strains neck, arms, shoulders.

Correct:
Sleeping on back is restful and correct when knees are properly supported.

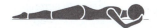

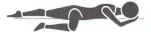
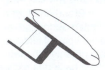

Incorrect:
Sleeping face down exaggerates swayback, strains neck and shoulders.

Correct:
Raise the foot of the mattress 8 inches to discourage sleeping on the abdomen.

Incorrect:
Bending one hip and knee does not relieve swayback.

Proper arrangement of pillows for resting or reading in bed.

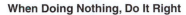

When Doing Nothing, Do It Right

Rest is the first rule for the tired, painful back. The following positions relieve pain by taking all pressure and weight off the back and legs. Note pillows under knees to relieve strain on spine.

For complete relief and relaxing effect, these positions should be maintained from 5 to 25 minutes.

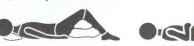

A straight-back chair used behind a pillow makes a serviceable backrest.

Exercise — Without Getting Out of Bed

Exercises to be performed while lying in bed are aimed not so much at strengthening muscles as at teaching correct positioning. But muscles used correctly become stronger and in time are able to support the body with the least amount of effort.

Do all exercises in this position. Legs should not be straightened.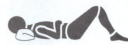

Bring knee to chest. Lower slowly but do not straighten leg. Relax.

Exercise — Without Attracting Attention

Use these inconspicuous exercises whenever you have a spare moment during the day, both to relax tension and improve the tone of important muscle groups.

1. Rotate shoulders forward and backward.
2. Turn head slowly side to side.
3. Watch an imaginary plane take off, just below the right shoulder. Stretch neck, follow it slowly as it moves up, around and down, disappearing below the other shoulder. Repeat, starting on left side.
4. Slowly, slowly, touch left ear to left shoulder; right ear to right shoulder. Raise both shoulders to touch ears, drop them as far as possible.
5. At any pause in the day—waiting for an elevator to arrive, for a specific traffic light to change—pull in abdominal muscles, tighten, hold for the count of 8 without breathing. Relax slowly. Increase the count gradually after the first week. Practice breathing normally with abdomen flat and contracted. Do this sitting, standing, and walking.

Bring both knees slowly up to chest. Tighten muscles of abdomen, press back flat against the floor. Hold knees to chest 20 seconds. Then lower slowly. Relax. Repeat 5 times. This exercise gently stretches the shortened muscles of the lower back, while strengthening abdominal muscles. Clasp knees, bring them up to chest at the same time coming to a sitting position. Rock back and forth.

Rules to Live By — From Now On

1. Never bend from the waist only; bend the hips and knees.
2. Never lift a heavy object higher than your waist.
3. Always turn and face the object you wish to lift.
4. Avoid carrying unbalanced loads; hold heavy objects close to your body.
5. Never carry anything heavier than you can manage with ease.
6. Never lift or move heavy furniture. Wait for someone to do it who knows the principles of leverage.
7. Avoid sudden movements, sudden "overloading" of muscles. Learn to move deliberately, swinging the legs from the hips.
8. Learn to keep the head in line with the spine when standing, sitting, lying in bed.
9. Put soft chairs and deep couches on your "don't sit" list. During prolonged sitting, cross your legs to rest your back.
10. Your doctor is the only one who can determine when low back pain is due to faulty posture and is the best judge of when you may do general exercises for physical fitness. When you do, omit any exercise that arches or overstrains the lower back: backward or forward bends, touching the toes with the knees straight.
11. Wear shoes with moderate heels, all about the same height. Avoid changing from high to low heels.
12. Put a footrail under the desk and a footrest under the crib.
13. Diaper a baby sitting next to him or her on the bed.
14. Don't stoop and stretch to hang the wash; raise the clothesbasket and lower the washline.
15. Beg or buy a rocking chair. Rocking rests the back by changing the muscle groups used.
16. Train yourself vigorously to use your abdominal muscles to flatten your lower abdomen. In time, this muscle contraction will become habitual, making you the envied possessor of a youthful body profile!
17. Don't strain to open windows or doors.
18. For good posture, concentrate on strengthening "nature's corset"–the abdominal and buttock muscles. The pelvic roll exercise is especially recommended to correct the postural relation between the pelvis and the spine.

One person slaps the ball at various positions while the other person tries to maintain body position. (See Chapters 7 and 9 for more stability ball exercises.) The unstable environment forces you to use numerous muscles at one time, much as you do when you carry out similar movements in daily life.

Unfortunately, many people are unaware of how to engage their core muscles. You can begin to become aware by lying on your back with your knees bent and feet on the floor. Without moving your back, try to "put your belly button on your back" or think of pulling your abs "in and up." Focusing on your trunk muscles when you cough is another cue teachers use. Now try a curl-up, but first engage the deep muscles and then use the abdominal muscles to pull you up. Kegel exercises (tightening the muscles that would stop urination) also help locate deep muscles. It takes time and often help from an instructor to become good at locating and using your deeper muscles, but once you do, you will be amazed how it changes how you move.

Here are two quick tests you can do to test your core strength. Try to hold these positions for a minimum of 20 seconds without visible shaking.

1. Lie face down. Brace yourself up on your forearms (forearms on the floor). Pull your toes under and lift up your body until you create a straight line from your feet to your head.
2. Lie face up. Brace yourself up on your forearms. Lift up your body until you create a straight line from your feet to your head.

When performing the following alignment checks, concentrate on stabilizing your posture by using core muscles. These positions are good beginning core exercises.

EXERCISE ALIGNMENT CHECKS

You can perform some alignment checks using a mirror. Some of the following can be checked in a normal full-length mirror. Others will require a larger mirror you might find on campus in a dance room or a weight room. If a mirror is not available, you can work with a partner and evaluate each other. During class, your instructor will also check your alignment and give you helpful suggestions and positive feedback on correct positioning.

During an aerobic dance exercise class, you will perform a lot of exercises in a standing posture. It is important to maintain good trunk stabilization during these exercises so that the back stays in a healthy position. This can be achieved by pulling in the abdominal muscles and holding the pelvis in a neutral

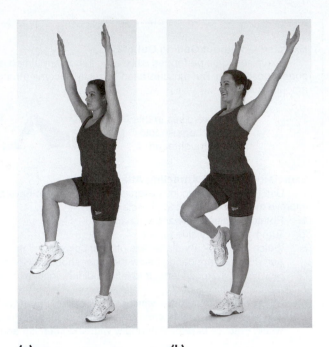

(a)   **(b)**

Figure 6.2(a) Correct knee lift alignment. **(b)** Incorrect knee lift alignment. Poor back alignment.

position. "Soft" or slightly bent knees help relieve pressure on the low back as well. See the Your Back and How to Care for It box on pages 55–57 for more information on standing and other postures. The illustrated information from Schering does an excellent job of presenting good body alignment for daily activities such as driving, sleeping, and picking up objects.

Stand sideways in front of a full-length mirror. Assume a good standing posture as described above. Pay special attention to the stabilizing effect your abdominals have. Now try the following moves while watching in the mirror to see whether you are able to maintain good back and neck alignment.

- Raise both arms overhead without arching your back. Now, one at a time, extend your legs to the back, side, and front and see if you can maintain a good back position.
- Perform knee lifts, first with the right and then the left leg. (See Figures 6.2a and 6.2b for examples of good and bad alignment.)
- Kick straight legs (one at a time) to the front. (See Figures 6.3a and 6.3b for examples of good and bad alignment.)
- Bend your right knee and touch your right foot behind your back with your left hand. Then try touching your left foot with your right hand. (See Figures 6.4a and 6.4b for examples of good and bad alignment.)

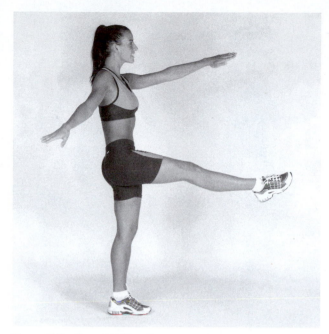

Figure 6.3a Correct kicking alignment.

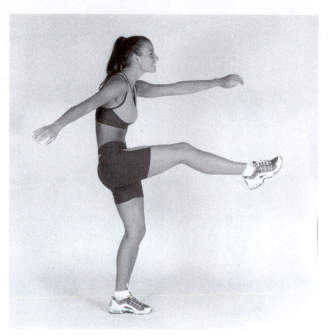

Figure 6.3b Incorrect kicking alignment.

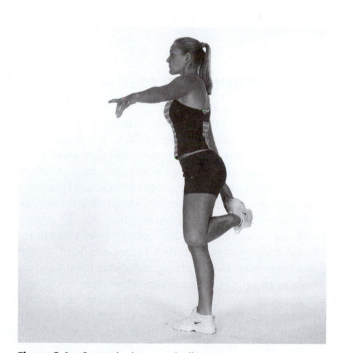

Figure 6.4a Correct back toe touch alignment.

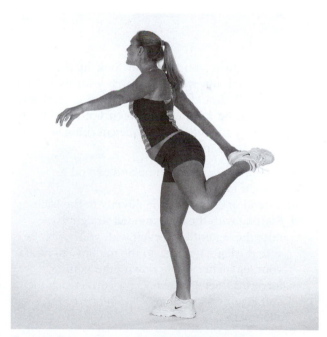

Figure 6.4b Incorrect back toe touch alignment.

- With your feet shoulder width apart, stretch directly to the side. (See Figures 6.5a and 6.5b on page 60 for examples of good and bad alignment.)
- Jog in place. (See Figures 6.6a and 6.6b on page 60 for examples of good and bad alignment.) In addition to a neutral back,

you want to keep your arms and legs moving forward and back without angling away from your body or crossing over your body.

Back stabilization is also very important in exercises performed on the hands and knees. Position yourself sideways to a mirror or partner. This will

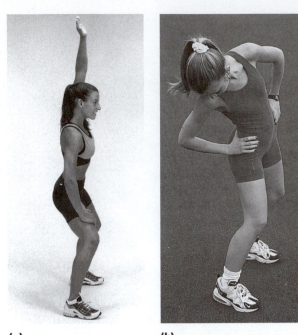

(a)   **(b)**

Figure 6.5(a) Correct side stretch alignment. **(b)** Incorrect side stretch alignment.

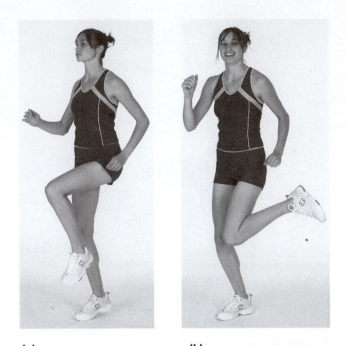

(a)   **(b)**

Figure 6.6(a) Correct jogging alignment—back neutral, knees forward. **(b)** Incorrect jogging alignment—back arched, knees down, feet to the side.

allow you to turn your head to look in the mirror rather than look up, which will arch your back. Your back and head should form a straight line, and your weight should be balanced between both hands and knees. Now try the following while checking back and neck/head alignment:

- Pick up one arm at a time and extend it straight forward.
- Extend one leg at a time directly to the back.
- Starting with the leg extended straight back, raise the leg until it is even with your back. Be sure the leg stays close to the midline. To raise your leg higher, lower down onto your forearms. (See Figure 6.7a for correct alignment and Figures 6.7b and 6.7c for *incorrect* alignment.)

OTHER INFLUENCES ON POSTURE

Poor posture is not always born of a lack of attention to alignment or to weak inflexible muscles. In some cases, posture or muscular tension reflects a psychological state, an emotional issue, and/or physical pain from injury or a chronic condition. While stretching exercises may be helpful in identifying tight muscles and teaching some relaxation, other approaches to finding the source of the stress and releasing tension may also be highly beneficial. Sometimes we don't need to "do" something like stretch or strengthen, but rather we need to *stop* doing something like worrying or looking up at a movie screen or computer monitor that is too high.

Another source of muscle tension is a cold environment. When people are chilled, they usually pull up their shoulders and drop their chin. All the

---

POSTURE QUICK TIP

If you regularly carry out posture checks and realignments, over time they will become unconscious habits. Misalignments will start to "feel" wrong, and you will automatically make adjustments. To build good standing and walking posture, try standing up tall every time you walk through a doorway. You will always make a grand entrance!

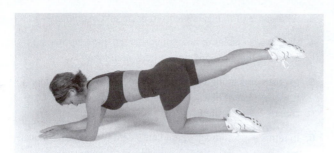

Figure 6.7a Correct leg and back alignment.

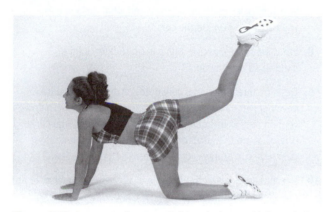

Figure 6.7b Incorrect alignment. Raising the leg too high results in back arch.

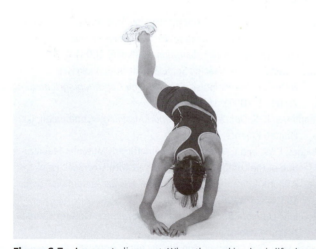

Figure 6.7c Incorrect alignment. When the working leg is lifted out to the side instead of directly upward, the body's weight has to shift away from center to maintain balance. This poor alignment can stress the back as well as interfere with the toning effect of the exercise.

strength and flexibility exercises in the world will not remove this tension, but turning up the heat or putting on more clothing will. Also, exercise will not improve poor posture brought on by self-consciousness or shyness. Other times, we try too hard and tense too many muscles. A beginning swimmer tenses many unnecessary muscles in an attempt to stay afloat.

The experienced swimmer uses only the muscles needed for buoyancy and movement. It may be that identifying and relaxing muscles that are not needed during an activity can bring relief. The next time you walk somewhere, see if your upper body is fully relaxed. How about your inner thigh muscles? Your hip muscles? Your gait will become much easier when you learn to release unnecessary tension. The important thing is to look for the source of muscle tension and detrimental postures, and work to change or relieve the root cause. If the source is disease or injury, be sure to consult the proper medical authority before embarking on posture-correcting exercises.

POSTURE AND SPORTS AND DANCE

Sometimes we elect to use postures and body alignments that are stressful to the body but helpful for sport or dance movements. For example, the flat back position (Figure 6.8) is used in dance to create an aesthetic line. Deep knee bends, the hurdler's position, and back arching are just a few of the movements used in athletics that are not recommended for normal health and fitness. If you participate in activities that use these types of movements, it is even more important to develop strong, long muscles to help ease the strain to your body. Dancers and athletes also try to minimize their use of such positions because they, too, want healthy, pain-free bodies.

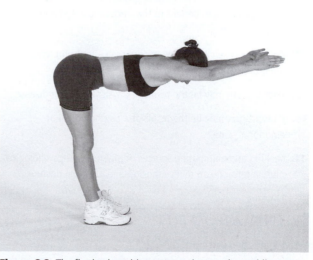

Figure 6.8 The flat back position stresses the muscles and ligaments of the lower back. It may, however, be used in dance for aesthetic reasons.

SUMMARY

The word "posture" conjures up images of a mother or army sergeant barking out orders to "stand (or sit) up straight!" It is easy to dismiss posture as something you should do for the sake of appearance and as something you need worry about only during static sitting and standing activities; in fact, posture is a dynamic concept. Every movement we make should be done with the best possible body alignment. This reduces strain to unneeded muscles and applies mechanical force to its best advantage. Whether you are removing boxes from the trunk of the car, cleaning, sleeping, or exercising, it is smart to pay attention to, and make automatic, good body postures. And, of course, someone with good body mechanics, strong core muscles, and nice alignment looks good moving.

KNOWLEDGE TIPS

1. Posture is a dynamic process whereby individuals try to select the posture and body alignment best suited to the activity in which they are engaged.

2. Posture is the position of the body in space.

3. Body alignment refers to how the body segments relate to one another.

4. Inflexibility can cause postural misalignments.

5. Muscular strength imbalances can result in postural misalignments.

6. Strengthening the "core" muscles will enhance posture and make you a better, stronger mover.

7. Proper exercise alignment during muscle strengthening ensures maximum benefit to the target muscle(s) and prevents injuries.

8. Awareness exercises can help correct postural problems that are due to inattention.

9. Poor posture may be the result of physical injury or disease.

10. Poor posture may be the result of a psychological or emotional state.

11. Seeking and eliminating sources of physical and psychological muscle tension can relieve tension and enhance posture.

THINK ABOUT IT

1. What is dynamic posture?

2. What is the difference between body posture and alignment? Give an example of each.

3. What kinds of things influence posture and alignment?

4. Give two examples of how strengthening and lengthening opposing muscles can improve body alignment.

5. In terms of posture and alignment, identify a stationary position (i.e., sitting) that you would like to improve. What changes would you make?

6. In terms of posture and alignment, identify a dynamic movement (i.e., leg kick) that you would like to improve. What changes would you make?

7. Which muscles make up the core and what are some exercises you can do to develop the core?

8. What are some exercises one can do to help build or maintain a healthy back?

9. Describe three abnormal curvatures of the spine and how development of these curvatures can be prevented. (The prevention part of this question is referring to functional curvatures that are the result of poor posture and alignment vs. structural curvatures with which a person may be born.)

10. Describe an activity that might encourage development of an imbalance in musculature and/or posture.

REFERENCES

Barr K. P., M. Griggs, and T. Cadby. "Lumbar Stabilization: Core Concepts and Current Literature, Part 1." *American Journal of Physical Medicine and Rehabilitation* 84 (No. 6, 2005): 473–80.

Chiu, Loren Z. F. "Are Specific Spine Stabilization Exercises Necessary for Athletes?" *Strength and Conditioning Journal* 29 (No.1, 2007): 15–7.

Clippinger, K. S. *Dance Anatomy and Kinesiology.* Champaign, IL: Human Kinetics, 2007.

Hodges, P. W., and C. A. Richardson. "Inefficient Muscular Stabilization of the Lumbar Spine Associated with Low Back Pain. A Motor Control Evaluation of Transversus Abdominis." *Spine* 15 (No. 21, 1996): 2640–50.

McGill, S. *Ultimate Back Fitness and Performance.* Ontario, Canada: Wabuno Publishers.

Segal, D. D. "An Anatomic and Biomechanic Approach to Low Back Health: A Preventive Approach." *Journal of Sports Medicine* 23 (1983): 411–21.

Thompson, C. W., and R. T. Floyd. *Manual of Structural Kinesiology.* 12th ed. St. Louis, MO: Mosby, 1994.

7

Flexibility: Warm-Up/ Cool-Down

"A muscle is like a car. If you want it to run well in the morning, you have to warm it up."

FLORENCE GRIFFITH JOYNER

- Why do I need to warm up and cool down?
- I've heard there is more than one way to stretch. Is that true?
- Are some stretches bad for you?
- Can you be too flexible?

An aerobic dance exercise class consists of four components (parts): (1) the warm-up, (2) an aerobic workout, (3) muscle strength and endurance exercises, and (4) a cool-down. Although opposite in purpose and at opposite ends of the class, the warm-up and cool-down are actually very similar in content and technique. The warm-up starts off with low-intensity movements and easy stretching and builds to moderately vigorous activity. The cool-down begins as the moderate to vigorous activity of the aerobic segment ends and slowly reduces the intensity, finishing with stretches and relaxation exercises. Both activities are composed of two similar parts: the first increases or decreases overall body activity, while the second stretches the muscles. Stretching during the warm-up helps prepare your muscles for action, and stretching during the cool-down helps increase flexibility and reduce muscle soreness.

This chapter teaches you general techniques for warming up and cooling down. It explains the principles of flexibility, provides examples of recommended stretches, and indicates stretches that may be harmful or cause unnecessary soreness for the "average" participant. Discussions for the other two components of class (aerobic workout and muscle strength and endurance exercises) are presented in subsequent chapters.

WARM-UP

The purpose of the **warm-up** is to prepare your body and mind for activity. Most people arrive at class after a

relatively inactive day. Muscles can be tight from sitting in class or a car, from working at a computer, or from bending over machinery. You need to ease into a workout, and a good warm-up is the way to do it. If you exercise early in the morning, the warm-up is even more important, because your muscles have been inactive all night. The warm-up is also a time to prepare mentally, increase your body awareness, concentrate on posture and movement technique, and rehearse, at a slower speed, some of the steps you will be using during the aerobics segment.

The first step in a warm-up is to literally make your body warm. This is the **general warm-up.** It may also be referred to as the standing warm-up. Easy, active movements to energizing music get your blood circulating and raise your body's internal, or core, temperature 1 to 2 degrees. This increase makes most people break a sweat.

The second part of the warm-up consists of stretching exercises. There is some professional disagreement about how much and what type of stretching should be included in the warm-up. This will be discussed in more detail shortly. When warm-up stretches are performed, they are usually done standing, but they may include floor work, and they are usually held for less time (about 10 seconds) than those performed during the cool-down. Stretches may be performed in combination with active warm-up movements, such as inserting a calf stretch between some jogging in place, as long as enough general warm-up has occurred prior to this to fully warm the muscles. A warm-up generally takes 5 to 10 minutes. More time may be needed if you are a beginner, are an older adult, or have a medical condition such as asthma.

GENERAL WARM-UP

It is important to start your workout slowly and easily and build up to a moderate pace. Warming up your muscles allows them to:

- become more elastic
- execute more forceful, rapid movements
- receive more oxygen because of increased blood flow
- increase metabolism
- become less vulnerable to injury

Starting slowly also gives the cardiorespiratory system a chance to adjust to the increasing oxygen demand of the muscles. Sudden, vigorous activity is hard on your body, and the quick shunting of blood to the muscles can leave you light-headed. Think about how you feel when you sprint to catch a closing door or leap out of the way of danger. To prevent this jarring feeling, start gradually and give your heart and muscles a chance to adjust.

Warm-up activity stimulates the secretion of synovial fluid. This fluid, secreted into the joints, acts as a lubricant. Much like the Tin Man in *The Wizard of Oz*, you need to "oil up" your joints. Start out with small movements, and as the joints and muscles respond, work up to bigger ones. Wearing high heels keeps the Achilles tendon in a shortened position all day. The transition from high heels to flat-soled aerobic shoes should be made carefully. Too often, people who are late to class skip the warm-up and jump directly into vigorous activity. If you are late, take a few extra minutes to warm up. Your heart, muscles, and tendons will all benefit.

The warm-up is a good time to mentally prepare yourself for exercise. Set aside the worries of the day, and release yourself to a fun-filled hour of invigorating exercise. Concentrate on the following five technique tips during the general warm-up.

1. *Move from general to specific.* Start with general whole-body movements such as walking, marching in place, light jogging, or easy dance steps with light arm work. When space permits, add traveling steps. After you are warmed up, you can move on to more specific movements such as new steps for class, sports movements, or dance isolations.
2. *Start with smaller ranges of motion and work up to bigger ones.* For example, start a shoulder warm-up by just lifting and rotating your shoulders while your arms hang relaxed at your sides. Next, do a circling motion with

your arms, letting your elbows draw the circle. Last, work the circles with straight, but not locked, arms. Start with low arms and eventually use above-the-shoulder arm movements. Start with step touches, and work up to stepping wider and using a deeper squatting position.

3. *Use movements that stay in a comfortable range of motion.* Wait until your muscles are warmed up before you put a lot of stretch and pull on them. For example, reaching one arm overhead and then the other is good, but stretching your arm way up and as far across your body as possible is too much right away. Similarly, use easy knee lifts and kicks as opposed to higher leg movements until your muscles are warm.
4. *Work with smooth movements.* This is not a time for bouncing or jarring your muscles and joints. Use flowing, sustained movements, and allow your body to make the transition from a sedentary day to an active class.
5. *Start slowly and work up to a moderate pace.* This will gradually increase your heart rate, raise your core temperature, activate the synovial fluid, and increase metabolism.

A **dynamic warm-up** consists of a series of exercises that include general mobility exercises, dynamic stretching, and balance and coordination movements. A typical dynamic warm-up would progress through some stationary general body warm-up movements like jogging in place and jumping jacks, to low-intensity transit movements like skipping and jogging across the floor, then to muscle activation exercises like squats and arm presses, followed by dynamic flexibility exercises such as walking (single) knee hugs and straight leg marches, and finally moderate and high-transit movements like butt kicks and power skips. If preparing for a sporting event, sport-specific movements can be added at the end of a dynamic warm-up. The advantages to this kind of warm-up are that they are similar to everyday movements that occur in more than one plane and that they prepare you neuromuscularly for a dynamic workout. They also improve coordination and balance when movements like standing on one leg and bending down to touch the ground are included.

WARM-UP STRETCHING: STATIC OR DYNAMIC

Stretching is an important part of warming up. You may have heard that stretching before an exercise is bad. This comes from a misunderstanding. The question is not whether stretching is good or bad, but rather which type of stretching should be used during the warm-up. Traditionally, static stretching (holding one position without movement) has been used. However, some research suggests that dynamic flexibility exercises more effectively prepare the body for dynamic movements. There is also some research evidence, stemming from running and weight-training studies, that static stretching calms the muscle rather than exciting it, and that in so doing may diminish the amount of force a muscle can exert in the activity following the stretch. This calming effect may also result in less muscular stabilization of joints, which could then lead to soreness or injury. Based on this, some professionals feel that dynamic stretching should be used in warm-ups and that static stretching is best left to the end of class. Dynamic flexibility research is still in its infancy, and as a result, there is not enough evidence yet to say that dynamic stretching is the best way to warm up for all individuals and for all sports events. Considerably more research is needed before we can reach definitive conclusions. In the meantime, knowing about the two types of stretching will allow you to understand the debate and perhaps try different types of warm-up stretches to see how they feel to you.

Dynamic stretching is when you use the pull of a muscle or group of muscles and the body's momentum to move through a full range of motion. **Dynamic flexibility** is how much range of motion you have at a joint during a dynamic movement. This is different from static flexibility, which is the stretch obtained in a held position. It differs from traditional ballistic stretching, in which the momentum of the body is used, but in a way that accentuates the endpoint of the movement, and the stretching is more "ballistic" or "bouncy" in nature as opposed to dynamic flexibility stretches that are done using smooth controlled and fluid movements. Dynamic stretches are also designed to move the body through functional (typical daily) movements, such as reaching for something on the shelf or bending to pick something up, and if desired, through sport-specific movements, such as throwing or striking a ball. It is fairly easy to see how certain aerobic dance warm-up movements can be dynamic flexibility exercises. Here are a few examples:

- The front lunge stretch can become dynamic by stepping into the lunge and then either returning to a stand or walking forward into a front lunge with the opposite foot forward.
- A knee-up (lifting one knee up in front while standing), which is dynamic to begin with, can become a dynamic stretch by lifting the knee high, hugging it with your arms, lowering it, and step hugging the opposite leg.
- The shoulders can receive a dynamic stretch by performing controlled arm circles forward and

backward and by swinging both arms across the front of the body at chest height to one side and then the other.

As with all aspects of exercise, it is important to start off easy and progress gradually with dynamic flexibility exercises. For some individuals, high knee skips and a series of squats can feel like a workout, not a warm-up.

At this time, aerobic instructors are using general warm-up movements (dynamic in nature) with either dynamic or static stretches. Special consideration is usually given to warming up and stretching out the calf and leg muscles. There is lots of agreement that performing longer, sustained stretching is best done at the end of class, when the muscles are really warm and flexibility can be developed. Static, ballistic, PNF, active, and passive stretching will be explained in more detail later in this chapter, followed by a number of flexibility exercises.

COOL-DOWN

Like the warm-up, the **cool-down** has two sections. The first part, often called the standing cool-down, is done right after the aerobic portion to reduce the body's exertion level gradually. The second portion of the cool-down is the developmental stretch, which follows either the standing cool-down or a final set of muscle-toning exercises. The purpose of this stretch is to elongate the muscles and improve range of motion. The standing cool-down usually lasts 3 to 5 minutes, and the developmental stretch about 5 to 10 minutes. If time permits, some instructors will follow the stretch with a few minutes of quiet relaxation.

STANDING COOL-DOWN

During exercise, a large portion of the blood (usually 30 to 50%, but it can be as much as 70%) is shunted (circulated out) to the limbs to supply the big working muscles with oxygen. At the end of a workout, it is important to keep moving so the blood is returned to the heart and lungs to be reoxygenated instead of being pooled out in the limbs. If you stop exercising suddenly, you may find yourself feeling light-headed because of a lack of oxygenated blood in the brain. If the lack of oxygen in your brain is significant enough, you will faint. This is your body's way of bringing you horizontal so that oxygenated blood can travel to your head more easily. There is no need to feel light-headed or faint in an aerobics class; simply keep moving and gradually reduce your activity level.

When you move the big muscles of your arms and legs during the standing cool-down, the muscles contract around the veins and help push or massage the

Table 7.1   Summary of Warm-Up and Cool-Down

	ACTIVITY	PURPOSE	DURATION
Warm-Up			
	Core Warm-Up: Start with easy, active, whole body movements; move from small to larger ranges of motion.	• Raise core temperature 1–2 degrees • Increase blood circulation • Stimulate secretion of synovial fluid • Prepare mentally	5–10 minutes total
	Warm-Up Stretch: Hold static stretches 15–30 seconds or perform a series of dynamic flexibility exercises.	• Prepare muscles for action and prevent injury	
Cool-Down			
	Standing Cool-Down: Start with big, active movements, and slowly wind down to smaller, easier movements.	• Reduce the body's exertion level • Return blood to the heart and lungs	3–5 minutes
	Developmental Stretch: Hold static stretches for 15–30 seconds, 2–4 times.	• Increase flexibility • Prevent muscle soreness	5–10 minutes

blood upward. This aids the **venous pump,** the system of moving blood up through the veins against gravity. Blood is pumped up the **veins** by the pressure created from the heart's contractions. Between heartbeats (contractions), blood is held in its newly elevated position by one-way valves inside the veins. Muscle contractions added to the heart's contractions help move the blood more quickly, which, in turn, helps you recover from exercise more quickly.

When you first start exercising, your aerobic system takes about 3 minutes to reach a point where it is producing as much energy as you are using. During this time, the anaerobic systems produce energy without the use of oxygen. At the end of exercising, you have to replenish these systems. During the post-exercise time, you continue to operate at a high level of oxygen consumption—that's why you continue to breathe hard and sweat after you finish exercising. As everything gets caught up and reset, your breathing and heart rate slow down, and you begin to cool off.

The actual movements and technique required for the cool-down are just like the warm-up, only you reverse the process. Start with big, active movements, and slowly wind down to smaller, easier movements. The cool-down can be as simple as a light jog that winds down to a brisk walk and, finally, normal-paced walking. The cool-down should continue until your heart rate is below 120 bpm.

DEVELOPMENTAL STRETCH

The end of class is the best time to work on developing flexibility because your body temperature is high and muscle tissue is elastic. In addition to standing stretches,

this final stretch often includes stretches sitting or lying down. The closing stretch differs from the opening stretch in the opportunity to hold stretches for up to 30 seconds, 2 to 4 times (sets). See Table 7.1 for a summary of the warm-up and cool-down.

PRINCIPLES OF FLEXIBILITY

Flexibility is defined as the range of movement you have around a joint or group of joints. Sometimes this flexibility is taken for granted, and it's not until you lose flexibility that you realize how much it affects your daily life. Flexibility is required to raise your arms to take off a shirt, to throw a ball, or to do the tango. These movements are effortless when you have good range of motion, painfully difficult when you don't. To appreciate flexibility, imagine that you have a stiff neck and try to go a few hours without turning your head independently of your body.

As you get older, your independence is, to a large degree, dependent on your flexibility. (I recently cringed while I watched one of my older relatives try, and fail, to bend over far enough to pick up her purse from the floor.) Regardless of your age, you can always improve your flexibility. However, it is easier to develop and maintain flexibility when you are young than to start to develop it when you are older. Now, let's look at how the principles of exercise introduced in Chapter 3 are applied to flexibility.

PRINCIPLE OF SPECIFICITY

Flexibility is specific to a joint or group of joints. This means that you can't perform just one exercise to develop body flexibility; you must select a variety of exercises for all of the body's major muscles and joints. This is also true for assessing your flexibility. On Worksheets 12 and 13, you will find a series of tests to determine the flexibility of your shoulders, back, hips, and so forth.

PRINCIPLE OF INDIVIDUALITY

Flexibility of a joint depends on a combination of factors, including bone shape, muscle and connective tissue properties, aging effects, the presence of disease such as arthritis, and other factors. Some individuals are born with looser joints than others. What is a healthy stretch for one may be injurious for another. For example, a loose joint would benefit more from strengthening of the muscle, which stabilizes the joint, than more stretching. People will also progress at different rates as they attempt to increase muscle flexibility. The one thing we all have in common is that (except for some cases involving disease or disability) we can all improve the flexibility of muscles and the range of motion of joints that need it.

PRINCIPLE OF REVERSIBILITY

If you do not perform flexibility exercises on a regular basis, you will gradually become less flexible. Aging has some effect on the elasticity of tissues, but overall much flexibility can be retained through a regular stretching program.

FITT PRINCIPLE

The flexibility target zone is described by four variables: frequency, intensity, time, and type of stretch (FITT). The American College of Sports Medicine (ACSM) recommendation is to perform a general stretching routine that exercises the major muscle and/or tendon groups using static or PNF (proprioceptive neuromuscular facilitation) techniques:

- a minimum of 2 to 3 days a week, ideally 5 to 7 days a week (frequency)
- stretching to a position of tightness, without inducing discomfort (intensity)
- holding the stretch for 15 to 30 seconds for static stretches, using a 6-second contraction followed by 15 to 30 seconds of assisted stretch for PNF
- repeating each stretch 2 to 4 times (time: combination of time held and repetitions)

PRINCIPLES OF PROGRESSION AND OVERLOAD

A progressive overload is achieved in stretching by manipulating the variables in the FITT principle. You can increase your frequency until you are stretching 5 to 7 days a week. You can increase the intensity by stretching a little further than normal, but remember to back off if you feel pain. And you can hold stretches for longer periods of time or increase the number of times you hold a shorter stretch (a 15-second hold, repeated 3 times). Whether you are adding frequency, time, or intensity, be sure to add on slowly to what you are presently doing.

TYPES OF STRETCHING

Types of stretches include static, ballistic, and PNF. Another way to classify stretching yields two additional ways of stretching: active and passive (or assisted) stretching. These may be used in combination with the first. For example, one can perform an active static stretch. You may want to build several different methods of stretching into your program. Each type of stretch facilitates flexibility in a different way. See Table 7.2 for the benefits and drawbacks of the different types of stretches, including previously discussed dynamic stretching.

In Chapter 1, you were introduced to special sensors located in the muscle tissue that monitor muscle tension. In the following discussion on stretching, you will see the roles these sensors and the nervous system play in flexibility development. Here is a quick review of these mechanisms. When a muscle is rapidly stretched, the muscle spindle sends a message to contract; this is called the "stretch reflex." The inhibitory Golgi tendon organ (GTO) reflex tells the muscle to relax when it feels too much tension from either a strong contraction or a rapid, forceful lengthening of the muscle. And finally, "reciprocal innervation" is the neuromuscular message to relax the muscle(s) opposite the one(s) being stretched. Now lets look at how the different types of stretching are affected by these mechanisms.

ACTIVE AND PASSIVE (ASSISTED) STRETCHING

Passive stretching is when something or someone else creates a stretch in your muscles. Because an outside force is helping you stretch, this is often referred to as **assisted stretching.** If you are the one being stretched, it is important to relax your muscles as your partner, gravity, or another part of your body creates the stretch.

A partner creates a static passive stretch by moving your muscles into a stretch position and holding you there. While the partner does the holding, you can relax and let the muscle lengthen. This works well if you have a trustworthy partner. Passive ballistic stretching is not recommended, as it carries a much greater risk of injury.

You can assist your own stretch by using muscles that aren't being stretched. For example, you can

Table 7.2   Types of Stretching

TYPE OF STRETCH	ACTION	BENEFITS	DRAWBACKS
Static	Move slowly into stretch position, and hold for at least 15 seconds. Performing a series works best.	Easiest safe way to increase flexibility	Possible muscle soreness May result in less force production in movements following the stretch May decrease joint stability
Ballistic	Place the muscle rapidly in and out of stretch position by bouncing or pulsing.	Increases flexibility Recommended after static stretching for those performing quick, explosive movements	Increased potential for injury May cause muscle to contract during the stretch Possible muscle soreness
PNF	Contract–relax (CR): isometrically contract muscle then passively stretch it.	Most effective type of stretching	Possibility of increased muscle soreness Requires a partner and more time
Dynamic	Move the muscle(s) and joints through a full range of motion using controlled active movements.	Increases dynamic flexibility; helps maintain joint stability Prepares body for dynamic movement	Many of the exercises require a degree of fitness (muscular endurance) to do repetitiously (e.g., squats or lunges). Primarily for warm-up; more research needed to assess overall effectiveness.

create a passive calf stretch by wrapping a towel around the ball of your foot and using your arms to pull your toes toward your shin. Gravity can also supply the assist. For example, a passive calf-muscle stretch is achieved when you stand on your toes on the edge of a platform and allow your heels to drop below the platform surface. Machines that put you in traction also provide a passive stretch. Passive stretching can help you break through "sticking points" and assist in an active stretch when the contracting muscle is weak.

In an **active stretch,** you are required to contract one muscle in an effort to stretch another. This type of stretch takes advantage of reciprocal innervation. This works well as long as the contracting muscle is strong enough to pull the other muscle through a full stretch. If it is not, additional stretching can be achieved by adding a passive assisted stretch. For example, an active stretch of the hamstring is achieved by lying on your back and contracting your quadriceps muscle to pull your leg toward your head. If your quadriceps muscle is too weak to create an effective stretch, maintain the quadriceps contraction and add an assist by pulling gently with your hands. Some people also like to follow an active stretch with a passive one.

STATIC STRETCHING

To perform a **static stretch,** move slowly into the stretch position and then hold (without moving) for a minimum of 15 seconds. Holding a stretch position "quiets" the stretch reflex and elicits the Golgi tendon organ reflex. This combination relaxes the muscle and allows it to stretch with little risk of injury. The stretch should be held at a point of mild discomfort but not

pain. If you feel pain, either release the stretch entirely and begin again, or ease the stretch until the pain is relieved. Performing a series of static stretches works even better because the GTO's thresholds are reset at a less sensitive level following the first stretch. This allows you to stretch further before encountering resistance. These relaxation effects are purposely elicited during developmental stretching and are avoided in dynamic stretching.

BALLISTIC STRETCHING

A **ballistic stretch** is one in which you put the muscle rapidly in and out of a stretch position by bouncing or pulsing during the stretch. Ballistic stretching may improve flexibility but has a couple of significant drawbacks. First, the rapid lengthening of the muscle elicits the stretch reflex, thus causing the muscle to contract—the opposite effect desired in a stretch. Second, because the movement is more forceful, it has more potential to injure the muscle and connective tissue. Thus, static stretching is generally recommended over ballistic stretching.

There is a time, however, when ballistic stretching may be beneficial. If you are going to be involved in a activity that requires quick explosive movements, then you need a final warm-up that is specific to that movement. After you have warmed up and done some dynamic and/or static stretching, you can start gently with ballistic stretching and build up to performance-level ballistic movements. For example, a softball player uses an explosive movement to throw the ball. After warming up and doing some dynamic and/or static stretches, the athlete can perform a series of bounce stretches, pulling the arm backward in the arm preparation position (elbow up, hand behind head). This is an example of an active stretch as the shoulder muscles pull the arm backward. For the full throw, easy throwing (dynamic action) precedes harder more ballistic throwing. Before a player takes the field, the athlete should practice all-out throwing for several repetitions.

PNF STRETCHING

Proprioceptive neuromuscular facilitation (PNF) stretching was originally developed as a rehabilitation tool. PNF stretching is the most effective type of stretching, but it requires a trustworthy and patient partner and considerably more time, and can result in more muscle soreness. Static stretching is almost as effective and is usually easier to perform. PNF stretching might be worth trying if you feel you are at a sticking point in your flexibility. Or you may want to include a few PNF stretches in a predominantly static stretching routine. There are a number of ways that PNF can be performed. The easiest one to incorporate into an aerobic dance exercise class is called contract–relax (CR). You must first isometrically contract the muscle you want to stretch for 6 seconds. Then, using a passive stretch, stretch the previously contracted muscle. For example, place your left hand on your left cheek and then try to rotate your head to the left. Hold this isometric contraction for 6 seconds. (During an isometric contraction, nothing moves. Your left hand does not allow your head to rotate.) Then relax and gently push your head through rotation to the right. To use CR with a hamstring stretch, lie on the ground and raise one leg up in the air. Have a partner place his or her hands on the back of your leg and resist you when you try to push your leg toward the ground. Hold this isometric contraction for 6 seconds and then, while you relax, have your partner gently push your leg toward your head. To do this same exercise by yourself, push your raised leg against a door jamb or use your own arms to resist the downward push of your leg. Then relax your leg and pull with your arms.

STRETCHES TO AVOID

Someone once said that "a weed is a flower out of place." So it is with some exercises; they are "weeds" in a health/fitness program but "flowers" in certain sports settings. A back bend is a good example. Gymnasts need a lot of hyperextension flexibility for tumbling stunts and to accent dance moves. But for most people, back bends place an unnecessary amount of stress on the back, particularly on the vertebral discs. The hurdler's stretch is another example. In track and field, hurdlers must use this position to clear the hurdles, but stretching in this position places an unhealthy torque on the knee. Because there are other exercises that effectively stretch the same muscles, even hurdlers limit their use of this position. Similarly, some positions that are performed in yoga and pilates classes can cause injury when attempted without the guidance of a well-trained instructor and preparation through lead-up exercises. Some exercises that are *not* recommended for general fitness are pictured in this chapter, along with healthier alternatives.

There is often more than one way to stretch (and strengthen) a muscle. If one particular exercise does not feel good to you, select a second one that will achieve the same effect. Sometimes simply doing a stretch lying down instead of standing can make it more comfortable. There are also some stretches that can be performed with the back supported against a wall to relieve back strain. Certain exercises, like a seated straddle stretch, are difficult when you are inflexible but become more comfortable as you develop flexibility. If you do not see an alternate stretch in this text, consult your instructor, physical therapist, or a stretch-specific text. If the class is performing an exercise that you know will hurt your body, don't do it; modify the exercise or perform a different one. It is tempting to want to look like the rest of the class, but it is important to listen to your body and individualize your exercise to suit it.

FLEXIBILITY EXERCISES

The following is a series of stretches for the body's major muscle groups. These stretches are appropriate for the warm-up and cool-down. Only the major muscles being stretched are listed; however, a number of smaller muscles will also be stretched during these exercises. The stretches are described for one side only (the side pictured), but they should be done on both sides. Emphasis is placed on body alignment. When performing standing stretches, be sure to maintain good abdominal tone, a neutral spine (natural curves), and slightly flexed knees. It takes practice to develop good exercise technique. Use the help of instructors, classmates, and mirrors to check your alignment and technique. When you change your technique, it may feel funny or awkward at first, but after a while you will feel better. Be sure to learn both the look and the feel of correctness.

To make the following stretches active, contract the muscles opposite those you are trying to stretch. You can add a passive assist by pulling with your hands or by having a partner work with you. For more ideas on PNF stretching, talk to your instructor or consult a more in-depth text.

Neck Stretches

Muscles stretched: sternocleidomastoideus (Figures 7.1a–d), erector spinae (Figures 7.1c, 7.1d only)

1. Rotating or holding the head to the sides and front provides a nice stretch of the neck muscles (Figures 7.1a, 7.1b, 7.1c). Rolling or laying the head to the back (Figure 7.1d) places pressure on the cervical vertebrae, so avoiding this position is probably healthier over the long run. (However, it may be necessary to stretch and strengthen the neck in hyperextension for certain sports.)

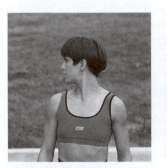

Figure 7.1a

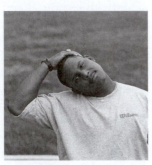

Figure 7.1b

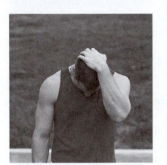

Figure 7.1c

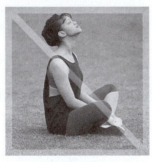

Figure 7.1d Hyperextending the neck places unnecessary stress on the cervical vertebrae.

VARIATIONS

a. Lifting the chin after fully rotating the head adds a little extra stretch to the neck muscles.

b. Dropping the chin and then looking to the right shoulder adds another angle to the stretch. Repeat to the left.

2. Pull the chin from a protruding position (Figure 7.2a) in toward the centerline of the body as if to create a double chin (Figure 7.2b). Hold for 2 to 3 seconds and release. Do 5 to 10 neck glides. This exercise helps counter the tendency to let the chin protrude and can be performed throughout the day to improve posture and prevent neck fatigue.

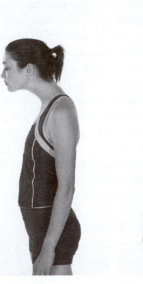

Figure 7.2a   **Figure 7.2b**

Arm and Shoulder Stretches

Muscles stretched: triceps, posterior deltoid (Figure 7.3), triceps, anterior deltoid (Figure 7.4), biceps brachii, forearm flexors (Figure 7.5)

1. Stretch the left arm across the front of the body parallel to the floor. Place the right hand above the left elbow and gently apply pressure across and in toward the chest (Figure 7.3).

2. Reach the right arm straight up. Bend at the elbow, and try to touch the right hand to the middle of the back. Place the left hand just above the right elbow, and push the arm into a stretch position (Figure 7.4). Drop the head forward slightly for comfort.

3. Extend the arm you wish to stretch in front of you with the palm facing the ceiling. Hyperextend the wrist of the extended arm by pulling down and back on the fingers with the opposite hand (Figure 7.5). Maintain good back alignment and soft knees during the stretch.

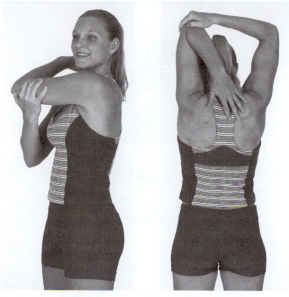

Figure 7.3   **Figure 7.4**

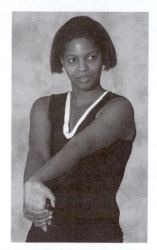

Figure 7.5

Shoulder and Chest Stretches

Muscles stretched: pectorals, anterior deltoids

1. Grasp the hands behind the back, interlacing the fingers. Try to raise the arms upward. Bend forward slightly at the waist with the knees bent (Figure 7.6).

2. Extend your arms behind you, and have a partner grasp your upper arms very gently and smoothly pull your arms together and slightly upward (Figure 7.7a). Your palms can be facing each other or rotated outward for more stretch through the chest and front of the shoulder. Be sure the partner grasps your arms between elbows and shoulders to avoid putting pressure on your elbow joint.

3. Bend your arms and have a partner pull them backward gently (Figure 7.7b).

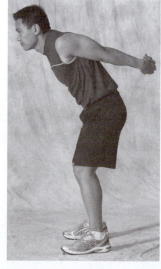

Figure 7.6

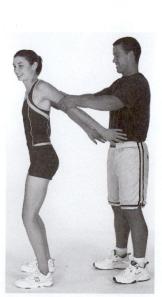

Figure 7.7a

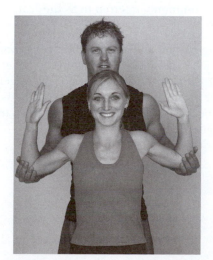

Figure 7.7b

Shoulder and Upper Back Stretch

Muscles stretched: deltoid, rhomboids

Stability ball: Kneel down with the ball in front and slightly to the left of your body. Place the back of your right hand on top of the ball. Roll the ball out to your left using the right arm. As your arm extends, bend forward at the waist (Figure 7.8). Keep your head facing front. Your chin may touch your upper arm. Keep your lower body stable with the hips square.

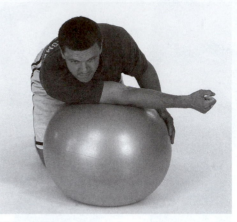

Figure 7.8

Back Stretches

Muscles stretched: erector spinae

1. Stand with feet shoulder width apart and knees bent. Tuck the pelvis under by contracting the abdomen. Grasp the hands in front of the body with palms facing outward. Try to cave in or hollow out the chest and abdominal areas (Figure 7.9). The back should appear rounded. Allow the head to follow the natural line of the curve.

   VARIATIONS

   a. You can also perform this standing exercise with the hands on the knees, rounding and flattening (or slightly arching) the back.

   b. In an all-fours position (on hands and knees), alternately round and arch the back. This is commonly referred to as the "cat stretch."

2. Lie on the ground and draw both knees toward the shoulders, grasping underneath the knees (Figure 7.10a). This exercise specifically targets the lower back. The "plow" position should be avoided because of the pressure it places on the neck (Figure 7.10b).

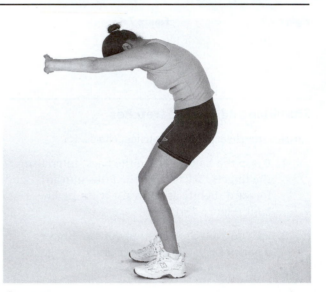

Figure 7.9

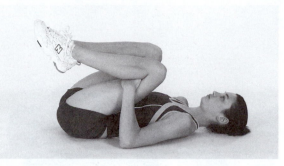

Figure 7.10a

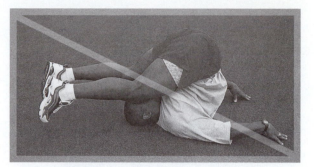

Figure 7.10b The "plow" position puts the weight of the entire body on the cervical vertebrae. This is very stressful to the upper spine. See the discussion concerning yoga positions in the Stretches to Avoid section on page 69.

Back/Abdominal Stretches

Muscles stretched: abdominals

1. Lie face down with hands up by the ears. Gently press up, supporting your weight on the forearms. Elbows should be under or slightly in front of the shoulders (Figure 7.11a). Hold for 5 to 10 seconds. If you experience pain, discontinue this exercise and consult a physician. Hyperextension of the spine to the extent involved in a back bend is not recommended for normal health and fitness (Figure 7.11b).

2. *Stability ball:* Sit on the ball. Walk your feet forward until the natural curve of the low back is over the ball (Figure 7.12a, on page 74). Hands can be by the ears with elbows out and laying on the ball or extended sideways. Press your feet into the floor and extend the legs, causing the ball to roll backward (Figure 7.12b). The farther back the ball rolls, the greater the stretch. If dizziness occurs, try holding this stretch for a shorter time or select a different stretch.

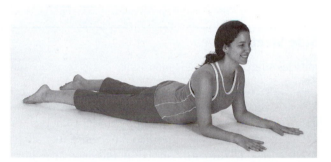

Figure 7.11a

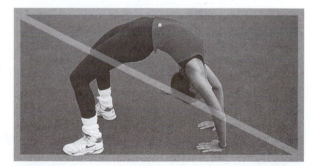

Figure 7.11b Hyperextension of the back is stressful to the spine. See the discussion on yoga positions in the Stretches to Avoid section on page 69.

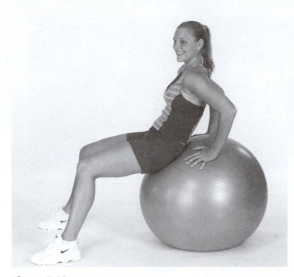

Figure 7.12a

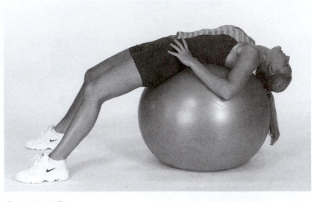

Figure 7.12b

Side Stretch

Muscles stretched: obliques, intercostals

1. Place the feet shoulder width apart. If you are stretching to the right, be sure that the right foot is angled outward and the right knee is bent. This keeps the torso, knee, and foot all going in the same direction and decreases the chance of knee soreness. Bend directly to the right side. The left arm can be relaxed by your side or extended for balance (Figure 7.13a) or, for a more advanced stretch, extended up by the left ear (Figure 7.13b). Incorrect alignment is shown in Figure 7.13c. For added support, place the right hand on the thigh of the bent right leg. If this position is held for an extended amount of time, pressure is put on the vertebral discs. Controlled movement into and out of the position is recommended.

2. *Stability ball:* Sit with one hip on the ball. Move your inside leg forward and outside leg backward for stability. Lay your torso down sideways on the ball. Keep one hip directly over the other. One arm is placed on the ball for stability; the other reaches overhead to add stretch. It may be necessary to place your feet against a wall to prevent yourself from rolling forward.

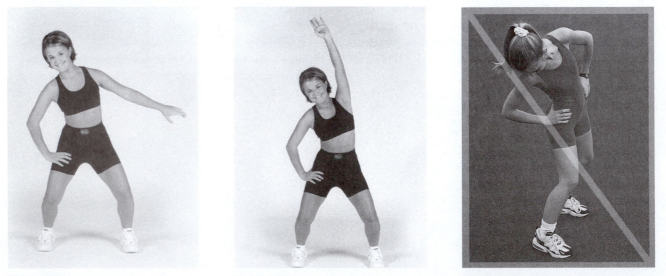

Figure 7.13a   **Figure 7.13b**   **Figure 7.13c** Poor back alignment.

Trunk Stretches

Muscles stretched: internal oblique, external oblique, piriformis, erector spinae

To do the pretzel stretch, first sit with your right leg extended forward and your left leg bent. Now lift and place your left foot against the outside of your right knee. Turn your torso gently, and position your extended right arm so that the back of your right elbow is against the outside of your left knee. Place your left hand on the floor comfortably behind your buttocks. Gently press your right arm against your right leg, and turn your body to the left. Look over your left shoulder (Figure 7.14).

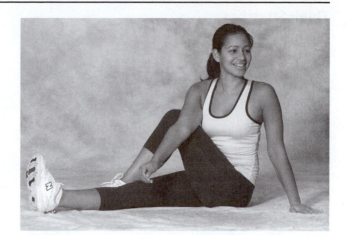

Figure 7.14

Buttocks Stretches

Muscles stretched: gluteals

1. Lie on the floor on your back with knees bent. Place the left foot on the right knee. Grasp the right thigh, and gently pull the right thigh toward the chest (Figure 7.15).

2. Kneel with the hands on the floor close to the knees. Lean over to one side until you feel a stretch in the buttocks muscles on that side (Figure 7.16). If this hurts the knees, use a different stretch.

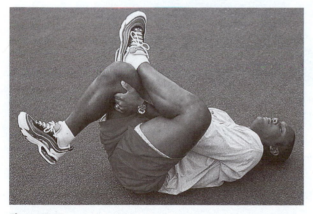

Figure 7.15

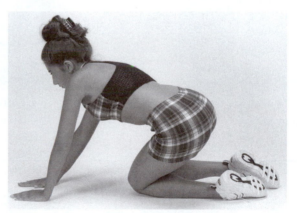

Figure 7.16

Thigh Stretches

Muscles stretched: quadriceps

Stand on the left leg. Bend the right leg, and grasp the ankle (not the foot) with the same arm. Keep the knee pointed downward. Allow a comfortable knee bend, and pull gently backward at the ankle. (The right foot should not be forced to the right buttock.) Maintain good posture and alignment by pulling in the abdomen and keeping the pelvis straight. Avoid arching the back or leaning forward. More strectch is not achieved by leaning forward, but a slight forward lean may relieve back pressure for some individuals. To keep your balance, extend the free arm to the side or overhead, look at something stationary, and keep the abdomen pulled up (Figure 7.17a). You can also place the extended hand against a wall or on a partner's shoulder. This same stretch can be performed lying on your side on the floor (Figure 7.17b). Stretching the thigh by leaning back in the hurdler's position (Figure 7.17c) is not recommended.

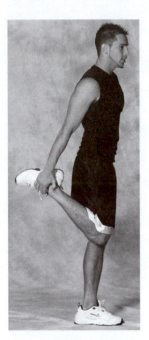

Figure 7.17a

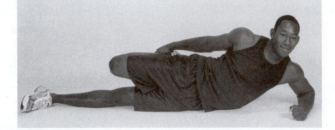

Figure 7.17b

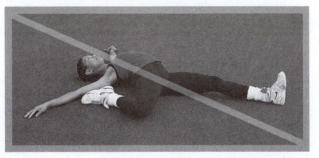

Figure 7.17c Leaning back in the hurdler's position stresses knee ligaments on the bent leg and may irritate the lower back.

Back-of-the-Leg Stretches

Muscles stretched: hamstrings

Exercisers have traditionally stretched the muscles at the back of the legs by performing a standing toe touch (Figure 7.18). Today, sports medicine professionals are concerned that hanging in this position stresses the ligaments that support the back, which could result in lower back pain. When the knees are straight, most of the major muscles in the hip and lower back area cannot function effectively to support the back. Bending the knees helps relieve the pressure on the lower back and allows the muscles to aid the ligaments. But, like the side stretch, hanging in one direction for an extended amount of time places stress on the intervertebral discs. Rather than hang in forward flexion, the toe-touch position, you can use some alternative methods of

stretching the hamstrings. Some of these alternatives include the following.

1. Sit on the floor with the legs extended forward. Bend the left knee, and place the left foot flat on the floor. Hold the bent leg, and pull yourself gently forward (Figure 7.19a). If this is uncomfortable, place the hands behind the buttocks for support and try sitting up straight. This sitting position is good for inflexible people. (More flexible people may not feel a stretch in this position.) This stretch is preferable to the hurdler's stretch, which strains the knee (Figure 7.19b).

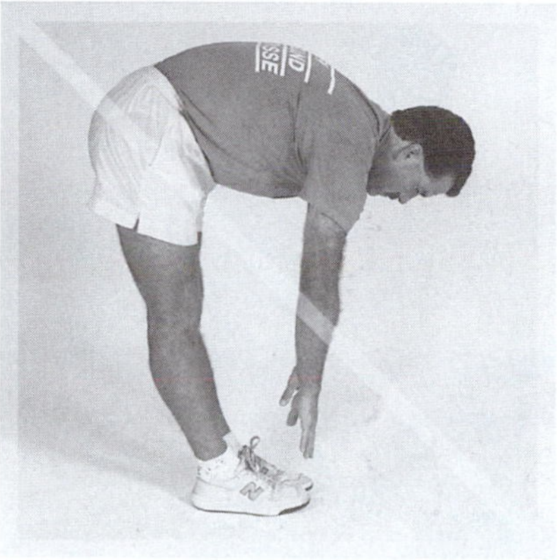

Figure 7.18 The straight-leg toe touch (standing or sitting) places stress on the ligaments in the lower back region. Bending the knees will take some pressure off the low back.

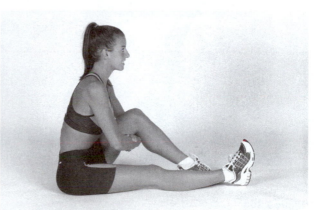

Figure 7.19a

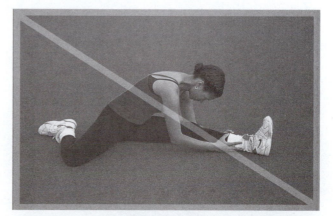

Figure 7.19b Stretching forward in the hurdler's stretch stresses the knee ligaments of the bent leg.

2. Lying flat on the back, extend the right leg straight out, bend the left leg, and place the left foot flat on the floor. Lift the right leg up until you feel the hamstring stretching. Keep the knee facing the chest; don't turn it out (Figure 7.20a). For an active stretch, use the thigh and hip muscles to pull the right leg toward your head. By contracting the quadriceps muscle, you are allowing the hamstrings to relax. The hands should assist as needed. In a passive stretch, the hands pull and the leg muscles are relaxed.

Use a towel if you have difficulty reaching the leg (Figure 7.20b). Assisted stretching can also be achieved by having a trustworthy partner push slowly and steadily against the leg. Partners must listen carefully to each other and push the leg only to a point of mild discomfort. The lower leg can also be straightened along the floor as long as this does not cause the lower back to strain or lift up off the floor.

3. Stand with the right leg bent and the left leg extended forward with the heel resting on the floor, stability ball, or step (bench). With hands on the thigh of the right leg, bend forward at the waist (Figure 7.21).

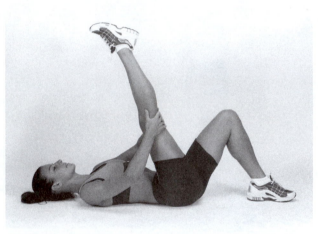

Figure 7.20a

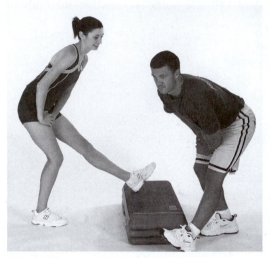

Figure 7.21

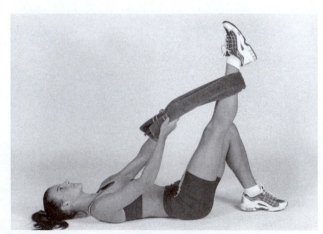

Figure 7.20b

4. *Stability ball:* Sit on the ball with one foot close to the ball and the other extended farther out in front. Put both hands on the knee of the close foot, and curl the body down over the knee (Figure 7.22). This stretches the calf muscles (gastrocnemious, soleus) of the near leg. Then push backward extending the front leg until only the heel is touching. This stretches the back of the leg (hamstrings) of the extended leg.

5. *Stability ball:* Lie down near a wall. Place the ball up on the wall, and hold it there with the bottoms of your feet. Your knees are bent and your torso flat on the ground. Roll the ball up the wall by slowly extending your legs. The closer your bottom is to the wall, the greater the stretch. Keep the hips square and the pelvis flat throughout (Figure 7.23).

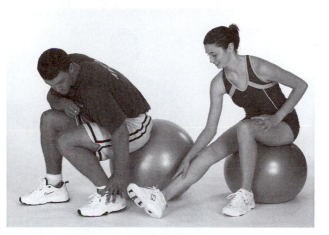

Figure 7.22

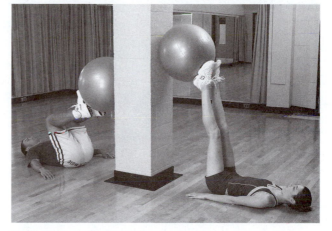

Figure 7.23 A pillar is used here to allow the reader to see both positions simultaneously. A flat wall is recommended for this exercise.

Inner Thigh Stretches

SIDE LUNGE POSITION (LEGS TO THE SIDES)

Muscles stretched: adductors, gracilis

1. With your body facing forward, assume a lunge position with right knee bent and left leg extended. Both feet should be comfortably aligned with the knees. Hands are placed on the upper thighs (Figure 7.24a). Hands can also be placed on the floor in front of the body for support (see Figure 7.24b on the next page). Try to lower hips. When a bench (step) is used, straddle the bench and place hands on top. Less flexible individuals may find this position more comfortable (Figure 7.24c). This stretch can also be performed with the trunk upright (standing) and hands on thighs. The bent right knee should not extend beyond the right instep (Figure 7.24d).

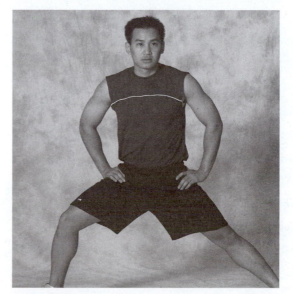

Figure 7.24a

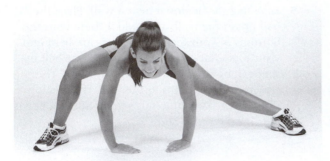

Figure 7.24b

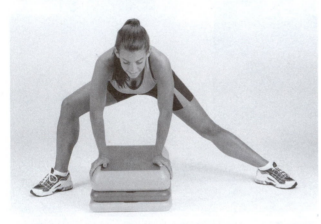

Figure 7.24c

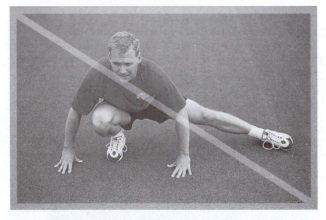

Figure 7.24d Extending the knee beyond the instep results in stress to the knee ligaments.

BUTTERFLY POSITION

Muscles stretched: adductors, gracilis

1. Sit on the floor with the soles of the feet together. Grasp the ankles. (Grasping the toes and pulling may stress the ligaments of the feet.) It is usually most comfortable to grasp the right ankle with the left hand and the left ankle with the right hand. Sit up tall, and lean forward until you feel a stretch in the groin area (Figure 7.26). Touching the head to the feet stresses the lower back instead of stretching the groin area.

2. *Stability ball:* Sit on the ball with legs apart and feet flat on the floor. Your respective feet and knees should be pointing in the same direction. Place your hands on your knees. Roll the ball to one side while extending the opposite leg to the side (Figure 7.25).

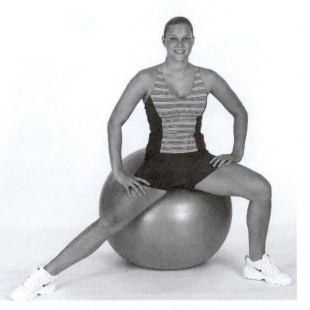

Figure 7.25

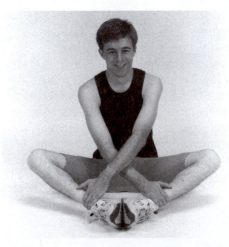

Figure 7.26

MODIFIED STRADDLE POSITION

Muscles stretched: adductors, gracilis

Sit on the floor with the left leg extended and the right leg bent in front. Stretch forward from the base of the spine (Figure 7.27). Think of putting your nose on the floor as far in front of you as possible.

You can also use this exercise to stretch the back of the legs by turning the hips to face the extended left leg and stretching forward. This is called the modified hurdler's stretch.

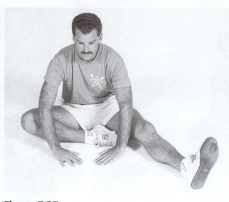

Figure 7.27

Combination Leg and Hip Stretch

FRONT LUNGE POSITION (ONE LEG FORWARD, ONE BACK)

Muscles stretched: quadriceps, hamstrings, hip flexors

1. Pretend you are straddling a straight line. Place the left foot out in front of your body just to the left of the imaginary line. Bend the left knee. Extend the right leg straight back with the right big toe just to the right of the line. Keep the hips absolutely square. Place your hands on the floor (or bench), one on each side of the bent leg, to support your weight. Try to lower the hips toward the ground (Figures 7.28a, 7.28b). This stretch can also be performed with the trunk upright (standing) and the hands on the front thigh. The bent front knee should stay above or behind the instep. (When the knee is pushed forward and the heel of the front foot lifts, stress is placed on the knee ligaments [Figure 7.28c].) When you want more stretch, move the rear foot back.

2. *Stability ball:* Take a front lunge position on the ball. Sit down on the ball. Place your hands on the ball on either side of you. Place the front foot far enough forward to maintain a 90-degree angle in the knee. Allow the heel to lift on the back foot (Figure 7.29, on page 82). For additional stretch, roll the ball forward (move the front foot forward as needed). Keep the hips square throughout.

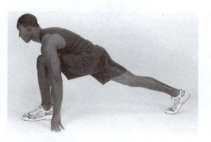

Figure 7.28a

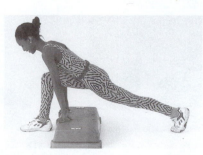

Figure 7.28b

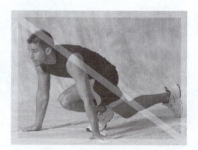

Figure 7.28c When the knee is pushed beyond the instep, pressure is placed on the knee ligaments.

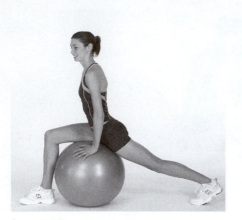

Figure 7.29

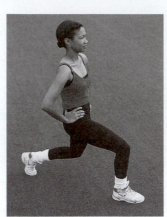

Figure 7.30a

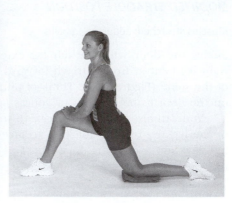

Figure 7.30b

HIP STRETCHES

Muscles stretched: hip flexors, quadriceps, hamstring

1. Place the legs in a front lunge position with the right foot in front. The back toes face straight ahead. The front foot may be turned slightly inward for balance. The back heel is off the ground. Keeping the hips square and the pelvis tucked under, try to lower the hips. Be sure the front foot is far enough out in front to do this comfortably. To avoid ligament stress, the bent front knee should stay directly above or behind the instep. The hands can be placed on the hips or on the front leg (Figure 7.30a). This same stretch can be achieved in a kneeling position (Figure 7.30b). You may want to pad the knees with a towel or mat.

2. *Stability ball:* Take the same position as described in Step 1 but with the hip resting on the side of the ball.

3. You can also stretch the hip flexors while lying on your back. Grasp under the knee, and pull one leg to the chest while keeping the other leg straight along the floor (Figure 7.31a). The extended bottom leg results in a greater stretch to the iliopsoas muscle (versus the quadriceps) than the previous two positions. Both the quadriceps and iliopsoas are hip flexors. Even more iliopsoas stretch can be achieved using a bench (Figure 7.31b).

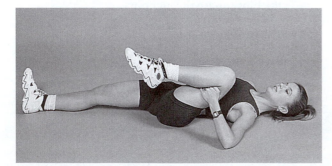

Figure 7.31a

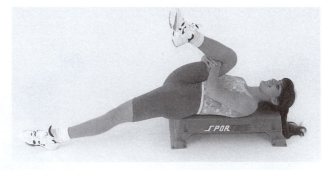

Figure 7.31b

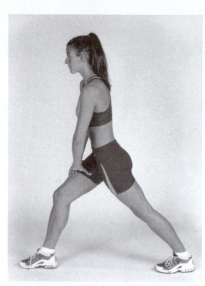

Figure 7.32a

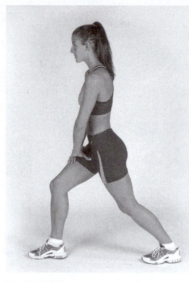

Figure 7.32b

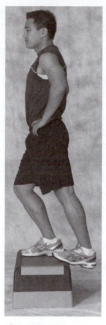

Figure 7.32c

CALF STRETCHES

Muscles stretched: gastrocnemius, soleus

1. Stand in the same front lunge position used for the hip stretch, but adjust the stance so that the back heel touches down. Support or balance yourself by placing hands on the forward knee. Be sure to keep the back foot facing directly front, and keep the abdomen pulled in. A straight back leg stretches the calf muscle called the gastrocnemius (Figure 7.32a). When you bend the back leg but keep the heel on the ground, you stretch the underneath calf muscle called the soleus (Figure 7.32b).

   To perform a calf stretch using a bench (step), stand on top of the step. Put weight on the right foot, bending the right knee slightly. Place the left foot so that the ball of the foot is on the step but the heel is over the edge. Gently press the heel down (Figure 7.32c).

VARIATION

You can also stretch the calves in a sitting position. Extend one leg forward, keeping the knee slightly flexed. Reach forward, grasp the ball of the foot, and gently pull back. If you can't reach your foot, loop a towel around the ball of your foot and pull.

2. *Stability ball:* See Figure 7.22 on page 79.

SUMMARY

A well-planned 50- to 60-minute class should include the following segments: a 5- to 10-minute warm-up, a 20- to 30-minute aerobic workout, a 5-minute standing cool-down, a 10- to 15-minute muscle-toning workout, followed by a 5- to 10-minute final (developmental) stretch. If you are late to class, take the time to prepare your body for vigorous exercise. If you must leave early, step out of class with enough time to cool down. The warm-up and cool-down are similar in the exercises and movements they incorporate, even though one is preparing the body for exercise while the other is bringing the body back to a resting state. Both the warm-up and cool-down promote flexibility. There are a number of ways to stretch, each with its advantages and disadvantages. A combination of methods may be the most effective. Finally, flexibility adds to the quality of your life and is something that can be maintained throughout your life.

KNOWLEDGE TIPS

1. The warm-up prepares the body and mind for physical activity. Warm-up movements raise the body's core and muscle temperature.

2. Warm-up movements work within comfortable ranges of motion, move from general to specific exercises, and raise the

heart rate gradually moving from slow to moderate intensity activity.

3. The standing cool-down is used to bring down your activity level gradually. This activity helps bring blood shunted to the limbs back to the heart.

4. The developmental stretch, which occurs at the end of class, develops flexibility and helps prevent muscle soreness.

5. The ACSM guideline for flexibility is to stretch a minimum of 2 to 3 days a week, ideally 5 to 7 days a week, at an intensity best described as holding to a point of tightness without discomfort, holding the stretch for 15 to 30 seconds for a static stretch; a 6-second contraction followed by 15 to 30 seconds of assisted stretch for PNF, with 2 to 4 repetitions for each stretch.

6. A stretch can be active (using contraction of the opposing muscle) or passive (using an outside force like a partner to elongate the muscle).

7. There are four types of stretches: static (sustained hold), ballistic (bounce stretch), dynamic, and PNF (combination of muscle contractions and stretches).

8. Good technique during a stretch ensures that you will receive the full benefit of the exercise.

9. Some exercises are appropriate in sports settings and inappropriate in health/fitness settings.

10. The step (bench) and stability ball can be used as effective tools for stretching.

THINK ABOUT IT

1. Why is it important to perform a warm-up? cool-down?

2. When in an aerobic dance exercise class is the best time to work on *developing* flexibility? Why?

3. Each type of stretching has advantages. Explain the advantages associated with static, dynamic, and PNF stretching.

4. Describe the FITT principle for flexibility.

5. A static stretch can be passive or active. Explain the difference and give an example.

6. What is the stretch reflex and what role does it play in each of the types of stretching (static, ballistic, dynamic, and PNF)?

7. Identify a range of motion you would like to improve and identify a stretch you can use to achieve this goal.

8. What are some stretches that are considered unhealthy for normal health-enhancing activity?

REFERENCES

Alter, J. *Stretch & Strengthen.* Boston: Houghton Mifflin, 1986.
——. *Surviving Exercise.* Boston: Houghton Mifflin, 1983.
Alter, M. J. *Science of Flexibility.* 2nd ed. Champaign, IL: Human Kinetics, 1996.
American College of Sports Medicine. *ACSM's Guidelines for Exercise Testing and Exercise Prescription.* 8th ed. Media, PA: Lippincott Williams & Wilkins, 2010.
American Council on Exercise. *Aerobics Instructor Manual: ACE's Guide for Fitness Professionals.* San Diego, CA: American Council on Exercise, 2000.
Åstrand, P. O., and K. Rodahl. *Textbook of Work Physiology.* 2nd ed. New York: McGraw-Hill, 1977.
Barnard, R. J. "The Heart Needs a Warm-Up Time." *The Physician and Sportsmedicine* 4 (No. 1, 1976): 40.
Corbin, C. B., and M. L. Noble. "Flexibility." *Journal of Physical Education and Recreation* 51 (No. 6, 1980): 23–6; 57–60.
Faigenbaum, A.D., M. Bellucci, A. Bernieri, B. Bakker, and K. Hoorens. "Acute Effects of Different Warm-Up Protocols on Fitness Performance in Children." *Journal of Strength and Conditioning* 19 (No. 2, 2005): 376–81.
Gerson, R. "Point-Counterpoint: Calisthenics Before Aerobics." *Dance Exercise Today* (May/June 1985): 26–8.
Holt, L. E., T. M. Travis, and T. Okita. "Comparative Study of Three Stretching Techniques." *Perceptual and Motor Skills* 31 (1970): 611.
Jones, A. "Point-Counterpoint: Aerobics Before Calisthenics." *Dance Exercise Today* (May/June 1985): 27–8.
Paraskevi, M., S. Rokka, A. Beneka, G. Mavridis, and G. Godolias. "Reducing Risk of Injury Due to Warm Up and Cool Down in Dance Aerobic Instructors." *Journal of Back and Musculoskeletal Rehabilitation* 20 (No. 1, 2007): 29(7).
Schultz, P. "Flexibility: Day of the Static Stretch." *The Physician and Sportsmedicine* 7 (No. 11, 1979): 109–14, 117.
Shellock, F. G. "Physiological Benefits of Warm-Up." *The Physician and Sportsmedicine* 11 (No. 10, 1983): 134–9.
Silvestri, L., and J. Oescher. "Use of Aerobic Dance and Light Weights in Improving Measures of Strength, Endurance, and Flexibility." *Perceptual and Motor Skills* 70 (April 1990): 595–600.
Taylor, D., J. Dalton, A. Seaber, and W. Garrett. "Viscoelastic Properties of Muscle-Tendon Units: The Biomechanical Effects of Stretching." *American Journal of Sports Medicine* 18 (No. 3, 1990); 300–9.
Wiktorsson-Moller, M., B. Oberg, J. Ekstrand, and J. Gillquist. "Effects of Warming Up, Massage and Stretching on Range of Motion and Muscle Strength in the Lower Extremity." *American Journal of Sports Medicine* 11 (No. 4, 1983); 249–52.

8

Rhythmic Aerobics: Variations and Styles

The sound of many sneakers dancing . . .

- I tried to sign up for a class but got confused by all the different names (styles). What do they mean?
- Do I have to do high-impact, running, jumping moves to get or stay fit?
- Will one style of aerobics make me more fit than another?
- Can I use interval training to train aerobically?
- Is the target heart-rate zone different for water aerobics?

THE term "aerobic dance," which usually conjures up an image of high-impact aerobics, is too restrictive for the great variety of rhythmic activities being done today. Perhaps better described as rhythmic aerobics, the aerobics scene now includes high-impact, low-impact, step, circuit, slide, martial arts, dance, and water (aqua) aerobics. And this list doesn't even begin to describe all the styles that have developed—everything from funk to combat aerobics. Instructors pull from their expertise and choreograph routines that are as varied and exciting as the instructors themselves. What follows is a brief description of some of the many fun styles loosely grouped into three categories: dance exercise aerobics, combat and martial arts aerobics, and cardio-machine aerobics. After that is a more in-depth discussion of high- and low-impact, step, circuit, interval, and water aerobics.

If you have the opportunity to choose from among these different types of rhythmic aerobic programs, first watch the one(s) you are thinking of joining, or take a free trial class. Make sure the class suits your fitness level and that the instructor is knowledgeable. You may find that one style feels right for you, or with all these possibilities (and more), you may decide to mix it up using a variety of styles. Maybe high-impact or step aerobics gets you in shape for some fall hiking, a low-impact class gives you a change of pace and a workout with less impact stress on your legs for the

winter, a salsa aerobics gets you set for that spring vacation to Cancún, and water aerobics keeps you cool and fit during the hot summer.

DANCE EXERCISE AEROBICS

Founders Jacki Sorensen (Aerobic Dancing—workout) and Judi Sheppard Missett (Jazzercise) both draw on their dance backgrounds to choreograph dancelike routines that have had great appeal for three decades. Following their lead but definitely in their own style are Victoria Johnson and Christy Lane, both well known for their funky fitness routines done to pop-funk and rap music. Funk is a mixture of ballet, jazz, modern dance, street dancing, maybe some line dancing, and a whole lot of "attitude." You can perform funk steps in a style that gets "down and into the floor" or in one that is up, light, and bouncy, called hip-hop. Funk can be fast moving and thrilling when you start picking up the moves. (Usually, moves are taught at a slower pace and then performed at a fast pace.) Country line dancing, upbeat and wildly popular, has also expanded into the aerobic arena. You can get fit doing the Electric Slide or the Achy Breaky. Salsarobics and Zumba are just two of the many companies exploring Latin moves on the aerobics floor. These forms of dance aerobics use steps from the merengue, cha-cha, rumba, samba, lambada, and more. If it's African you like, or Gospel . . . you can find that, too. Instructors are pulling from their strengths and producing all kinds of specialty classes.

For those who want to jump less, at least two companies have developed nonimpact aerobic styles. Debby and Carlos Rosas introduced NIA (nonimpact aerobics), a flowing, undulating, rising-and-falling form of dance that sustains training zone heart rates with nonimpact changes of feet on the floor. Another company, called Yogarobics, has used yoga and tai chi to develop a style that involves moving from a state of quiet or stillness to one of chaotic (vigorous) movements and back to stillness. And, of course, there is step aerobics, started by Gin Miller, which is more comfortable for individuals who prefer a class with less dance emphasis.

COMBAT AND MARTIAL ARTS AEROBICS

As rhythmic aerobics has grown, nondancelike styles have also emerged with a punch and a kick. Some, like Boot Camp and Fit Camp, use military basic training movements and rope jumping to develop aerobic fitness to music. Other styles have applied expertise in boxing to rhythmic aerobics. Programs such as Boxercise, Boxerobics, Box Aerobic, and Cardio Knockout use boxing footwork and punches, rope jumping, shadow boxing, and bag and focus mitt workouts to develop strength and aerobic conditioning.

There are also many martial arts–based aerobic programs. The first, Cardio Kickboxing, started in 1992 by Frank Thiboutot, set out to promote the sport of kickboxing through kickboxing for fitness. His objective has been to safely mainstream the workout of a fighter to the general public for its fitness and self-defense benefits. His program is now joined by a number of others, such as Cardio-karate, Karatics, Kempocise, Tae-Bo, and TKO Aerobics. This style of group fitness uses jogging; calisthenics; rope jumping; a number of punches, jabs, and kicks, alone and in combination; shadow boxing; and self-defense moves (Figure 8.1). When equipment is available, these programs use a variety of hanging or free-standing bags, focus pads, and punch mitts. The philosophy behind the workout will vary depending on the particular type of martial art from which the program draws.

CARDIO-MACHINE AEROBICS

Some of the newest trends in group fitness have made rhythmic aerobics jump off the aerobics floor onto a variety of cardio equipment. Fitness specialists are

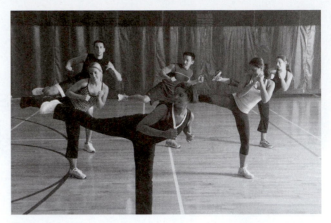

Figure 8.1

taking advantage of the growing number of aerobics machines available at fitness facilities, including those at colleges and universities. People who don't like traditional aerobics, or people looking for a new group-oriented cross-training activity, are eagerly signing up for these classes. You can go "spinning" on a stationary cycle, "stomp" on a stair stepper, or go "trekking" or "treading" on a treadmill. Even rowing machines are getting into the act. What all these group fitness classes have in common is an instructor who leads, educates, and motivates participants through a shared event. Music is used to energize and, in most cases, set a cadence for the workout. These classes appeal to both men and women of all ages. Since they are low-impact to nonimpact in nature, they are excellent choices for people prone to impact-stress injuries or who are rehabilitating after an injury. They are also perfect for overweight individuals who want to spare their joints. Some classes include the use of small weights to promote upper body muscle development.

A number of fitness levels can be easily incorporated into one class. But as these activities have grown in popularity, more classes are being offered for specific fitness levels and fitness objectives. The intensity can range from a high-level athletic workout to an endurance fat-burning workout. For example, indoor group cycling, dubbed "spinning" (Figure 8.2) by its founder Johnny G. (John Goldberg), now offers four different kinds of classes. (Similar programs are also offered by companies like Body Bike, Cycle Reebok, and Keiser Power Pacer.) There is the medium-resistance flat ride for endurance and fat burning. Then there is a cardio workout with an emphasis on leg strengthening, in which the cycle's resistance is set to make it feel as though you were riding steadily uphill at a relatively high but still aerobic intensity. The all-terrain or race day workout includes both aerobic and high-intensity anaerobic riding while traversing through flat and

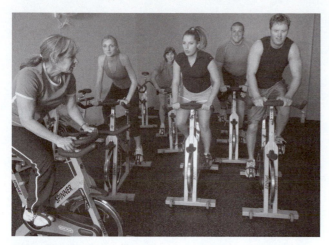

Figure 8.2

hilly terrain and performing sprints, jumps, and recovery rides. The fourth type of class is a recovery workout, which uses light resistances and is intended for off days; its purposes are loosening up the muscles, focusing on breathing, and "centering the psyche."

Whichever cardio equipment you choose to use, be sure to have a qualified instructor show you how to set the machine to "fit" you and go over some of the basics before you start. With all this innovation, one has to wonder what the next five years will bring to group fitness and rhythmic aerobics.

THE AEROBICS PORTION OF CLASS

All aerobics classes, regardless of type or style, use continuous, rhythmic, large-muscle movements to condition your cardiorespiratory system. The training strengthens your heart, reduces the risk of coronary heart disease, reduces your percentage of body fat, and provides you with a sense of well-being. Some evidence even suggests that aerobic training can lengthen your life, and it definitely can improve the quality of it. (For a complete discussion of the benefits of aerobic dance exercise, refer back to Chapter 1.)

The aerobic part of class follows the warm-up and/or any muscle-toning exercises that follow the warm-up. The most commonly used cardiorespiratory workout uses a sustained aerobic approach. The first part of the routine is 5 to 10 minutes of moderately paced activity to gradually bring you up to a training intensity. Instructors often use low-impact aerobics for this. Once in your training zone, you sustain this level of exertion for 20 to 30 minutes and then taper down as you reach the end of the workout. (The aerobic portion of class may be slightly longer in a low-impact or nonimpact style of rhythmic aerobics or advanced classes.) The aerobic section is followed by the standing

cool-down (postcardial section) during which the activity level continues to decrease until you are well below your training zone and sufficiently recovered (a heart rate of 120 beats per minute [bpm] or lower) to go on to muscle-toning exercises or a cool-down stretch. A cardiorespiratory workout may also be obtained using short segments of high-intensity exercise alternated with lower intensity (but still in the training zone) recovery exercise periods. See Circuit and Interval Training for Aerobics on page 101 for more information. Many people do not find this type of workout as comfortable and, as a result, more people drop out. Highly fit, highly motivated individuals, however, may enjoy it.

TECHNIQUES FOR ALL FLOOR-BASED RHYTHMIC AEROBICS

1. Maintain good standing or sitting posture. Pull your chin back to prevent jutting the head forward. Pull back gently on your shoulders, pull in your abdomen, keep your hip joints released (relaxed) and vertically aligned, soften your knees, and avoid unnecessarily rounding or arching the back. Pretend you are being pulled up by a string that attaches to the top of your head. Good alignment relieves pressure in your lower back and prevents unnecessary exercise stress.

2. Breathe! Some people have a tendency to hold their breath when they pull in their abdomen. Breathe normally. This means breathing more deeply and quickly as the oxygen demand increases.

3. Keep your feet and knees going in the same direction to prevent rotation soreness, and bend the knees when landing from a jump. Try to absorb the impact of a jump or step by bending your knees instead of arching your back. (Some people lose their alignment by arching their backs when they land.)

4. Maintain good neutral spine back alignment during straight-leg kicks. Enthusiastic aerobicizers tend to exceed the limits of their flexibility by kicking too high. To compensate, the lower back will round. Kick only as high as your hamstring flexibility allows. Correct and incorrect kicking alignment are shown in Chapter 6, Figures 6.3a and 6.3b, on page 59.

5. Limit repetition of a movement to a healthy number. This concept is discussed more as it applies to each type of aerobics. For example, in step aerobics, you switch lead legs after

1 minute, and in high-impact aerobics, you should limit yourself to four consecutive hops. Repetitions should be limited anytime overuse is a concern. If you are recovering from an injury, the number of repetitions may need to be fewer than normal.

6. Control your arm movements. Momentum from flinging an arm can carry the arm beyond its normal range of motion and hurt the joint. Arm movements can and often should move above shoulder level, but the arms should not be held above the shoulders for extended periods of time. The isometric contractions performed by the shoulder muscles will increase blood pressure and may add to unnecessary soreness. Instead, arms should frequently move between low, middle, and high positions.

7. Do not wear ankle weights during the aerobic portion of class. Extra weight attached to the ankle increases the risk of impact injury to the lower leg.

8. Handheld and wrist weights are generally not recommended during the aerobic phase of class. Even small weights can pose a risk in a fast-moving activity.

9. Use an intensity that is high enough to create an overload but low enough to allow oxygen delivery and let aerobic metabolism dominate.

10. Elevate or lower intensity by increasing or decreasing range of motion, arm movements, the amount or height of jumps (high-impact aerobics, step), or the amount of knee bend (low-impact aerobics).

When your movements demonstrate good positioning, alignment, and control, you are said to have "clean lines." It is always fun to watch people with clean lines because they make the movements look crisp and effortless. Strive for this in whichever form of aerobics you select.

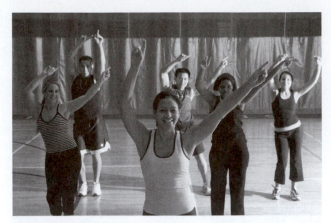

Figure 8.3 Aerobics with "attitude."

HIGH-IMPACT AEROBICS

High-impact aerobics (HIA) classes consist of large-muscle movements such as jogging, jumping, hopping, skipping, knee lifts, dance steps, and calisthenics. Some routines are highly choreographed; others are improvised. Choreographed routines are not necessarily more dancelike but are planned routines that closely follow the music and can be repeated exactly the same way each time. Because they are planned, well-choreographed routines usually provide a more balanced workout. The advantage of freestyle routines is their spontaneity and easy adjustment to class ability (Figure 8.3).

Planting the foot is probably the most important skill to perfect, since many HIA steps require you to land on the balls of your feet. A dancer counts four different positions between being on the ball of the foot and standing flat. Although you don't need to be able to identify the four positions, you do need to learn how to roll down through all of them as you land from a jump. To land, roll down through the balls of your feet (Figures 8.4a and 8.4b), and bend your knees as you touch down your heels (Figure 8.4c). When you forget

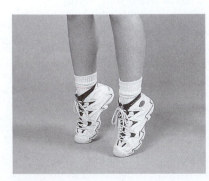

Figure 8.4a

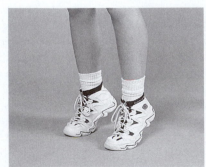

Figure 8.4b

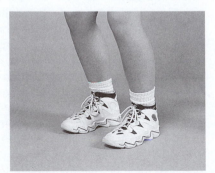

Figure 8.4c

to touch your heels down, your calf muscles remain contracted. Constant contraction for 20 to 30 minutes makes for very tight calf muscles. Rolling your feet all the way down will also help prevent shinsplints.

Moderation is the key. Since you are bringing about 3 times your body weight down on your foot each time you hop, it is a good idea to limit the number of consecutive repetitions on one foot to four hops. This moderation will help prevent overuse injuries such as **shinsplints** and **tendinitis.** Similarly, overdoing two-footed movements can be hard on the lower legs. Switch off two-footed steps with steps that involve alternate feet. Lateral leg movements, such as jumping jacks, press the knee and ankle in an outward direction. They are good exercises, but you should limit the number you perform in a row, and you should bend your knees as you land. If at any time you feel overuse occurring, modify the routine you are doing. Most instructors will be glad that you took the initiative to individualize your workout.

A forward running stride results in less impact stress than more vertical movements such as hopping or jumping. Therefore, whenever there is enough room, high-impact choreography should include use of the regular running (jogging) stride. Jogging with heel-toe mechanics also stretches and therefore provides relief to the calf muscles. Instructors will often have the class jog in place while working on arm movements. During this time, pay special attention to foot plant and leg position. Letting up on technique—kicking your heels out to the side or letting your knees turn out—is easy. Instead, concentrate on technique—lift your knees directly to the front and roll down through your foot with each step.

HIA is exciting and upbeat. Faster music (150 to 170 bpm) can be used with it than with step aerobics or low-impact aerobics. When fast-paced music is used, however, use smaller movements so that you stay with the beat comfortably, or you can perform movements to every other beat. Conversely, slow music can be double-timed.

LOW-IMPACT AEROBICS

Low-impact aerobics (LIA) is designed to provide an aerobic experience without the risk of impact injury that may result from the stress of high-impact movements. To accomplish this goal, one foot must touch the floor at all times. Keeping one foot on the ground effectively cuts the impact stress in half. In place of the jumping movements of HIA, LIA substitutes bending movements that lower and then raise the body's center of gravity. Because it lessens impact shock, LIA is a good activity for people who are prone to shinsplints, but both the bending and the lateral steps often associated with LIA may irritate a knee joint that is prone to injury.

LIA is low-impact but not necessarily low-intensity. Participants can increase their workout intensity by moving their body's center of gravity upward against gravity. When you jump, you move your center of gravity up the number of inches you jump. In LIA, you bend your knees, lowering your center of gravity, and then lift it upward by returning to your starting position or perhaps higher by rising up on the balls of your feet. The sinking and rising motions of LIA are one way in which work is created. Large, controlled arm movements also increase intensity. Extended limbs (long levers) are also more challenging to move than are bent limbs (short levers). For example, swinging the arms out to the side and then overhead is more difficult when the arms are extended than when they are bent at the elbow. Finally, large moving patterns are effective for raising the heart rate. Think of the energy expended in long, striding steps such as those used in power walking. Traveling moves can go side to side, forward and back, on the diagonal, or in a circle. The larger the space in which you work out, the more you can take advantage of traveling steps. Traveling steps help LIA achieve similar intensities and benefits as HIA. Stationary choreography with a lot of over-head arm movements appears to reach the same intensities, but the arm work elevates heart rate without a corresponding rise in oxygen consumption and metabolic costs. In other words, your circulatory system works harder, but you don't get corresponding aerobic benefits.

The following will help you prevent injuries.

1. Turn your feet and knees out during large (wide) steps to the side—this placement helps maintain hip, knee, and foot alignment.
2. Make sure knee flexion does not exceed 90 degrees.
3. Avoid too many steps that cross the foot in front while moving to the side (such as that which can occur in "grapevine" step), because this type of movement can promote foot pronation. This can be prevented in the grapevine by crossing the foot behind.

The music for LIA is moderately paced (120 to 140 bpm) to allow sufficient time to execute larger movements. Occasionally, instructors use slightly faster music for which they may increase the speed of dance

ON THE BEAT!

Understanding the way music is organized and used can help you know what to expect in a routine. For example, most movements are done an even number of times. If an instructor works with songs in their original form, there may be musical irregularities (such as bridges) that result in odd numbers of steps or some recovery marching while waiting for the chorus. If, however, the instructor is working with music produced for exercise classes, the music is much more predictable. There are advantages to working with both kinds of music.

UPBEATS AND DOWNBEATS

The strong beat of the music is the downbeat; the softer one that follows is the upbeat. Most aerobic dance exercise movements will start on the downbeat. For example, during a jumping jack, you move your arms and legs outward on the downbeat and back to center on the upbeat. Funk and hip-hop movements often emphasize the upbeat, which makes them a little trickier for people to learn. Putting the accent off the beat like this is a form of syncopation. But when you get the hang of it, it is a lot of fun.

TEMPO

Tempo is how quickly the beats are played, usually expressed in beats per minute. Different styles of aerobics use different tempos. Low-impact and step require slower tempos than high-impact aerobics.

TIMING

Regular or single timing means to make one movement per beat. To jog in single time means to land on the right foot for one beat and then the left foot on the next beat. When you perform a step in double-time, you must make two movements per beat. To double-time the jog, you must land on the right and then left foot within one beat. To half-time the same movement means to take twice as long. So with our jogging example, you would land on the right foot and hold there for a second count before jumping to the left foot. Half-timed movements are slower; double-timed movements are faster. In a routine you might do single-time marching, double-time marching or jogging, and then half-timed squats.

RHYTHM

Rhythm is the pattern of the music. Much of the music used today is created for exercise classes and uses a very strong and regular beat pattern. Different rhythmic step patterns can be put to the beat pattern.

Three typical rhythm patterns, each with an example of a corresponding step pattern, are shown on the opposite page. Note that all of them use 4 beats. When an "and" is used, the movement must occur quickly between the beats.

steps and decrease the size of steps or movements. LIA choreography should follow natural movement patterns and be performed with good muscle control.

One of the advantages of LIA is its emphasis on arm work. Most women lack good upper-body strength, as is evident by the small percentage of women who can perform just one pull-up. LIA and some good upper-body resistance exercises can improve upper-body strength. However, the arms should not remain raised above the shoulder for too long. This results in a sustained isometric contraction for the shoulder muscles, which, in turn, can result in pain, fatigue, and a sharp increase in blood pressure.

Another advantage of LIA is that more people can do it than HIA. LIA is ideal for people who are overweight, because it does not involve jumping, which in overweight people can place excessive strain on joints. It is also good exercise for older people who no longer enjoy jumping and for those who experience

incontinence with jumping. Large-breasted women and women in a prenatal or postnatal condition may also prefer this less bouncy exercise. People who tend to have chronic impact stress injuries as well as people returning to exercise after an injury may prefer LIA. In addition, HIA exercisers may enjoy LIA for a change of pace. It is also a less stressful class for individuals who demonstrate poor biomechanical technique or who have poor structural leg alignment. And it provides a comfortable way for beginners to start exercising, because LIA is easy to adapt to a low-intensity workout. Under a physician's care, people with high blood pressure, heart problems, orthopedic problems, or physical disabilities can enjoy an LIA class, although participants with a special medical condition should check with their physicians before beginning a class. LIA may also be a good way for people with diabetes and asthma to start exercising, because it can enable them to increase their workout intensity gradually.

ON THE BEAT! (continued)

1, 2, 3, 4 (STEP TOUCH)

Count 1:   Step sideways to the right onto the right foot.

Count 2:   Touch the left foot next to the right foot.

Count 3:   Step sideways to the left onto the left foot.

Count 4:   Touch the right foot next to the left.

1 AND 2, 3 AND 4 (PONY)

Count 1:   Step forward or sideways onto the right foot.

Count and: Move the left foot next to the right instep, and briefly place weight on the ball of the left foot.

Count 2:   Return the weight to the right foot.

Count 3:   Step forward or sideways onto the left foot.

Count and: Move the right foot next to the left instep, and briefly place weight on the ball of the right foot.

Count 4:   Return the weight to the left foot.

1, 2, 3 AND 4 (MAMBO, CHA-CHA)

Count 1:   Step forward onto the right foot.

Count 2:   Shift the weight back to the left.

Count 3:   Step right.

Count and: Step briefly on the left foot.

Count 4:   Step right.

PHRASING

Music is grouped into units called phrases. The most common phrase length for aerobic dance exercise is 32 beats. During these 32 beats, the instructor can build choreography in a variety of ways. One way is to introduce a step for 8 counts, such as a march/jog. Keep the step going for another 8 counts but add an arm movement such as biceps curls to it. Then change to another step, such as a grapevine, for 8 counts (4 to the right, 4 to the left), and finally add upright row arms to this movement during the last 8 counts. A new 32-count pattern may then be started or may simply be added on to this one. Movements are generally repeated 2, 4, or 8 times in a row. Instructors often count backwards to let you know how many steps you have left to go. They reserve the last couple of beats in an ongoing pattern to call out the next move. For example, "8 more, 7, 6, 5, 4, 3, grapevine right." The instructor may also count up and not voice 7 and 8 so that he or she can call the next move.

When these individuals know how exercise will affect them, they can work up to a high-intensity LIA or HIA class. Because LIA is so adaptable, it appeals to people of all ages, often bringing together one, two, or even three generations.

COMBINATION HIGH-/LOW-IMPACT AND MODERATE-IMPACT AEROBICS

Combination high-/low-impact aerobics (also known as **combo-impact, CIA,** and **hi/lo-impact aerobics**) is a form of aerobic dance exercise that uses both LIA and HIA in one class, with a tempo range of 130 to 170 bpm. This can be done three different ways. One whole song can be LIA and another HIA. Or a set of movements (a phrase) within a song can be LIA, and another sequence HIA. Or each sequence of steps can contain both LIA and HIA steps. These combinations add some terrific variety, eliminate some of the impact stress, and produce routines that are easily adjusted to people's fitness levels.

Moderate-impact aerobics (MIA) keeps one foot on the floor at all times like LIA, but it moves the center of gravity by emphasizing going up and down on the ball of the foot. The emphasis is not on getting lower to rise up like LIA, but rather on moving upward from a normal bend of the knees onto the ball of the foot. For example, march, and as your right knee goes upward, rise up on your left toe. Or rise up and down on the ball of your left foot as you move your right leg in and out of a side lunge position. MIA is less "bouncy" than HIA and can cut down the impact stress by about a third. MIA can constitute its own class, but more often MIA movements are incorporated into higher-intensity (or power) LIA classes and used to gradually increase or taper down intensity during HIA classes.

STEP AEROBICS

Step aerobics (also called bench), a form of aerobics that involves stepping up and down on a bench using a variety of step patterns, was invented and popularized by Gin Miller in the late 1980s. It became very popular when she teamed up with Reebok to create the Step Reebok program. Stepping up and down on a bench, however, dates much further back. Bench stepping has been used for rehabilitation purposes and for screening individuals for cardiovascular fitness for many years. In fact, it was when Miller was recovering from an injury and prescribed therapeutic bench stepping that she conceived the idea of using a variety of stepping patterns for general fitness. It caught on, not only with the regular aerobics crowd, but also with those who had been uncomfortable with some of the "danciness" of aerobic dance.

Step aerobics uses a bench or "step" that is between 4 and 12 inches high. Bench height is adjusted according to the participant's fitness level: lower for beginners and higher for more advanced students. Higher platform heights are associated with knee discomfort. A person's height, particularly leg length, should be considered in this decision. In general, most people should use a bench height that results in knee flexion of 60 degrees or less when the foot is placed on the bench. The 60-degree angle provides a good workout and limits knee soreness. A 30-degree knee angle provides the most comfort and the least impact stress, but the corresponding step height may be insufficient to produce the desired training intensity. For safety and injury prevention reasons, the knee angle should never be more than 90 degrees. Bench heights of 4, 6, and 8 inches work for most people.

One of the biggest advantages to step training is that people of different fitness levels can perform the same steps to the same tempo side by side—the bench height, the amplitude at which steps are performed, and arm movements determine the intensity. This is one of the most popular forms of aerobic dance exercise for men. Some instructors use very linear, almost military-looking movements, while others use more dancelike movements. Stepping patterns start out very simple and build in complexity. Some instructors even use two or more benches per person and take the steps up and down across both. Although this practice adds a lot of fun variations, it does not increase the aerobic effect, and it often requires more equipment and space.

Step aerobics can be performed on the floor (lowest intensity), on a low step, or on a higher step for higher intensity (Figure 8.5). Step aerobics use a range of tempos, from 118 to 122 bpm (beginners) to a maximum of 128 (advanced). Combination bench mixes patterns of steps on and off the bench with patterns that stay on the floor

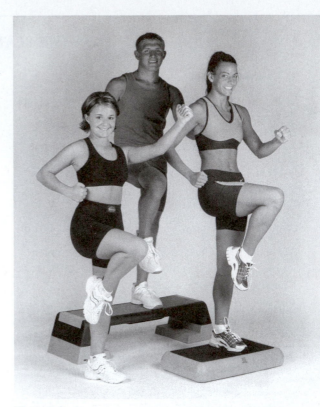

Figure 8.5

or stay on top of the bench. This combination lowers the number of step (up and down) repetitions, which will reduce knee discomfort and overuse for some people. For advanced students, higher intensities can be achieved by adding power moves. The use of weights and step is still somewhat controversial. The existing evidence indicates that it is preferable to restrict the use of weights to a separate muscle training segment of class during which slow, controlled movements with the proper technique can be ensured.

BASIC STEPS FOR STEP AEROBICS

The leg you step with first is referred to as the "lead leg." Usually, you begin a new step with the right leg. Because it's best not to lead off with the same leg for more than 1 minute of stepping, you can use a "tap change" to change from one lead leg to the other. The tap change is explained and diagrammed on page 93.

Tapless step is a newer version of step aerobics that doesn't use tap changes. The choreography is designed to use steps that naturally change the lead leg rather than inserting numerous tap changes. This allows the routine to flow more, but in some cases it also makes the routines more complex. After you have learned the basic steps presented in the next section, try performing the two routines in the Step Aerobic Routines box on page 98. One is a traditional-style step routine, and the second is tapless. Often instructors use a combination that uses some tap changes but also takes advantage of other transition steps.

In these diagrams, all steps are presented with an initial right-leg lead. The right foot has been shaded to help you distinguish between right and left legs. When necessary, an aerial view of the step has also been included. Most steps are performed in 4 counts, although positions between counts are also shown for clarification. The positions you should be in on the count are labeled. The names for the steps are fairly standard, but there may be some variation between instructors.

Classes begin with an off-the-bench warm-up and then slowly bring up the intensity. The progression pattern most often used is one of learning the step pattern, adding arms, and then adding a direction change. For example, you might begin with a basic pattern of stepping on and off the bench, add arm curls with each step, and then turn the stepping so that you

are stepping on the diagonal (corner to corner). Depending on the level of the class, the instructor may stop the arm motion until the new direction is established and then may restart the arm motion or begin a new arm motion. The stepping portion of class is followed by an aerobic cool-down, which finishes with off-the-bench steps and then some strength and flexibility work. The bench is a useful tool for strength and flexibility moves such as the triceps push-ups (Figure 10.23 on page 130) and hamstring stretch (Figure 7.21 on page 78).

A visual and written description of some of the basic movements for step aerobics follows. Another good source is the website www.turnstep.com, which offers an excellent dictionary of step aerobic steps with animated step patterns that make step aerobics easy to learn. Individuals can also post their routines, but be aware that they are not professionally screened for correctness.

Basic Step

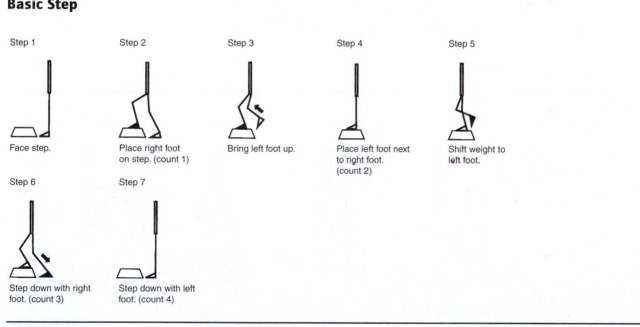

Step 1 — Face step.

Step 2 — Place right foot on step. (count 1)

Step 3 — Bring left foot up.

Step 4 — Place left foot next to right foot. (count 2)

Step 5 — Shift weight to left foot.

Step 6 — Step down with right foot. (count 3)

Step 7 — Step down with left foot. (count 4)

Tap Change

The basic step above was performed with a right-foot lead. To change to a left-foot lead, perform the tap change with this alternate Step 7. This tap allows you to lead with the left foot for the next basic step. Tap changes may be used to change the lead leg after one step or after a series of different steps.

Step 7 alternate

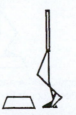

Tap left toe on floor without putting weight on it, then lead with left foot in next step.

V-Step

The V-step step is the same as the basic step, but the feet are positioned further apart on the bench and closer together on the floor. An aerial view helps demonstrate this.

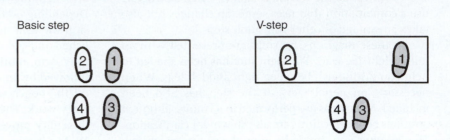

Basic step   V-step

Note: A Turnstep can be accomplished by turning one-quarter to the right as you step off the bench. This will put you sideways to the bench.

A-Step

The A-step step is similar but opposite to the V-step. The feet are close together on the bench and wide apart on the floor.

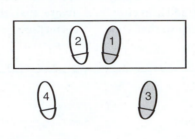

Knee-Up

The basic step can be performed with a knee-up as shown, or a leg curl, a forward leg kick, or a side leg lift.

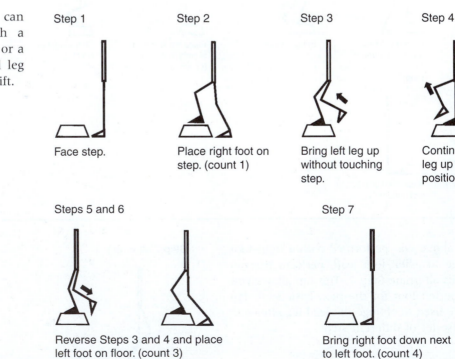

Step 1

Face step.

Step 2

Place right foot on step. (count 1)

Step 3

Bring left leg up without touching step.

Step 4

Continue to draw left leg up to keep knee-up position. (count 2)

Steps 5 and 6

Reverse Steps 3 and 4 and place left foot on floor. (count 3)

Step 7

Bring right foot down next to left foot. (count 4)

Note: To make this a Repeater step, only touch the ball of the foot down in Step 6, then draw the knee back up. Repeat twice more and then perform Steps 5 and 6 as normal. (8 counts)

Tap Up, Tap Down

This step is also known simply as "tap up."

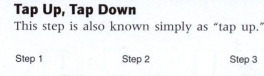

Step 1	Step 2	Step 3	Step 4	Step 5
Stand sideways to step.	Place right foot on step. (count 1)	Bring left foot up and tap it on step. (count 2)	Step down with left foot. (count 3)	Step down with right foot and tap it on floor. (count 4)

Over the Top

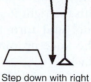

Step 1	Step 2	Step 3	Step 4	Step 5	▲ = Right foot △ = Left foot
Stand sideways to step.	Step up with right foot. (count 1)	Step up with left foot and shift weight onto it. (count 2)	Step down with right foot. (count 3)	Step down with left foot. (count 4)	

Across the Top

This step is similar to over the top, but it starts on the end of the bench and travels the length of it.

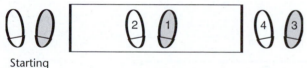

Starting position

Straddle Down

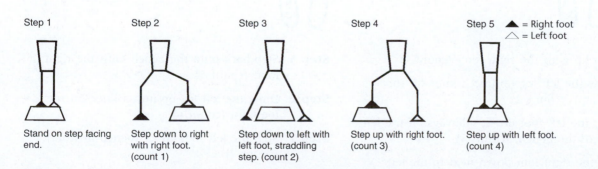

Step 1	Step 2	Step 3	Step 4	Step 5	▲ = Right foot △ = Left foot
Stand on step facing end.	Step down to right with right foot. (count 1)	Step down to left with left foot, straddling step. (count 2)	Step up with right foot. (count 3)	Step up with left foot. (count 4)	

Note: To make this a Lunge step, perform Steps 1 and 2 and then step the right foot back up onto the bench. Repeat to the right or perform alternating left and right lunges.

Corner-to-Corner

Perform Steps 1–7 with a right-foot lead. To continue the corner-to-corner pattern, use the opposite corner (right) and a left-foot lead as follows: Count 1, place the left foot diagonally on the corner of the step. Count 2, draw the right leg into a knee-up position. Count 3, step down with the right foot. Count 4, step down with the left foot and turn toward the left corner of the step. (The knee-up can be substituted with a leg curl or leg kick.)

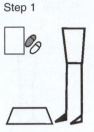

Step 1
Face left corner of step.

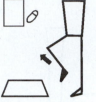

Step 2
Lift right (inside) leg.

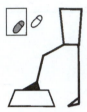

Step 3
Place right foot diagonally on corner of step. (count 1)

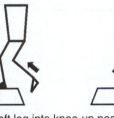

Steps 4 and 5
Draw left leg into knee-up position. (count 2)

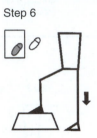

Step 6
Step down with left foot. (count 3)

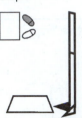

Step 7
Step down with right foot and turn toward right corner of step. (count 4)

L-Step

⌐ = Knee-lift
↓ = Toe touch

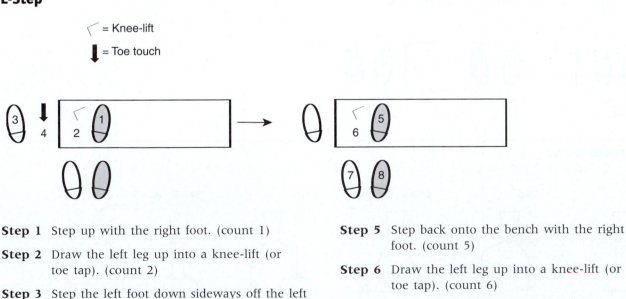

Step 1 Step up with the right foot. (count 1)

Step 2 Draw the left leg up into a knee-lift (or toe tap). (count 2)

Step 3 Step the left foot down sideways off the left end of the bench. (count 3)

Step 4 Tap the right foot down next to the left foot (or raise it in a knee-lift). (count 4)

Step 5 Step back onto the bench with the right foot. (count 5)

Step 6 Draw the left leg up into a knee-lift (or toe tap). (count 6)

Step 7 Step the left foot down (bench in front). (count 7)

Step 8 Step the right foot down. (count 8)

K-Step

Starting position is standing sideways behind the bench near the right end. (Bench is on your right.)

Step 1 Right foot steps forward and up onto the middle of the bench. (count 1)

Step 2 Left foot toe taps next to the right foot. (count 2)

Step 3 Left foot steps forward and down off the bench. (count 3)

Step 4 Right foot toe taps next to the left foot. (count 4)

Step 5 Right foot steps back onto the middle of the bench. (count 5)

Step 6 Left foot toe taps next to the right foot. (count 6)

Step 7 Left foot steps backward and down off the bench. (count 7)

Step 8 Right foot steps down beside it. (count 8)

Note: This pattern looks more like the letter K when it is done with a left-foot lead. The bench is the straight line of the K, and the arm and foot of the K are drawn by the step pattern.

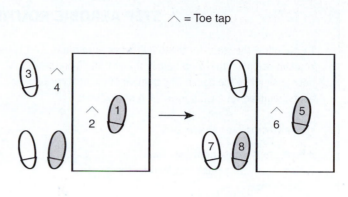

∧ = Toe tap

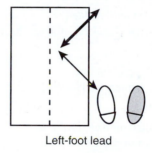

Left-foot lead

Hop Turn (Pivot Turn)

Starting position can be facing the bench or from a sideways position with the bench on the right. You can execute the rotation of the turn (1) while in the air during the hop or (2) by pivoting with the foot in contact with the bench.

Step 1 Step the right foot up on the bench. (count 1)

Step 2 Hop and turn (pivot) to the right until you are facing the opposite end of the bench.

Step 3 Land the hop on the right foot. (count 2)

Step 4 Step the left foot down off the bench (opposite side from the starting position). (count 3)

Step 5 Step the right foot down. (count 4)

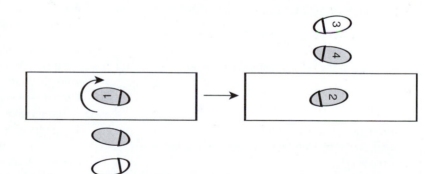

AROUND THE WORLD

This pattern can be accomplished by performing two hop turn steps using the same lead foot. This will result in a 360-degree turn in the same direction.

STEP AEROBIC ROUTINES: TWO STYLES

Try to follow the steps for these two types of routines. You can use an actual step bench or a rectangle on the floor to simulate the bench. The number of counts (musical beats) required for each pattern is in parentheses.

STEP ROUTINE: TAP TRANSITIONS

3 basic steps with a right-foot lead.
1 basic step with a right-foot lead finishing with a tap change. (16)

3 basic steps with a left-foot lead.
1 basic step with a left-foot lead finishing with a tap change. (16)

3 V-steps with a right-foot lead.
1 V-step with a right-foot lead finishing with a tap change. (16)

3 V-steps with a left-foot lead.
1 V-step with a left-foot lead finishing with a tap change. (16)

1 turnstep (V-step turn) with a right-foot lead. Finish with a tap change.
1 turnstep (V-step turn) with a left-foot lead. Finish with a tap change. (8)

Repeat above turnstep pattern 2 more times. (You will finish with the bench on your right.) (8)

4 over-the-top steps alternating right- and left-foot leads.
Use a tap change to change the foot-leads. (16)

4 K-steps with a right-foot lead. (36)
1 turnstep with a right-foot lead. Tap change. (4)

4 K-steps with a left-foot lead. (36)
1 turnstep with a left-foot lead but finish facing the bench. (4)

*A mambo-cha-cha-cha pattern may be substituted.

STEP ROUTINE: TAPLESS TRANSITIONS

4 basic steps with a right-foot lead. (16)
1 cha-cha step to transition to a left-foot lead. (2)
(Step right for count 1; step left and right more quickly for count 2.)

4 basic steps with a left-foot lead. (16)
1 cha-cha to transition to a right-foot lead.
(Step left for count 1; step right and left more quickly for count 2.) (2)

4 V-steps with a right-foot lead. (16)
2 jumping jacks. (4)
4 V-steps with a left-foot lead. (16)
2 jumping jacks. (4)

4 knee-lifts with alternating right- and left-foot leads. (16)

4 corner-to-corner knee-lifts starting with a right-foot lead to the left corner and transitioning to a left-foot lead to the right corner. Repeat right and left. Finish facing square to the bench. (16)

1 L-step with a right-foot lead finishing with a big step to the right.
1 L-step with a left-foot lead finishing with a big step to the left.
Repeat left and right. Finish with a step that centers you on the bench. (32)

1 hop turn with a right-foot lead and turning to the right. You will end on the far side of the bench, weight on the right foot.
4 marches in place, turning 180 degrees to the right, starting with the left foot (LRLR).*
1 hop turn with a left-foot lead and turning to the left. You will end on the original side of the bench, weight on the left foot.
4 marches in place, turning 180 degrees to the left,* starting with the right foot (RLRL). (16)

Step training is fun and easy to do. Here are some technique tips to get you started.

1. Place your whole foot on the bench. Be careful that the heel of your foot is not hanging over the near edge.

2. Lean from your ankles, not your waist. (This helps keep the pressure off your lower back.)

3. Step down near to the bench. (This helps prevent Achilles tendinitis.)

4. Roll down through your foot (toe, ball, heel) unless you are doing lunge steps or repeaters, in which case touch only the ball of your foot down. (This helps prevent tight, sore calf muscles, and plantar fasciitis.)

5. Look where you are stepping by keeping your head up and using your eyes to look down.

6. Wear shoes that have a heel notch to avoid irritation of the Achilles tendon.

7. Before stepping, warm up calf muscles well.

8. Adjust the step height to match your fitness level. Never use a step that bends your knee more than 90 degrees.

9. Adjust workout intensity by increasing or decreasing arm use and extension and the number of propulsion or power moves.

10. Decrease intensity by performing steps off the bench if you become fatigued.

11. Change lead legs after a maximum of 1 minute.

12. On repeater steps, perform a maximum of 5 repetitions. Here is an example of a repeater step: Step onto the bench with the left foot, draw the right knee up in a knee-lift, touch the ball of the right foot to the floor, draw the right knee back up in a knee-lift, touch the right ball of the foot to the floor, knee-lift again, step down right, step down left. The 3 knee-lifts constitute 3 repetitions.

13. If you are working at an advanced level and are using power/propulsion moves, perform the moves for approximately 1 minute (or less) and then alternate with a less stressful step.

14. When performing a kick or a lunge to the back, be careful about placing your arms high overhead, because this movement may lead to back arching.

15. Step quietly. Stamping or stomping on the step will increase impact stress—unless, of course, you are so mentally stressed that the release is well worth the added leg stress!

Caution: Step aerobics is *not* recommended for people with knee joint problems unless prescribed by a physician.

WATER AEROBICS

Water aerobics (aqua aerobics) is a great way to get all the benefits of an aerobic workout with motivating music, a comfortable environment, and little or no impact stress. And anyone, of any age and fitness level, can do it. The routines can be easily modified so that people of different abilities can exercise together. Unlike swimming, in water aerobics you do not have to get your hair wet—unless the weather is very hot, in which case wetting your hair will help keep you cool. Water aerobics has a distinct advantage for those who are body conscious or who worry about being seen making mistakes; the water provides a certain degree of anonymity. It is also an excellent form of aerobic exercise for individuals who are overweight, have joint problems, or are recovering from an injury.

Two types of water aerobics have developed. Shallow-water aerobics are performed in standing-depth water. Deep-water aerobics uses flotation devices to suspend individuals in a vertical position in water over their heads. Deep-water aerobics is generally for swimmers, whereas shallow-water aerobics can be enjoyed by swimmers and nonswimmers alike. Both types of water aerobics classes are similar to other forms of aerobics in their class format. Class begins with a warm-up (which is usually done in the water but may be performed on the deck), an aerobic workout, an aerobic cool-down, a muscle-toning section, and finally, flexibility work. Water provides buoyancy; the deeper the water you work out in, the more buoyancy you experience. This buoyancy decreases the impact stress you experience as you push off the bottom of the pool. This means that the aerobics workout can be extended (for those who want a longer workout) with less risk of injury. Impact stress is lessened about 50% when working out in water waist deep and as much as 90% when working at the shoulder/neck level. Most instructors prefer to have students exercise in chest/armpit-deep water because water deeper than this makes it difficult for participants to control their movements. Deep-water aerobics, in which a student does not use the bottom of the pool at all, is impact-free.

Water aerobics benefits from the fact that water is 12 times more resistive than air. For example, because it is 12 times harder to walk through water than air, you burn more calories walking through water. Water aerobics programs also take advantage of the fact that both directions of a movement meet with resistance. There is no rest phase as there is in land-based resistance exercises. For example, on land, a leg lift to the side works the abductor muscles (outer thigh), whereas the same exercise in water provides resistance not only to the abductors but also the opposing adductor muscles (inner thigh) as they draw the leg back to its starting position. Water aerobics, as a result, is an excellent medium for achieving a balanced muscle workout.

Monitoring exercise intensity with heart rate is not as straightforward for water-based activities such as swimming and water aerobics as it is for land-based activities such as running, biking, and aerobic dance exercise. People who perform both land and water exercises often find that their heart rate is lower during water exercise even when the aerobic benefits are the same. Several theories are being tested about why heart rates vary in relation to oxygen consumption during water-based activities. Remember, heart rate is only a good indicator of workout intensity when it correlates with oxygen consumption. In water, this relationship seems to be affected by a number of factors, including water depth and temperature. Anything that reduces the workload of the circulatory system will result in a reduced exercise heart rate. Body heat generated through exercise is more easily dissipated in water. The cooler the water, the greater the cooling effect and the lower the heart rate. The greater the percentage of the body submerged in cool water—the deeper the water—the more pronounced the effect. Water exercise performed in warmer water can produce heart rates similar to land-based exercise. Aerobic exercise in hot water is not recommended, because this prevents body cooling. Wearing a wet suit or a bathing cap in a warm environment can also interfere with body cooling and can drive the heart rate up. Heart rate changes due to temperature conditions are independent of the amount of oxygen being used during exercise.

Deep water offers more buoyancy. When gravity is affected this way, blood is more easily transported back to the heart. Water also acts to compress the blood vessels, which is believed to aid in venous return. This compression factor is also thought to help oxygen diffuse into the blood. The deeper the water, the greater the compression effect. Exercise in water lowers the demand on the heart, which results in lower exercise heart rates.

One important point should be stressed. Even though most people experience lower exercise heart rates in water versus land workouts, the benefits they receive from the exercise are usually the same. The question then is, "How much lower a heart-rate results in the same benefits?" Research has documented reductions in water-based heart rates ranging from 10 to 20 bpm. The Cooper Institute for Aerobic Research recommends lowering the target heart-rate zone by 17 bpm. Others would argue for less of a reduction, and some claim that healthy participants can safely attain and benefit from the same heart rates during water exercise as they attain during land-based exercise. Much, no doubt, depends on the environment in which you are exercising. If you decide to participate in water aerobics, work with your instructor to determine how best to monitor your intensity.

The principles of exercise presented earlier in this book apply to exercise in the water. And many of the exercises you are already familiar with can be used in the water. But, in addition to heart-rate monitoring, there are some significant differences between water- and land-based exercise, a few of which are described here.

1. If you are supplying the music, be sure your music box runs on batteries or that the electrical outlet you are using is above the deck and meets both state and local bathing codes. Burn fat, not the rest of you!

2. Music tempo is slower for water movements, usually between 124 and 136 bpm. When instructors use music with a tempo greater than 136 bpm, they use it at half time (that is, they use every other beat).

3. Optimum water temperature is between 83 and 86° F. Cool water is good for people with multiple sclerosis, whereas warmer water is good for people with arthritis. Hot water would be good only for a class performing stretching movements.

4. Dehydration may occur more easily. Most classes are held outdoors in warm weather or indoors in a heated area. Because you are in water, you may not realize how much you are sweating. Drink water from a plastic container (glass is not allowed in pool areas) throughout class. Much of the body's heat is lost through the head, so be careful about wearing a swimming cap that traps heat, since it may cause heat stress in warm weather. If you are in a pool that requires a cap (to help keep hair from clogging the pool filter) and you don't mind getting your hair wet, you can wear a Lycra cap and get it wet periodically.

5. Pool attire might seem obvious, but here are a few tips to consider. If you get cold easily, wear tights and a bathing suit or leotard in the pool. Wash out clothing immediately after changing—chlorine is very hard on fabrics. Lycra blends tend to hold up better in pools. Women may prefer one-piece suits with a good built-in bra for support when jumping. Wearing a pair of aqua shoes can help prevent abrasions caused by pushing off the pool bottom, provide cushioning, and supply traction in and out of the pool.

6. A variety of movements and movement speeds results in a good overall workout. When speed is added to a movement, the

water resistance increases, which means the workout is more intense. For example, it is much more difficult to run through water than walk through it. When speed is reduced, intensity decreases, but larger ranges of motion with more extended limbs can occur. For more discussion on methods of increasing and decreasing resistance in the water, see Chapter 10.

7. Special equipment is available for water aerobics. Webbed gloves and plastic or foam barbells can be used to increase resistance. For deep-water work, you can use flotation belts, jogging vests, kickboards, and other devices to support your body while you perform running-type exercises. Some devices are contoured better than others to fit comfortably under your arms.

Water aerobics is popular, and it has expanded into a variety of forms. Some classes resemble land aerobic dance exercise, some use a weighted step for aqua step aerobics, others have participants run in deep water, and some use circuit- and interval-training principles. As a side note, racehorses have been doing deep-water running in harnesses for years. Trainers know that they can train the horses longer and harder without risking stress fractures. So you see, you, your family, and your horse can all perform water aerobics together!

CIRCUIT AND INTERVAL TRAINING FOR AEROBICS

Circuit training is the use of a series of exercise stations through which an individual progresses in a specified order. The participant progresses from one station to the next, with or without a rest, depending on the type of training desired. The circuit can consist of stations of any type: aerobic, anaerobic, flexibility, muscular strength, or endurance. If the purpose of the circuit is to train the aerobic system, then an all-aerobic circuit is desirable. This way, continuous, large-muscle, rhythmic activity occurs throughout. Such a circuit might have in it an exercise cycle, a rowing machine, a stair machine, a jump rope, a mini-trampoline, a dance mat, and a treadmill. Or it might be composed completely of aerobic dance exercise step patterns. For example, one station might be knee-lifts, the next might be four jumping jacks and four kicks, and the next might be a series of steps onto a bench.

A mixed circuit might consist of resistance training (muscle-toning) stations such as lunges and squats interspersed between aerobic stations. Although this can be effective training, be careful that the resistance exercises do not require you to drop your head below your waist after vigorous aerobic work, because lowering your head may cause light-headedness. You should also be careful that fatigue from previous stations does not result in poor technique, especially if you are using weights or other resistance equipment. Muscle strength and endurance can also be increased using a circuit composed of resistance training stations. At one time, it was believed that moving through a series of stations composed of weight-training equipment with only 30-second intervals between stations would result in aerobic fitness gains. Research has shown that while the heart rate may be in the training zone, oxygen consumption does not increase proportionately. Although all individuals receive muscular strength benefits, only low-fit individuals will increase their aerobic fitness using this type of circuit.

Interval training consists of a series of short bouts of high-intensity activity alternated with rest intervals or lower-intensity activity. Interval training that alternates activity intensities between the high and low ends of the heart-rate target zone will develop aerobic fitness and may be referred to as interval aerobics. Intervals that use intensities that exceed the target heart-rate zone will emphasize anaerobic work. This type of training will improve the cardiorespiratory system but does not target the aerobic system. Anaerobic training is uncomfortable for most people, increases the risk of injury, and results in a greater exercise drop-out rate. For this reason, anaerobic interval training is recommended for advanced students who like this kind of demanding workout.

AEROBICS VIDEOS

Some excellent videos are on the market, but some that promote ineffectual or even harmful exercises are also available. Ask your instructor for guidance in selecting one. Also, please be aware that an instructor on a screen can't see and correct your body position and technique, whereas live instructors can provide you with this valuable feedback. A combination of live and taped instructors may be the best solution.

COMMONLY ASKED QUESTIONS

Am I working hard enough if I don't sweat much?

Sweat is not a good measure of exercise intensity. Different people sweat different amounts and in different places. Some sweat profusely before they even cross the training threshold. Others hardly sweat at all. Heart rate and ratings of perceived exertion are better indicators of intensity.

Men usually sweat more than women because they have more sweat glands and more muscle. When muscle is working, heat is generated—the more muscle, the more heat. Sweat is a good thing. The evaporation of sweat cools the body.

Is it good to "go for the burn"?

The burn is the feeling you get when your muscles are working so hard that oxygen cannot be supplied to them fast enough to produce energy. This ischemia (lack of oxygen) and the accumulation of lactic acid make your muscles feel heavy and sometimes cause a burning sensation. If you are trying to work aerobically, the burn is counterproductive because it is a product of heavy anaerobic exercise. Muscle-toning exercises are anaerobic, and it is during these exercises that you are most likely to feel the burn. If you feel the burn during the aerobic portion of the class, you should reduce the intensity or change the exercise until you no longer feel it. For example, if your arms are burning in an overhead position, bring them down and do an easier motion at or below waist level. When you have recovered, you can return to the original exercise or intensity or continue with the modification.

Sometimes I get bored with aerobic dance exercise. Is that normal?

Yes; everyone can experience burnout. You can take a break from aerobic dancing by getting involved with another kind of aerobic exercise. The important thing is to continue exercising!

What is cross-training, and should I do it?

To cross-train is to use two or more types of exercises to train. For example, you can train aerobically using both swimming and aerobic dance exercise. Because each activity uses your muscles differently, you will get a more complete workout. But you do not need to cross-train to achieve health-related fitness—each activity by itself provides a good aerobic workout. Cross-training can help combat boredom and prevent overuse injury, two reasons that people drop out of programs. Cross-train if it appeals to you and if you want to increase your skill and ability in more than one activity.

To avoid confusion—or add it!—be aware that cross-training can also refer to using different types of activities to make up a complete workout, such as combining stretching, dumbbell exercises, and step aerobics.

I don't feel like I'm getting a workout when I exercise in my training heart-rate range (THR). Why?

There may be several reasons for this. You may have calculated your THR incorrectly. Check your figures. Or you may not be counting your pulse accurately. Have someone else take your pulse, and compare it to your count. If you have calculated and counted correctly, it might be that the formulas are not working for you. Remember, they are based on the average person. If you have the opportunity, run a treadmill or cycle test to find out your true range. You can also try working with the rating of perceived exertion scale (Chapter 4). It is also possible that you are used to competitive levels of training and need time to adjust to the feel of exercise just for the health of it. Discuss your situation with a health/fitness professional.

SUMMARY

Aerobic dancing has expanded into a family of rhythmic aerobic activities. Some of the newer variations have made it possible for a greater variety of people to get involved. Other variations have resulted in more coeducational classes, and still others have enabled friends of varying fitness levels to exercise together.

KNOWLEDGE TIPS

1. There are many excellent forms of aerobic exercise. Select one or more activities (styles or variations) that appeal to you.

2. Precede aerobic activity with a good warm-up, and follow it with a good cool-down.

3. Perform all aerobic movements with good alignment and control.

4. Aim to sustain a target heart rate throughout the aerobic portion of class.

5. The risk of injury in all forms of aerobic dance exercise is low; however, some forms have lower impact stress than others.

6. Handheld and wrist weights are better reserved for muscle-toning. Ankle weights are not recommended for use during the aerobic portion of class.

7. High-impact aerobics consists of large-muscle movements like jogging, jumping, hopping, skipping, knee lifts, dance steps, and calisthenics.

8. Low-impact aerobics is similar to high-impact except that jumping-type moves are not used, as one foot must always

be in contact with the floor. There is also usually a greater emphasis placed on arm work and movements that involve lowering and then raising the center of gravity.

9. Step aerobics involves stepping up and down on a bench with a variety of step patterns.

10. Water aerobics can be performed in either standing-depth or deep water. Both are effective aerobic exercises.

11. Exercise heart rates tend to be 10 to 20 beats lower during water workouts than during land-based exercise.

12. Circuit aerobics training involves a series of stations through which the participant moves either with no break or short breaks while sustaining a target heart rate.

13. Interval training consists of high-intensity bouts of work alternated with short rest periods or low-intensity activities.

14. Aerobic intensity can be increased or decreased by increasing/decreasing arm movements; by raising the step height in step aerobics; or by increasing speed, amplitude, or lever length in water or high-impact aerobics.

THINK ABOUT IT

1. Why are there so many different styles of "aerobic dance"?

2. Describe the differences between low- and high-impact aerobics.

3. What are some key technique points to remember while performing aerobic moves?

4. What are some key technique points to remember while performing step aerobics?

5. How can you make aerobic movements easier (less intense) and harder (more intense)?

6. What are some advantages to water (aqua) aerobics?

7. What type of group exercise appeals to you? Why?

REFERENCES

American Council on Exercise. *Aerobics Instructor Manual: ACE's Guide for Fitness Professionals.* San Diego, CA: American Council on Exercise, 2000.

Berry, M. J., C. C. Cline, C. B. Berry, and M. Davis. "A Comparison Between Two Forms of Aerobic Dance and Treadmill Running." *Medicine and Science in Sports and Exercise* 24 (No. 8, 1992): 946–51.

Blessing, D. L. "The Energy Cost of Bench Stepping With and Without One and Two Pound Hand-Held Weights." *Medicine and Science in Sports and Exercise* 23 (No. 4, 1991): S28 (abstract).

Bonelli, S. *Step Training.* San Diego: American Council on Exercise, 2000.

Bricker, K. *Traditional Aerobics.* San Diego, CA: American Council on Exercise, 2000.

Brooks, G. A., T. D. Fahey, and K. Baldwin. *Exercise Physiology: Human Bioenergetics and Its Applications.* 4th ed. New York: McGraw-Hill, 2004.

Brown, D. *Dawn Brown's Complete Guide to Step Aerobics.* Boston: Jones and Bartlett, 1992.

Calarco, R. M., J. Wygand, J. Kramer, M. Yoke, and F. D'Zamko. "The Metabolic Cost of Six Common Movement Patterns of Bench Step Aerobic Dance." *Medicine and Science in Sports and Exercise* 23 (No. 4, 1991): S140 (abstract).

Carroll, M. W., R. M. Otto, and J. Wygand. "The Metabolic Cost of Two Ranges of Arm Position Height With and Without Hand Weights During Low Impact Aerobic Dance." *Research Quarterly for Exercise and Sport* 62 (No. 4, 1991): 420–3.

Copeland, C., L. Francis, P. Francis, and G. Miller. *Power Step Reebok.* Boston: Reebok International, 1992.

Darby, L. A., K. D. Browder, and B. D. Reeves. "The Effects of Cadence, Impacts, and Step on Physiological Responses to Aerobic Dance Exercise." *Research Quarterly for Exercise and Sport* 66 (No. 3, 1995): 231–8.

Elder, D. "Cardio Combat." *Women's Sports and Fitness* 14 (January–February 1992): 55–6.

Francis, L., P. Francis, and G. Miller. *Introduction to StepReebok.* Boston: Reebok International, 1991.

Francis, L., P. Francis, and G. Miller. "Teaching Step Training." *Journal of Physical Education, Recreation, and Dance* 64 (March 1993): 26–30.

Francis, L. L. "Improving Aerobic Dance Programs: The Key Role of Colleges and Universities." *Journal of Physical Education, Recreation, and Dance* 62 (September 1991): 59–62.

Garber, C. E., J. S. McKinney, and R. A. Carleton. "Is Aerobic Dance an Effective Alternative to Walk-Jog Exercise Training?" *Journal of Sports Medicine and Physical Fitness* 32 (No. 2, 1992): 136–41.

Garrick, J. G., and R. K. Requa. "Aerobic Dance: A Review." *Sports Medicine* 6 (1988): 169–79.

Giddens, S. "Yogarobics." *Women's Sports and Fitness* 14 (January–February 1992): 54.

Gordon, J. "Jam Up for Jelly Bellies: Street Dancing Pumps New Life into Aerobics." *Newsweek* 117 (April 29, 1991): 57.

Grant, G. *Technical Manual and Dictionary of Classical Ballet.* New York: Dover, 1967.

Harste, A. "Bench Aerobics: A Step in the Right Direction?" *The Physician and Sportsmedicine* 18 (No. 6, 1990): 25–6.

Hooper, P. L., and B. J. Noland. "Aerobic Dance Program Improves Cardiovascular Fitness in Men." *The Physician and Sportsmedicine* 12 (No. 5, 1984): 132–5.

Hopkins, D. R., B. Murrah, W. W. K. Hoeger, and R. C. Rhodes. "Effect of Low-Impact Aerobic Dance on the Functional Fitness of Elderly Women." *The Gerontologist* 30 (April 1990): 189–92.

Hovell, M. F., M. M. Mulvihill, M. J. Buono, S. Liles, D. H. Schade, T. A. Washington, R. Manzano, and J. F. Sallis. "Culturally Tailored Aerobic Exercise Intervention for Low-Income Latinas." *American Journal of Health Promotion* 22 (No. 3, 2008): 155(9).

Hufhand, D., L. Crowe, M. Whaley, and P. Banning-Schaffner. "Metabolic Responses to Low-Impact Aerobic Dance." *Medicine and Science in Sports and Exercise* 20 (1988, Suppl): S88 (abstract).

Kennedy-Armbruster, C. K., and M. M. Yoke. *Methods of Group Exercise Instruction.* 2nd ed. Champaign, IL: Human Kinetics, 2009.

Koszuta, L. E. "Low–Impact Aerobics: Better Than Traditional Aerobic Dance?" *The Physician and Sportsmedicine* 14 (No. 6, 1986): 156–61.

Kravitz, L. "Getting in Step." *Women's Sports and Fitness* 12 (April 1993): 18.

Kravitz, L., V. H. Heyward, L. M. Stolarczyk, and V. Wilmerding. "Does Step Exercise With Handweights Enhance Training Effects?" *Journal of Strength & Conditioning Research* 11 (No. 3, 1997): 194–99.

Malanka, P. "Aerobics Rebound! From Sports Drills to Step Training, New Techniques Are Transforming the Way America Works Out." *Health* 22 (March 1990): 59–65.

Martin, K. "Soft Aerobics: Gain Without Pain?" *Ms* 14 (May 1986): 52, 54, 113.

Michaud, T. J., J. Rodrigues-Zayas, C. Armstrong, and M. Hartnig. "Ground Reaction Forces in High Impact and Low Impact Aerobic Dance." *Journal of Sports Medicine and Physical Fitness* 33 (No. 4, 1993): 359–66.

Neporent, L. "Aerobics: Watch Your Step." *Women's Sports and Fitness* 14 (September 1992): 71–2.

Nethery, V. M., and P. A. Harmer. "The Energy Cost of Slideboard Training and Cycle Ergometry." Unpublished ms. Department of Physical Education, Health Education, and Leisure Services, Central Washington University, Ellensburg, WA; and Exercise Science, Willamette University, Salem, OR, 1994.

Olson, M. S., H. N. Wiliford, D. L. Blessing, and R. Greathouse. "Cardiorespiratory Responses to 'Aerobic' Bench Stepping Exercise in Females." *Medicine and Science in Sports and Exercise* 23 (No. 4, 1991): S27 (abstract).

Otto, R. M., C. A. Parker, T. K. Smith, J. W. Wygand, and H. R. Perez. "The Energy Cost of Low Impact and High Impact Aerobic Dance Exercise." *Medicine and Science in Sports and Exercise* 18 (No. 2, 1986): 523 (abstract).

Pahmeier, I., and C. Niederbaumer. *Step Aerobics for Schools, Clubs, and Studios.* Meyer & Meyer Sport (UK) Ltd., 2001.

Paul, L. "Funky Fitness: Victoria Johnson's Technifunk Aerobics Mixes Exercise and Expressive Dance." *Women's Sports and Fitness* 14 (No. 1, 1992): 68–9.

Reebok International, Ltd. *Slide Reebok™ Professional Training Manual.* Los Angeles: Reebok University Press, 1993.

Reeder, S. "The New Aerobics: Now You Can Bop to the Beat Without Jarring Your Joints." *Women's Sports and Fitness* 7 (December 1985): 27–9.

Reeves, B. D., L. A. Darby, C. L. Moss, and C. Armstrong. "Energy Costs and Vertical Forces of High-Impact and Low-Impact Aerobic Dance Sequences." *Research Quarterly for Exercise and Sport* 63 (1992, Suppl.): A28 (abstract).

Seabourne, T. *Complete Guide to Cardio Kickboxing.* Boston: YMAA Publication Center, 1999.

Sekulic, D., N. Rausavljevic, and M. Zvan. "Characteristics and Differences in the Heart Rate and Blood Lactate Concentration Values Measured During Hi-lo and Step Aerobic Classes." *Kinesiology* 33 (No. 1, 2001): 27–36.

Smith, T. "Swing into Salsa." *Women's Sports and Fitness* 13 (March 1991): 60.

Stanforth, D., C. Hamman, and C. Senechal. "Relationship of Heart Rate and Oxygen Consumption During Low Impact Aerobic Movements." *Medicine and Science in Sports* 20 (No. 2, 1988): S88 (abstract).

Stanforth, D., K. Velasquez, and P. R. Stanforth. "The Effect of Bench Height and Rate of Stepping on the Metabolic Cost of Bench Stepping." *Medicine and Science in Sports and Exercise* 23 (No. 4, 1991): S143 (abstract).

Wilson, B. R., D. C. Nirwtsu, J. M. Lindle, and C. Winters. "Doing the Two-Step." *American Health* 12 (May 1993): 92.

Yoxall, P. "All the Right Moves." *Current Health 2* 20 (November 1993): 16–7.

9

Muscular Fitness: Building Strength and Endurance

"Look well into thyself; there is a source of strength which will always spring up if thou wilt always look there."

MARCUS AURELIUS ANTONINUS

- Why do I need muscular strength and endurance?
- What kinds of exercises build muscular fitness?
- What is the difference between training for muscular endurance and for muscular strength?
- How and when should I add resistance to my exercises?
- What are the advantages of training with equipment?
- Are there special techniques and safety tips I should know about?

MUSCULAR fitness: What does that mean? It actually means a whole range of things, and it is time to move past the singular image of a super-muscled individual. Although large, developed muscles might be the goal of a few people, the possibilities of toning, shaping, and firming muscles has a broader appeal that brings with it both health and appearance benefits. In this chapter, you will be introduced to exercise concepts underlying muscular fitness, and then you will learn more about ways to achieve it including the use of body weight, free weights, exercise bands, stability balls, and water.

Before diving into the specifics of muscular fitness development, let's take a brief look at the history behind it and define some terms that have been used to describe it. Prior to the aerobics movement, the main way to get "fit" was to perform calisthenics. The roots of this type of activity are found in the German and Swedish systems of gymnastics that emigrated to the United States with natives of those countries during the 19th century.

In the 1950s, body builder and fitness guru Jack LaLanne used television to popularize callisthenic-based workouts that included exercises like squats and push-ups to which he often added homemade weights like soup cans. Typically women performed "body-toning" exercises with the hope of eliminating the "jiggly stuff" on the backs of their arms and thighs, while men focused more on developing a muscular appearance, particularly with respect to their abdomens and chests. Although these appearance-oriented goals remain as strong motivators for people starting an exercise regimen, people who sustain muscle fitness activity quickly discover the benefits of additional strength and endurance as well as improvements in appearance. It is also important to note that muscular fitness will alter body composition primarily by increasing muscle; aerobic exercise is still the best way to take off fat. Getting rid of the "jiggly stuff" or unwanted "belly" requires fat loss but at the same time you can build up your muscles so that as the fat comes off nicely toned muscles are revealed.

The phrase "body toning" has historically been used to describe a series of muscle exercises performed predominantly by women. This term is still used occasionally today, but more current terms have taken its place. There has been a shift especially among women from the idea of "body toning" to the idea of muscular fitness (strength and endurance). Men who were not focused solely on muscle size have appreciated the increased opportunities provided by exercise programs intended to develop overall muscle fitness as well.

Body toning is more accurately expressed as "muscle toning," because it is the skeletal muscles that are firmed and shaped. When sufficient resistance is used, muscles not only become toned, they also increase in size, strength, and endurance. It is therefore more accurate to refer to them generally as "resistance exercises" or more specifically as "muscular strength" or "muscular endurance" exercises. These then, are the terms that will be used in this text. Another label you may hear is "floor exercises." This is what some aerobics classes call the resistance exercises that are performed sitting or lying down on the floor. There are also trade names such as Vertifirm™ that refer to resistance exercises performed standing up.

Most hour-long aerobic dance exercise classes incorporate 10 to 20 minutes of muscle-developing exercises. If you want to devote more attention to muscle development, you can perform additional resistance exercises on your own or take a specialized course. You may find resistance training courses offered under titles such as weight training, body sculpting, body building, body shaping, and power lifting. How the muscles are worked, and whether the emphasis is on body contouring, hypertrophy (increasing muscle size), muscular strength, or muscular endurance, will differ among these programs.

Muscular strength and endurance have always been important in the sports world, but for a time they were overshadowed in the public eye by the health-conscious aerobic movement. The idea that you are more likely to die prematurely from a poorly conditioned cardiorespiratory system than from weak skeletal muscles has been supported by research on lifestyle diseases. However, experts do agree that muscular strength and endurance play a vital role in physical health and wellness, and professionals have become more outspoken about incorporating exercises that develop muscle strength, recommending that individuals perform a series of resistance exercises at least twice a week (see the Benefits of Resistance Training box). Some activities such as running will develop the cardiorespiratory system and tone the legs but do little for upper-body strength and endurance, so it is important to supplement these activities with a balanced set of resistance exercises. Aerobic dance exercise is a wonderful package of both aerobic and total-body muscle conditioning. Classes almost always include resistance exercises, and today it is common to see exercise bands, weights, bars, weighted balls, and stability balls being used to develop greater strength and endurance.

BENEFITS OF MUSCULAR STRENGTH AND ENDURANCE

Good strength and endurance are important for getting through the day without muscle fatigue. This also means having enough "muscle" to enjoy recreational activities and deal with any emergencies that might arise. If you find yourself sitting down because your legs and back are tired, or stopping something because your arms feel heavy, you are suffering from weak muscles. The more physically demanding your daily and recreational activities, the more strength and endurance you will need. Being in good muscular shape also helps prevent injuries and is especially helpful in preventing back pain. Another important reason to perform resistance exercises is to prevent osteoporosis, a disease characterized by a weakening of the bones. When bones are stressed, they get denser and stronger. Both the aerobic and muscle-toning sections of an aerobics class will strengthen and/or maintain bones. Finally, if you enjoy sports activities, muscular strength and endurance play

---

BENEFITS OF RESISTANCE TRAINING

RESISTANCE TRAINING:

- increases your muscular strength and endurance

- enables you to do more work with less fatigue

- improves posture and trunk stability

- reduces your risk of injury, especially to the lower back

- helps increase or maintain bone density

- can create a more aesthetic body build (shape)

- provides the muscular energy for recreational activities in addition to normal life demands

- improves your ability to perform physical skills such as skills needed for specific sports

an important role in skill performance. For example, you can hit a softball farther with good strength, and you can keep up good footwork longer on the tennis court with good muscular endurance.

RESISTANCE EXERCISES: BEFORE, AFTER, OR DURING AEROBICS?

Resistance exercises may be performed at the beginning of class following a good warm-up, or they can be done closer to the end of class following the aerobics and aerobic cool-down. Doing them early in the class may do the following:

- help lower the body's store of glycogen, thus encouraging more fat burning during the aerobic part of class
- promote better resistance-exercise technique since the muscles are less fatigued
- lessen the chance of a person experiencing postural hypotension, the disorientation or dizziness that occurs when you go from one position to another, like sitting to standing. (Those who prefer to do resistance exercises after the aerobic section avoid postural hypotension by doing a thorough cool-down and starting with resistance exercises that don't drop the head.)

Performing resistance exercises after the aerobic cool-down may do the following:

- result in slightly more cardiorespiratory conditioning and calorie burning, because the heart rate remains higher for a longer period of time. This is most true if big-muscle endurance exercises are done first, such as a series of lunges.
- promote good technique during the aerobic portion of class, because the muscles are not fatigued from the resistance exercises

At this time, there is no conclusive evidence that it is better to perform resistance exercises before or after aerobic conditioning. In fact, many instructors do both by incorporating standing muscle-toning exercises after the warm-up and performing additional exercises that require a sitting or lying position toward the end of class. There have been some attempts to add resistance such as small weights to step or low-impact aerobic routines, but research indicates minimal advantage in doing this and a greater risk of injury. Resistance training can be performed with the best technique, concentration, and safety during its own segment of class. If you have a personal preference and schedule flexibility, select an instructor who does it in the order you like.

Individuals who are less fit can also increase their muscular endurance (and strength to a lesser degree) during the aerobic phase of class. Arm movements and stepping patterns for 20 to 30 minutes develop muscle endurance. Even if you are highly fit in one way (for example, if you are a runner), you may find that you are less fit in another way (for example, in upper body strength) and will benefit from the full-body workout of the aerobic section.

ACHIEVING RESISTANCE

You can achieve resistance in a number of ways. Calisthenic exercises use the pull of gravity and the weight of body parts to achieve resistance. For example, doing a push-up means extending your arms and lifting up your torso against gravity. To achieve more resistance, you can add weights, the pull of an exercise band, the instability of an exercise ball, or the drag of water. Exercises incorporating the use of weights, bands, and balls are discussed in Chapter 10. Sometimes you can also achieve more resistance by using a different body position both with and without a stability ball.

Here are some examples. The easiest push-up to do is one performed against a wall. Place your hands shoulder-height on the wall, and put your feet about 2 feet away from the base of the wall. Bend your arms. You can progressively increase resistance by doing a push-up (1) on your hands and knees, (2) on your hands and toes, (3) on your hands and toes with your toes up on a bleacher, step, or ball. You can make side leg lifts more difficult by beginning with a bent leg lift and progressing to a straight leg lift. Curl-ups are easiest when your arms are down at the sides of your body, harder when your arms are crossed over your chest, still harder with your hands up by your head, and most difficult when your arms are extended over your head. Curl-ups can also be made more difficult by putting your feet up on a step or ball or by performing them on a stability ball.

When an exercise is being performed in class, select the position and intensity that suits your personal needs. There are limits, however, to the amount of resistance you can achieve through body position. For more resistance and greater strength and endurance gains, you will have to use outside sources such as weights, weighted balls, exercise bands, or even a partner resisting your movements through a range of motion.

THE MUSCULAR STRENGTH–ENDURANCE CONTINUUM

To understand the relationship between strength and endurance, picture a continuum with strength at one end and endurance at the other. Exercises performed with heavy resistance (weight) exhaust muscles in just a few repetitions and build strength. Exercises with light to moderate resistance performed with many repetitions build muscular endurance.

STRENGTH	⟷	ENDURANCE
Heavy Resistance		Light-Moderate Resistance
Few Repetitions		Many Repitions

Because there is no definitive point along the continuum where strength ends and endurance begins, the target zones for these two fitness components overlap. For health-related purposes, resistance training intensities that fall in the middle, where the two target zones overlap, are used to develop muscular strength and endurance, collectively referred to as muscular fitness.

THE FITT PRINCIPLE

As mentioned in Chapter 3, the FITT principle, incorporating Frequency, Intensity, Time, and Type of exercise (the variables used in locating and exercising within your target zones), can be used to create an optimal muscular fitness program to achieve your desired outcome.

FREQUENCY

If you want to build muscular strength and endurance, you should incorporate resistance training (muscle toning, weight training) into your fitness program at least twice a week, and if possible, three times a week, on alternate days. You should not work the same muscle tissue twice in less than 48 hours because the tissue needs time to rest and rebuild. If you work out too frequently, your muscles will weaken over time. Serious weight trainers may work out more days of the week, but they use one set of muscles one day and a different set the next. This type of training is called working split sets. A person might do chest, back, and abdominals one day and arms and legs the next; a four-day-a-week schedule might consist of trunk on Monday and Thursday and limbs on Tuesday and Saturday.

INTENSITY

Intensity is determined by the amount of resistance involved in the exercise. The more resistance, the greater the force you will have to exert. As depicted on the continuum, muscle endurance activities work with lower levels of resistance than do strength exercises. Intensity is measured as a percentage of the maximum weight (resistance) you can lift, push, or pull one time. This weight is called one **repetition maximum (1 RM).** In general, strength gains occur when you work between 50 and 100% of 1 RM. Endurance increases when you work between about 20 and 70% of 1 RM.

These guidelines are easiest to put into use when working with measured weights and weight-lifting equipment. A good rule of thumb is to use an amount of weight or resistance that makes doing 8 to 12 repetitions difficult by the end of the set; this number of repetitions places you in the middle of the strength–endurance continuum. For example, if you can do 8 push-ups on your knees easily, but numbers 9, 10, 11, and 12 become progressively more difficult, then you are within the target zone for intensity. When you can perform 12 push-ups with relative ease, it's time to increase intensity. Intensity can be increased by adding resistance through body position or the use of resistance equipment.

TIME

Time or duration is the entire amount of time an exercise session lasts. In a typical 1-hour aerobic dance exercise class, the "time" or duration of the resistance exercise segment is about 20 minutes. Classes that are more than an hour long or that emphasize muscle development will have longer resistance training durations. The amount of time available is then divided into the number of exercises, and the number of repetitions, and the sets of each exercise you want to perform. Consecutive repetitions of an exercise make up a set. If you perform 10 squats in a row, for example, you have done 1 set of 10 repetitions ("reps"). If you do another 10 repetitions, you have completed a second set.

There is considerable debate among experts about the optimum number of repetitions and sets needed to build strength and endurance. But, in general, 1 to 5 sets of 3 to 8 repetitions builds strength, and 1 to 5 sets of 8 to 25 repetitions builds endurance. The American College of Sports Medicine (ACSM) recommends completing a minimum of 1 set of 8 to 12 repetitions (to near fatigue) of between 8 and 10 exercises that use the major muscle groups two or three times a week on nonconsecutive days. Research shows that two sets of each exercise is more effective in building strength. If you have the time, you can progressively overload by adding resistance to a single set or add a second (possibly third) set to your workout. You may also want to add more exercises to your routine. If you are older or deconditioned, the ACSM recommends working with 10 to 15 repetitions.

If you want to emphasize muscle endurance, you can increase the number of repetitions in a set. But how many repetitions are enough? For example, it is impressive to be able to do 100 push-ups in a row, but does that make you healthier than when you could do 25? To answer this question, you must consider the amount of endurance you need for the things you like to do (recreational activities, job requirements, competitions, etc.), the psychological benefits of being able to perform a certain number, the wear and tear on your body, and the amount of time you have to train. Usually, it is more effective to increase resistance and do fewer repetitions than to do a really large number of repetitions. Staying closer to the strength end of the continuum also has a hidden benefit for endurance. Increases in strength actually increase muscle endurance. An example will best illustrate this. Imagine two people, one who can lift 50 pounds (lbs), and another who can lift 25 lbs. When they each lift 5 lbs repeatedly, the first person is lifting only 10% of his or her maximum, whereas the other person is lifting 20%. It is easier to keep lifting a smaller percentage of your maximum.

The resistance exercises most often associated with aerobic dance exercise emphasize a combination of muscular endurance and strength. When you increase the number of repetitions, the emphasis shifts toward endurance. The introduction of equipment like weights, bands, tubing, and weighted balls has allowed group exercise settings to better target the strength end of the continuum. Stability balls can challenge even advanced-level participants and can be combined with handheld weights. Barbells can also be loaded with increasing weight to challenge advanced participants. If you are interested in pursuing high levels of strength, you will want to seek out additional sources of free or machine weights and use a spotter when appropriate.

TYPE: STATIC AND DYNAMIC TRAINING

There are two types of exercises for muscles: static and dynamic. Most people know static exercises as isometrics. During an **isometric contraction,** the muscle contracts, but it doesn't change in length. You perform isometrics by pushing against an immovable object (like a wall) or by holding a weight in one position. The weight can be the weight of your own limb, your whole body weight, or a weight you are holding. For example, you might hold yourself in a curl-up position for 10 seconds, or you might exert force by pressing one hand against the other. To increase strength, you would use short-duration holds of heavier weights or short-duration exertion using near-maximal force. To develop endurance, you would hold lighter weights or exert less force for longer durations. Isometrics can be very useful for strengthening a muscle in one position, which is particularly helpful for rehabilitating a weak point in a muscle's range of motion or strengthening postural muscles. One important word of caution: Isometric contractions can result in a rapid rise in blood pressure; therefore, people with high blood pressure and pregnant women should check with their physician before performing them.

In exercises that use **dynamic (isotonic) contractions** a force is applied through a range of motion. A curl-up is a good example of a dynamic exercise. Since most of our daily and recreational activities use a range of motion, dynamic exercises are usually the preferred way to train muscles. All of the resistance exercises in this chapter are dynamic in nature. However, there will be certain position-holding (stabilizing) muscles performing isometric holds. For example, during a regular push-up, the arms, chest, and shoulders perform dynamic contractions, but the abdominals, gluteals, and leg muscles perform isometric contractions. In more advanced weight training, you may find that isometric holds are incorporated within a dynamic movement to target specific parts of the range of movement.

You may also hear about isokinetic contractions. During these, the speed of movement is controlled, while the force exerted by the muscle can vary. These require special equipment that moves at a set rate and matches the force you apply with an equal resistance. Normally, if you push hard on a weight machine, the weights fly up. But this is not the case with isokinetic equipment. This type of exercise is especially good for rehabilitation, since you can push hard and receive high resistance during the healthy part of a movement and still push hard but apply less force and receive less resistance through the part of the motion where the muscle has been weakened by an injury.

ADDING RESISTANCE

Resistance training, now recognized as an important element of good fitness for everyone, has long suffered from myths and misunderstandings. Coaches once worried that an athlete who lifted weights would become muscle-bound and lose flexibility and coordination. Women worried that they would develop bulky, unseemly muscles. High-protein diets including amino acid supplements also have been touted to enhance muscle building. And at one time, circuit weight training was claimed to be a good aerobic workout. Today, we know that resistance training improves muscle performance, maintains and sometimes even improves flexibility, and does not cause women to develop bulky muscles (see Chapter 1). We also know that a high-protein diet is not needed to enhance muscle building; most resistance workouts require only a small increase in protein consumption in order to rebuild muscles and a lot of carbohydrate to fuel the exercise session. (See the discussion on protein in Chapter 12.) And although circuit weight training does increase heart rate into the training zone, it does not boost oxygen consumption to the same extent. Therefore, individuals who are less fit may receive some cardiorespiratory benefits, but for the most part, resistance training benefits muscles and aerobic exercise strengthens the heart and lungs.

More and more people have become aware of and are taking advantage of the benefits of resistance training. A normal program (moderate resistance for 1 to 3 sets of 8 to 12 repetitions) does not take long to complete, results in a firm physique, and develops a healthy combination of strength and endurance. Weights and bands were formerly reserved for more advanced students, but in most cases, beginners can start with light weights, easy resistance bands, and movements in the water. Remember, too, that although some people are beginners at cardiorespiratory conditioning, they may not be beginners in strength and endurance. A person may also have more strength in some muscles and less strength in others. For example, many women have weaker upper body strength than lower body strength.

As a safety precaution, individuals with injuries, joint disease, or other medical conditions should discuss resistance training with a physician. You will also want to review the technique tips presented in Chapter 10. Technique becomes increasingly more important as you increase resistance. (Chapter 10 has many examples of how to add resistance to your exercises using body weight, free weights, bands, and stability balls.)

TYPES OF RESISTANCE

Things that create a resistance to muscles as they move can be used to increase the muscle's strength and endurance. Today, a variety of approaches and equipment can be used to achieve resistance, but that was not always true. Group exercise classes have changed a lot over the years. The weights that were first introduced in aerobic dance classes were handheld weights (many of which were not dumbbell shaped), elastic weights that slid onto a limb, and weights that wrapped around the limb with Velcro® attachments. These weights were limited to 1–3 lbs. As resistance training has grown in popularity among the general public and as more women have become involved in it, the equipment has shifted toward the use of dumbbells, barbells, and weighted balls. The amount of weight available is now greater, although workloads are usually still in the low to moderate range because the main focus is on muscle endurance. Another important reason to keep the resistance moderately low is that more challenging levels of free weights (dumbbells and

weighted bars) should be performed only if a spotter is available. Group exercise classes do not usually involve paired activity with a spotter, although they can.

Resistance can be achieved in a number of ways, and each has its advantages. The simplest form of resistance is that of moving your body against gravity. When you want more resistance you can have a partner push or pull against you while you perform an exercise. To increase the resistance even more, you can use a variety of equipment. Resistance training machines are safe, usually do not require spotting, and can provide challenging loads without having to load weight plates. They do, however, restrict you to a certain motion, and they are designed for average-sized individuals. Newer machines allow for greater adjustments to accommodate body sizes. Unfortunately, they are not conducive to group exercise. The use of free weights—equipment that you hold, such as dumbbells, bars, and weighted balls—allows you to recruit more muscle fibers than machine exercises because you must stabilize the weight in addition to pushing or pulling it. Free weights are also more versatile in that they allow motions to be performed in more directions, angles, and planes. Free weights also prevent one body part from lifting for another. For example, during a machine bench press, the right arm can push more than the left. In a free weight press—especially with dumbbells, but also with a bar—this imbalance will become obvious (if one arm is capable of more, the bar tilts) and can be corrected. Smaller barbells are becoming popular. Some bars themselves are weighted, whereas others are very light and allow you to load and clip into place weight plates ranging from 1 to 10 lbs. This arrangement works nicely with a step bench in a group setting for a variety of resistance exercises set to music.

If you chose to use free weights that wrap on to the body or are elastic and slip onto the wrist or ankles, be sure to reserve this equipment for the muscle-toning portion of class; do not wear it during the aerobic portion. This type of weight works well for people who do not like to, or cannot physically, grasp a dumbbell. You can also position the weight along the limb and adjust the difficulty of an exercise. For example, during a side leg lift, it is more difficult to lift a weight at the ankle than one placed above the knee. Medicine balls and smaller weighted balls are also free weights, but they are softer and can be used in many ways. You certainly wouldn't want to throw and catch a dumbbell, but you can do so with a medicine ball. You can develop a specific kind of strength by moving a weighted ball through the motions you use in daily life, creative activities, sports, and recreation (Figure 9.1). Because they are weighted, they build strength in whatever range of motion you use them. You can use them on the go, such as tossing and catching while walking or jogging. You can balance on them with your feet or with your hands (i.e., push-up positions) for core strength, or turn and pass them to a partner to develop core stabilization during rotation (Figure 9.2). You can hold on to them and do many of the exercises described in Chapter 10 (lunges, squats, curl-ups, etc.), or if you are looking for explosive strength, you can use them in "give-and-go" motions with a partner. The possibilities are endless and, unfortunately, beyond the scope of this book, but there are other books and professionals who can share this information with you.

Exercise bands provide resistance in a somewhat different way than free weights do. They provide what is known as dynamic variable resistance, which means that as you stretch them, the resistance becomes greater. The disadvantage of this type of resistance is that at the end of a motion, the resistance may be more than you want, in which case you will have to use a less resistive band. But overall, they work very well. They are easily transported, easy to store, and inexpensive to buy. They also have the advantage of being able to stretch in many directions.

Two additional sources of resistance are stability balls and water. Stability balls take advantage of an unstable environment and body position to challenge the muscles. In addition to being fun, the balls are very versatile and easy to do at home. Pushing and pulling water can create resistance and offer the major advantage of being nonimpact; aqua or water aerobics is a very popular form of exercise for all ages.

FREE WEIGHTS

Weight should only be added to an exercise when the exercise is relatively easy to perform without weight, and you have established good technique. Start with light weights and work your way up in resistance. You will need to use lighter resistances with smaller muscles and heavier resistances with larger muscles. Fixed ends on dumbbells (as opposed to screw-on ends) are generally preferred because they cannot become loose and fall off accidentally. Dumbbells used in group exercise classes generally range in weight from 1 to 10 lbs. and bars weigh from 9 to 15 lbs.

Weighted limbs should always be moved with fluidity and control. When you add resistance to an exercise, it becomes even more important to maintain good alignment and control. When a weight is swung through the air, speed and momentum give it a force greater than its actual weight. The muscles, tendons, and ligaments around a joint have to stop the weight at the end of their range of motion. Too much weight, amplified by indiscriminate flinging of the arms or leg, can tear these tissues. (Think of the damage a wrecking ball can do when it is swung into a building.) An appropriate weight is one that you can move through a desired number of repetitions with the last few repetitions being difficult. If you find yourself recruiting extra muscles and losing your alignment for the last few repetitions, the weight is too heavy. Be sure to breathe comfortably throughout the exercises. With heavier resistance (difficult repetitions regardless of actual poundage), it is important to breathe out during the work phase and in during the recovery phase. This prevents a buildup of pressure in your chest.

RESISTANCE EXERCISES WITH FREE WEIGHTS

Exercise order and tempo are important components of a free weight workout. When performing a basic muscle workout, it is generally recommended to perform multi-joint and large muscle exercises first, followed by smaller muscle and single-joint exercises. Exercise order can also ensure that opposing muscle groups both achieve a workout and that the same muscle is not worked in back-to-back exercises, a technique reserved for more advanced workouts. For example, to fully balance the sample workout provided on page 117 in Chapter 10, add the toe flexion exercise with a band shown in Figure 10.85 (on page 155). If more emphasis on the inner and outer thighs is desired, leg lifts with wrapped weights (or band) can also be added. The tempo generally recommended is 2 counts on the work phase and 4 counts on the recovery phase. However, in an aerobic dance exercise setting, where only light to moderate weights are used and where an instructor is trying to use the rhythm of the music and/or the

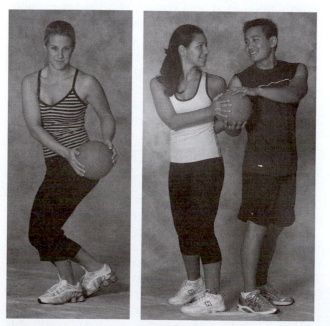

Figure 9.1   **Figure 9.2**

cadence of stepping up and down on a bench, it is common to see exercises counted with 2 (or 4) counts in both directions. When time is short, multi-joint exercise and exercises that provide the most balance for the aerobic workout and your personal weaknesses should be selected. Choreography or job-related or recreational activities can sometimes work one group of muscles more than its opposing group. Resistance exercises can restore balance. Perform 1 to 3 sets of 8 to 12 repetitions.

Here are some additional important tips for working with dumbbells and barbells.

- Always *breathe out* during the *work* phase. On an arm curl, the work phase occurs when you are bringing the weight to your body. On a chest press, it occurs when you are pushing the weight away from the body. On a squat or lunge, it occurs when you are coming back up. An easy way to remember this is to *Exhale on Exertion*.
- Grip the equipment firmly, but not so tightly that it causes hand and wrist tension.
- There are several different ways to grip the equipment. In a closed pronated grip, the palm faces downward when you first pick up the equipment, and the thumb is wrapped around. When you change the position of the dumbbells or the barbell for some exercises (such as a shoulder press), the palms will end up facing forward even though you are still in a closed pronated grip. In a closed supinated grip, the palms face upward and the thumbs are wrapped.
- If you sweat a lot and the equipment feels slippery in your hands, wear weight-lifting gloves.
- Stick to light to moderate weights with which you can perform a higher number of repetitions rather than very heavy weights you can only lift a few times. *Never* perform heavy, demanding loads (weights) without a spotter. It is best to do these exercises outside a group fitness setting.
- Technique is critical to your success. If you feel yourself breaking form, stop, take a break, perhaps lighten the load, and then begin again if it is appropriate. Exercising to **failure** means to go until you can't do another repetition or until you break form. In a group fitness class, you want to challenge yourself but avoid working to failure. (In strength training with excellent form and with a spotter, working to failure can be a good challenge to the muscle.)
- If you are using a barbell with weight plates, be sure to clip the weights in place.
- When lifting a barbell, make sure to keep the bar level.
- When lifting with two dumbbells, be sure to move them both through the action simultaneously.

- Perform one set of 8–12 (or 10–15) repetitions and build up to 2–3 sets.
- If you have a history of joint problems such as arthritis, bursitis, ligament damage, or knee surgery, you should not use weights unless cleared to do so by a physician.

EXERCISE BANDS AND CABLES

Exercise bands, sometimes referred to as resistance bands, are an inexpensive and versatile way to increase the resistance during a muscle-toning exercise. They come in a variety of forms, including colorful flat sheets of rubber 5 to 6 inches wide resembling strips of inner tubes, cables with handles, and surgical tubing. The first are produced commercially for aerobics classes and therapeutic clinics under several names such as Dyna-bands and Thera-bands®. They usually come in several colors; each color represents the amount of resistance, such as light, medium, or heavy.

Bands come in different widths and thicknesses. The wider or thicker the band, the more difficult it is to stretch. Some exercises require long bands that may be referred to as double bands. You can buy bands in different lengths and amounts of resistance. Most bands contain latex, but it is possible to purchase latex-free bands. Be sure to store latex-free bands in a separate bag.

If you choose to use a band, take off any jewelry that may cut into the band and always check the band for small cuts or tears before using it. (You can wear weight-lifting or bicycling gloves to take the pressure off your hands and to cover jewelry you do not want to remove.) Using the recommended range of 8 to 12 repetitions, you should change to a thicker or more resistant band when you can easily perform 12 repetitions and try a thinner or less resistant band if you can't do at least 8 repetitions. You may have to reduce band difficulty further if your goal is more endurance oriented and you intend to do more than 12 repetitions. For more resistance, you can use two bands at once and/or grasp the band farther from the end.

Bands and cables with handles can be interchanged in most exercises. If you are using a band, grasp or wrap the band. If you are using a cable, hold it by the handles. Many different cables are available in a variety of lengths and resistances, and some types of cables have loops built into them for inserting a hand or foot. If using a straight band, you can create a loop by tying the ends of the band together with a square knot.

If you have high blood pressure or have suffered a cumulative trauma disorder such as carpal tunnel syndrome, have a previous joint injury or chronic joint disease, check with a physician before using bands or cables. If you have knee problems, always work with the band above your knees. Bands may pull on leg hair, so socks, tights, or sweatpants are recommended. When pulling a band with your hand, be sure to keep the hand in line with the forearm. In other words, do not allow the wrist to "break" or "lay back."

RESISTANCE EXERCISES WITH BANDS

The band exercises in Chapter 10 are a representative sample of what can be done with bands. Note that each flexion exercise is presented with an opposing extension exercise and in some cases an additional lateral moving exercise. The large muscle, multi-joint exercises for a body area are presented before corresponding small muscle or single-joint exercises because this is usually the preferred order for performing them. In some cases, exercises for opposing muscles or muscle groups (for example, bench press and seated row exercises) are performed back to back with no rest period, a practice called **supersetting.** This method of training is more demanding and is therefore appropriate for more experienced and more fit individuals. The same order of exercises, but with a rest between exercises, is appropriate for all fitness levels. For more exercises and information on exercise bands, look for books written by qualified experts.

STABILITY BALLS

Stability balls are large, heavy-duty inflatable balls that are used as exercise equipment in many fun and effective ways. They are a versatile tool for developing strength, balance, and flexibility. (Some instructors are even using them in aerobic routines.) Just sitting on one of these large exercise balls makes all kinds of muscles work to keep you balanced. The ball creates an unstable environment in which your muscles, especially your core (trunk) muscles, have to work to stabilize you. This not only strengthens the muscles, but it also enhances the communication between the nervous system and the muscles. The improved neuromuscular efficiency results in better overall coordination. Stability balls have many aliases, including **exercise ball, physioball,** and resistance ball, but the name **Swiss ball** has historical importance because the balls were first introduced in Switzerland as a rehabilitation tool. The term stability ball will be used here to reflect their use for developing body stabilizing strength.

Unlike traditional resistance training programs that target one muscle or muscle group, stability ball exercises work a combination of muscles in the body. This more closely imitates normal body movement. During each of the stability ball exercises presented in Chapter 10, one or more muscles will be performing dynamic full range-of-motion contractions, while others will be busy making small stabilizing adjustments to maintain the body's position on the ball. One of the nice things about stability ball exercises is that the difficulty of the exercise can be easily adjusted by changing your body position on the ball. A softer, less inflated ball is also easier to work on than a harder, more inflated ball. As a result, stability ball exercises can be equally effective for beginners working on developing functional (everyday and postural) strength and for college athletes trying to maximize their strength and performance.

The benefits of using a stability ball include the following:

- improves muscular strength and endurance and is especially effective for increasing abdominal and back strength
- improves flexibility, including healthy motion ranges of the spine
- enhances balance and coordination of the muscles that are used to stabilize the spine and control proper posture
- helps you learn and maintain a healthy (and injury-preventing) neutral spine position to use during exercise
- improves core muscle strength, which translates into greater control for athletic skills

Stability balls can be made of vinyl or plastic. When purchasing a ball, be sure you are getting heavy-duty vinyl that is burst-resistant and will not tear if punctured; if a ball is punctured, it deflates slowly to prevent injury. The balls are inflated using a hand or electric pump. Some balls come with what looks like an udder (three-pointed extensions) on which the ball can rest. When using the ball, the udder is rotated out to the side so that the ball can roll properly during exercises. The udder is strictly a means of keeping the ball from rolling around when not in use.

It is best not to wear sharp items (jewelry, belt buckles, etc.) when working on inflated balls. Also be aware that plastic balls can be damaged by heat or excessive sunlight. Supplies that are useful for maintaining stability balls include a variety of hand or electric pumps, stands to keep the ball from rolling away, plug removers, carrying straps, and storage accessories.

RESISTANCE EXERCISES WITH A STABILITY BALL

The following are key technique points to keep in mind when using a stability ball.

- Use a ball that is large or small enough to allow you to maintain a 90-degree (or slightly greater) angle at the knees when you sit on it. Your thighs will be parallel to the ground or will point down slightly. Smaller and larger balls also may be used for different exercises to achieve different angles, but for the exercises depicted in Chapter 10, the 90-degree rule is a good one. A 45-centimeter (cm) ball is generally used for individuals under

5 feet (ft) tall, a 55-cm ball for 5-ft to 6-ft tall individuals, and a 65-cm ball for those over 6 ft tall. Most balls will hold up to 500 lbs.

- Always wear a shirt. A sweaty body can make you slide off the ball.
- Use progressions. When placing the lower body on the ball, the easiest position is to have the hips on the ball followed by the thighs and feet.
- Only perform exercises for which you have enough core strength to maintain a safe position. If you feel yourself losing alignment, select an easier version of the exercise or use one that doesn't involve the ball.
- Work with a neutral spine (natural curves) unless the exercise calls for spinal flexion or extension.
- Avoid scapular collapse (e.g., don't let your chest sag in a push-up position).
- The more external support you use, the less strengthening you will achieve, because the support stabilizes your position for you. One exception is presented in Figure 10.46 on page 139, where you will see that the student is using another student's feet to stabilize the side-lying position. This is done to keep the feet from sliding across the floor, not to control the person's position. On a non-slip floor this stabilization will not be needed.

You can make exercises more difficult by reducing the amount of your body that touches the ball surface, such as using only the lower legs instead of whole legs, or using one leg on the ball instead of two (advanced). Placing arms or legs farther apart on the ball makes holding positions easier, whereas placing them closer together results in a greater balance demand. (Ball exercises for posture control and flexibility have been included in Chapters 7 and 10.)

There are other types of balance and stability-challenging equipment available that are fun to use, such as foam rollers, Bosu balls, balance discs, and balancing boards. But because of the cost of these types of equipment, they are less often available for large groups.

WATER

To move your body through water, you have to move the water that is in your way. Pushing or pulling against the water provides a resistance that can be used for strength and endurance conditioning. Out of the pool, the air resistance you encounter during muscle toning is minimal, but the effect of having to work against gravity is significant. On the other hand, you are more buoyant in the pool (which lessens the effect of gravity), but the water offers 12 times more resistance to movement than does air.

You can increase water resistance using the following methods.

- Move the broadest body surface possible through the water. For example, moving a flat palm through the water creates more resistance than moving the edge of the hand through water. Moving a webbed glove or plastic barbell (Figure 9.3) through the water similarly increases the amount of surface and therefore the amount of resistance.
- Increase the length of the resistance arm of a lever. The arms and legs of the body act like levers. When the arm or leg is extended, it meets more resistance going through the water than when it is bent.
- Exert more force against the water. Moving a body part through the water quickly (with more force) is harder than moving it slowly through the water.
- Change the direction of moving water. Sweeping water in one direction and then reversing directions forces your muscles to work harder as they fight the current.
- Move as much water as possible. When you get a block of water moving, momentum will keep it moving and your limb will get to rest a little. Instead of continuing to push right behind the block of moving water, change the position of your arm up or down and pick up a new block of water. Circular and undulating movement patterns move more water than do straight-line movements.

Resistance exercises performed in water are similar to those on land, but aqua muscle toning has two distinct advantages. First, resistance is applied in both directions of an exercise. As the leg sweeps out to the side in a leg lift, the outer thigh muscles work against the water. As the working leg is brought back in, the inner thigh works against the water. As long as equal force is applied in each direction, muscle balance is

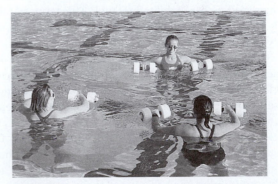

Figure 9.3

achieved. (It takes two exercises, an outer and inner leg lift, to accomplish the same thing on land.) Second, people of all abilities can exercise together, because it's simple to adjust the intensity of the exercise. For example, participants can perform a lower-body exercise of jumping off the bottom of the pool by pushing off with a little or a lot of force. Grandparent and grandchild can do this together and both benefit! The intensity can also be adjusted in very small increments, unlike using weights or bands that require you to jump to the next available resistance level. For more resistance, webbed gloves, bands, Styrofoam dumbbells and noodles, kickboards, and pull buoys can all be added to the workout. Kickboards and pull buoys are more often used in a deep-water workout than a shallow-water one.

RESISTANCE EXERCISES IN WATER

Many of the resistance exercises you perform on land can be performed in the water. Some have to be adjusted to account for body position and stability requirements in the water, and some can be adapted to take advantage of the floating environment. Still others are unique to water aerobics. Described here are a handful of exercises to help you see how muscle toning is achieved in the water. If you like the idea of exercising this way, consider taking a course or purchasing a good water aerobics book.

You can perform exercises such as triceps extension, biceps curl, toe raise, and lateral arm raise in the pool just as you do on land. Flies, instead of being done lying down, are performed vertically and you can do them while walking backward to increase the resistance against the water. Leg exercises like squats and lunges have to be modified because of the buoyancy factor—you actively push off the bottom of the pool when performing these exercises. This jumping is not hard on the body, since the landing impact is cushioned by the water. You can do leg lifts while bracing the body against the side of the pool.

You can also use exercise bands in the pool. Again, you can perform many of the exercises that use bands the same way that you do them on land. Side stepping and walking forward and backward with bands around the ankles are good ways to work the legs during a shallow-water workout. For deep-water work, two bands can be tied together in the middle with loops tied into each end. A person floating in a waist belt can then insert a foot and a hand in the loops and perform various exercises like leg extensions and arm curls. Figure-eight bands (with loops at each end) are also commercially available.

Deep-water workouts borrow movements from swimming strokes, water polo, and synchronized swimming. For example, you can develop leg endurance by kicking laps with a kickboard, treading water with an eggbeater leg kick (used in water polo), or performing scissor kicks under or on the surface of the water (used in synchronized swimming). You can also use the pool edge (deck) or gutter edge to advantage.

Depending on the depth of the water and strength of the participant, triceps push-ups can be performed by gently pushing with the legs off the bottom or by kicking to assist the arms. You can work on abdominal muscles by placing your back against the pool wall and stretching your arms up on the deck, and then, in this position, draw your feet up to your chest. Or you can perform similar curl-ups in deep water while holding a noodle across your upper back and under the arms for support. Finally, you will find that motions that are difficult to perform on land with resistance can be executed easily in water. For example, you can move your hands and arms in a figure-eight pattern or using a pattern that simulates a golf stroke. The possibilities are endless. Water aerobics can be a great stand-alone activity or an excellent way to cross-train.

SUMMARY

You can increase your muscular strength and endurance by progressively overloading. One way to achieve an overload is to increase the resistance against which the muscles work. You can increase resistance by adding weights or exercise bands to muscle-toning exercises, by performing the exercises in water, or by adjusting your body position. You can also use stability balls to add resistance or increase the number of muscles being used during an exercise.

KNOWLEDGE TIPS

1. As resistance increases, so does the importance of body alignment and movement control.

2. Beginners should start with low levels of resistance and use progressive overloads to achieve higher levels of fitness.

3. Light to moderate resistance loads develop muscular endurance and are appropriate in group fitness classes. Heavier loads or working to failure must, for safety, be performed on a machine or with a spotter.

4. Individuals of all fitness levels should overload gradually by increasing the resistance or the number of repetitions (or sets) being performed.

5. Resistance training, which involves a minimum of 1 set of 8 to 12 repetitions of 8 to 10 exercises for the major muscles, is recommended for all healthy adults.

6. Individuals with joint injury, high blood pressure, heart disease, orthopedic problems, or other health concerns should discuss resistance training with their health care provider before beginning.

7. Resistance can be increased through the use of free weights, exercise bands, or stability balls, by performing exercises in the water, or by adjusting body position.

8. Stability balls add the element of instability, which results in increased strength, balance, and coordination. Body position on the ball can increase or decrease the difficulty of an exercise.

9. Water exercises can be made more difficult by presenting the broadest body surface to the water, extending a limb, moving through water with greater force, changing the direction of moving water, and moving more blocks of water.

THINK ABOUT IT

1. What are the benefits of having muscular fitness?

2. What is the difference between muscular endurance and muscular strength?

3. Explain the FITT Principles for muscular endurance and muscular strength.

4. Explain how increasing strength can help increase muscular endurance.

5. Resistance can be created using machines, body weight, free weights (dumbbells, barbells, medicine balls), stability balls, exercise bands, and water. Explain the key advantages to each type.

6. Stability balls, Bosu balls, and core boards all create an unstable environment in which to exercise. Explain why an unstable environment can be an advantage.

REFERENCES

Aaberg, E. *Resistance Training Instruction.* Champaign, IL: Human Kinetics, 1999.

American College of Sports Medicine. *ACSM's Guidelines for Exercise Testing and Exercise Prescription.* 8th ed. Media, PA: Lippincott Williams & Wilkins, 2010.

——. "The Recommended Quantity and Quality of Exercise for Developing and Maintaining Cardiorespiratory and Muscle Fitness in Healthy Adults." *Medicine and Science in Sports and Exercise* 30 (No. 6, 1998): 975–91.

Brooks, G. A., Fahey, T. D., and K. Baldwin. *Exercise Physiology: Human Bioenergetics and Its Applications.* 4th ed. New York: McGraw-Hill, 2004.

Cassidy, C. "Should You Add a Little Weight to Your Workout?" *Women's Sports and Fitness* 8 (March 1986): 38–9, 47.

Delavier, F. *Strength Training Anatomy.* Champaign, IL: Human Kinetics, 2001.

Fardy, P. S. "Isometric Exercise and the Cardiovascular System." *The Physician and Sportsmedicine* 9 (No. 9, 1981): 42.

Fleck, S. J., and W. J. Kraemer. *Designing Resistance Training Programs.* 2nd ed. Champaign, IL: Human Kinetics, 1997.

Goldenberg, L., and P. Twist. *Strength Ball Training.* 2nd ed. Champaign, IL: Human Kinetics, 2007.

Hopson, J. L., R. J. Donatelle, and T. R. Littrell. *Get Fit, Stay Well!* San Francisco: Benjamin Cummings, 2009.

Kirk, E. P., J. E. Donnelly, B. K. Smith, J. Honas, J. D. Lecheminant, B. W. Bailey, D. J. Jacobsen, and R. A. Washburn. "Minimal Resistance Training Improves Daily Energy Expenditure and Fat Oxidation." *Medicine and Science in Sports and Exercise* 41 (No. 5, 2009): 1122–9.

MacFarlane, P. A. "Out with the Sit-Up, In with the Curl-Up." *Journal of Physical Education, Recreation, and Dance* 64 (August 1993): 62–6.

National Association of Sports Medicine, M. A. Clark, S. C. Lucett, and R. J. Corn (editors). *NASM Essentials of Personal Fitness Training.* 3rd ed. Baltimore, MD: Lippincott, Williams & Wilkins.

National Strength and Conditioning Association, T. R. Baechle and R. W. Earle (editors). *Essentials of Strength Training and Conditioning.* 2nd ed. Champaign, IL: Human Kinetics, 2005.

——. *NCSA's Essentials of Personal Training.* 3rd ed. Champaign, IL: Human Kinetics, 2008.

Page, P., and T. Ellenbecker. *Strength Band Training.* Champaign, IL: Human Kinetics, 2005.

Ricci, B., M. Marchetti, and F. Figura. "Biomechanics of Sit-up Exercises." *Medicine and Science in Sports and Exercise* 13 (No. 1, 1981): 54–9.

Rose, S. *exercise Ball.* Bath, UK: Parragon, 2005.

Santana, J. C. *The Essence of Stability Ball Training.* Vol. 1, *Chest, Shoulders, Back, and Balance.* Training Optimum Performance Systems, 1998. Videocassette.

——. *The Essence of Stability Ball Training.* Vol. 2, *Legs, Hips, and Core.* Optimum Performance Systems, 1999. Videocassette.

Seibert, R. J. *Group Strength Training.* San Diego: CA: American Council on Exercise, 2000.

Silvestri, L., and J. Oescher. "Use of Aerobic Dance and Light Weights in Improving Measures of Strength, Endurance, and Flexibility." *Perceptual and Motor Skills* 70 (April 1990): 595–600.

Thompson, C. W., and R. T. Floyd. *Manual of Structural Kinesiology.* 12th ed. St. Louis, MO: Mosby, 1994.

VanGalen, P. A. *Exercising with Dyna-band, Total Body Toner.* Hudson, OH: Thomas B. Gilliam Ent., 1987.

Veit, K. "Bodysculpt." *Women's Sports and Fitness* 14 (January –February 1992): 52.

Vincent, W. J., and S. D. Britten. "Evaluation of the Curl-up—A Substitute for the Bent Knee Sit-up." *Journal of Physical Education, Recreation, and Dance* 51 (1980): 74–5.

Webb, Tamilee. *Tamilee Webb's Original Rubber Band Workout.* New York: Workman Publishing, 1986.

Wellness Letter, University of California at Berkeley. *The New Wellness Encyclopedia.* Boston: Houghton Mifflin, 1995.

10

Resistance Exercises: Weight, Bands, and Balls

*"The undertaking of a new
action brings new strength."*

EVENIUS

- Which exercises work which muscles?
- Is there more than one way to exercise the same muscle or muscle group?
- What is the proper technique for each of the exercises?
- How can I maximize muscular fitness and minimize injury and soreness?
- Does it matter the order in which I perform the exercises?
- How many repetitions and sets do I need to do?

READY to build, shape, and tone your muscles? This chapter is filled with resistance exercises you can use to develop muscular fitness. You can perform many of these exercises with body weight alone, or you can add more resistance using weights, stability balls, and exercise bands. The technique for each exercise is detailed and illustrated so that you can perform the exercise correctly. However, if you perform these exercises without a careful plan, you may experience less than optimal results and unnecessary muscle soreness or injury. Therefore, it is important to team these exercises with the technique tips section of this chapter on page 118 and the information presented in Chapter 9. Muscle balance, for example, is important for appearance and to prevent injury. Someone not aware of this concept might select an array of exercises in this chapter that do not represent a well-balanced workout. Your instructor and/or courses specifically for muscular fitness are also excellent resources for putting together a muscular workout beyond the scope of the class in which you are presently enrolled.

The exercises in this chapter are organized by body part, starting with the upper body, then trunk and core exercises, then lower body. Each of these sections presents the multi-joint exercises first, followed by single-joint exercises. There are two reasons for performing combination (multi-joint) exercises before single-joint exercises. The first involves making the best use possible of your available exercise time—if you have limited time, you can get the most out of your workout by doing combination exercises that hit all the major joints and muscles with the fewest number of exercises. The second has to do with preserving the strength of specific, often smaller, muscles so that they don't limit combination exercises. For example, if you perform triceps kickbacks that isolate the triceps muscle, and then try to bench press or do push-ups, the fatigued triceps will give out before the larger pectoral (chest) muscles have been fully worked. You will have pre-exhausted the smaller muscle in the single-joint exercise and limited your ability to work the chest and shoulders adequately. Here are two more examples: (1) perform squats before doing leg extensions or leg curls and (2) do shoulder presses before lateral arm raises.

Following multi-joint exercises, you can choose to add single-joint exercises to further strengthen individual muscles. (Purposefully pre-exhausting specific muscles is a technique used in advanced training but is beyond the scope of this text.) So begin your workout with combination and large muscle exercises and then, time permitting, follow those with single-joint and small muscle exercises. Another important pairing consideration involves back exercises and abdominal exercises. Although both sets of exercises are multi-joint, you should do the back exercises first so that the abdominals are not too fatigued to help support the back during the back exercises.

Within body part sections (i.e., the upper body, core, and lower body), some exercises are grouped to show you how to work the same muscle(s) using different forms of resistance including body weight, dumbbells, barbells, exercise bands, and stability balls. Variety is good for muscle development, so when you are comfortable with one method, you may want to try another form of resistance. Switching up your exercise routine also keeps workouts mentally fresh.

The exercises in this chapter are not all inclusive; there are many variations and methods of training. The selected exercises provide a balanced muscle workout and are those commonly performed in group exercise classes. Many of the exercises require that you work first one side of the body and then the other. To save space, the exercise descriptions give the action for only one side (the side shown in the photograph, if provided), but be sure to work both sides equally. Because you need to include exercises that work opposing muscle groups, this chapter provides flexion exercises and extension exercises, abduction (away from the center of the body) and adduction (toward the center of the body) exercises, and pushing and pulling exercises. The names of the muscles being exercised and the function of the muscles are labeled for each type of exercise. When variations work slightly different muscles, this is indicated as well. To help you focus on where major muscles are located, there are icons accompanying many of the exercises that show the basic position of the muscles being worked by each exercise. In addition, you can refer to the more detailed diagram of the muscles in Appendix 1.

Finally, as you perform these exercises, do not confuse muscle toning with spot reduction. The idea that a toning exercise will remove fat from a specific body part is false. Toning and strengthening exercises work the muscle so that when good body composition is achieved (fat burned through aerobic exercise and energy balance achieved through good diet), toned muscles that were hiding under the fat will appear. And don't forget that developing muscular fitness has many benefits other than appearance!

TECHNIQUE TIPS FOR RESISTANCE EXERCISES

Look over the following technique tips before you try any of the exercises in this chapter, because your technique is important in performing the exercises in this chapter safely and effectively. These tips are even more important to remember when performing exercises with added resistance.

- Warm up thoroughly before beginning your workout.
- Perform multi-joint and large-muscle exercises before single-joint and small-muscle exercises (i.e., squats before hamstring curls; push-ups before triceps extensions).
- Isolate the muscle(s) you want to work. Some additional muscles will be used to stabilize your position; the rest should remain relaxed. It is very easy, but not advantageous, to recruit extra muscles to help do the work. For example, you can lift more weight in an arm-curl by leaning back, but the targeted biceps muscle doesn't receive any additional benefit, and your back may become sore.
- Maintain good body alignment throughout the exercise. When correct alignment and body position cannot be maintained, stop.
- Perform resistance exercises at a moderate pace. Fast movements mostly strengthen muscles in the positions in which a change of direction occurs. Momentum does most of the work between the turnaround points. Fast ballistic movements are required in certain power lifts, but they are not used for any of the basic resistance exercises presented in this text.
- Use fluid, controlled movements. Do not swing your limbs indiscriminately, especially if you are using weights.
- Use a full range of motion. This promotes flexibility and improves strength and endurance through the complete range of motion. Only use a range of motion in which you can maintain good technique. For example, less flexible individuals will have to use smaller ranges of motion until flexibility is improved.
- Avoid locking your joints. When a joint is locked, the potential for injury is greater.
- Breathe! Breathe during resistance exercises. Breathe naturally during repetitions with lighter resistance. With heavier resistance, breathe out during the work phase and in during the recovery phase. For example, breathe in as you bend your knees in a squat, and breathe out as you straighten your legs. Breathe out in an arm-curl when you draw your arms up, and breathe in as you lower your arms. Never hold your breath, since this can

create dangerous pressure in the chest, especially when heavier resistance is used.

- Rest muscle groups for 30 seconds to 3 minutes before exercising them again. Shorter rest breaks promote muscle endurance. Longer rest intervals are needed for recovery between heavy resistance strength exercises. While the muscle(s) are resting, you can exercise the opposing muscle(s) or perform a series of exercises repeating the series, starting with the first exercise.
- Exercise opposing muscle(s) to prevent soreness and maintain a balance between agonists and antagonists. (Examples of opposing muscles include biceps/triceps, hamstrings/quadriceps, pectorals/latissimus dorsi, and abdominals/erector spinae.)
- Stop if you feel pain at any time. Pain is your body's way of telling you that you have imposed too much of an overload. If pain persists, see a health care practitioner.
- Stretch the muscles following a resistance workout.

EXERCISES FOR THE UPPER BODY

The exercises in this section target your arms, shoulders, and upper back. Most women (and some men) lack upper body strength. If you are weak in this area, it is important to begin with light resistance and build up to more resistance. A stronger upper body can be empowering and protective. You are less apt to recruit low back muscles when your upper body and abdominals are strong. You will also experience less fatigue in a number of daily activities as well as in recreational and sport activities. You will be able to swing harder, push harder, and pull yourself up (i.e., out of a pool) more easily. Working the upper back also acts to balance the forward posture used in keyboarding.

UPPER BODY MULTI-JOINT EXERCISES

Shoulder Press

Muscles worked: deltoid, triceps brachii

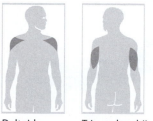

Deltoids   Triceps brachii

POSITION—BANDS

Sit on the floor with your legs crossed (or with your legs extended and knees bent), or sit straddling a step bench. Place the center of the band under your buttocks or under the step. Grasp the ends of the bands with your palms facing forward, elbows bent, and hands up by your shoulders. Sit up tall so that your back maintains a neutral posture (natural curvature of the spine). The band should have a little tension on it; if not, adjust the length of the band.

ACTION Extend your arms up over your head (Figure 10.1). Make sure your wrists stay firm and in line with your forearms and your palms stay facing front. Do not lean forward or arch the back. Slowly return your arms to the shoulder position.

VARIATION You can also do this exercise with just the weight of the arms.

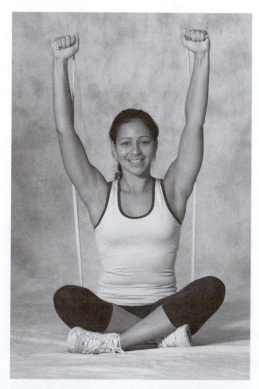

Figure 10.1

POSITION—WEIGHTS

DUMBBELLS Sit on the floor with your legs crossed (or sit on a step bench). Sit up tall so that your back is in good alignment. Hold the dumbbells with a closed pronated grip to the outside of the shoulders. (Palms will be facing forward, thumbs wrapped.) Keep your wrists in line with your forearms. (You can also do this exercise while standing.)

BARBELL Stand with your feet shoulder width apart, knees slightly flexed. Hold the bar with your hands slightly wider than shoulder width, with a closed pronated grip (palms down, thumbs wrapped). Balance the bar on your collar bones and across the front of your shoulders (deltoids). At this point your palms should be facing forward. Keep your wrists firm and inline with your forearms. (This exercise can also be done seated.)

ACTION Press the weight overhead (Figure 10.2), extending your arms fully but without locking your elbows. Keep your wrists firm with palms facing front. Do not lean forward or arch the back. Slowly lower the weight.

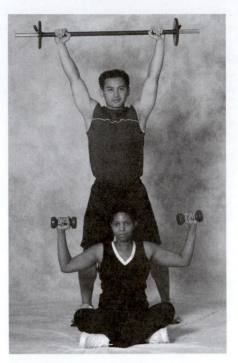

Figure 10.2

Push-up

Muscles worked: pectoralis major, deltoid, triceps brachii

Muscle action: elbow (arm) extension, shoulder horizontal flexion

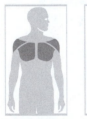 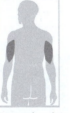

Pectoralis major

Triceps brachii

Deltoids (anterior)

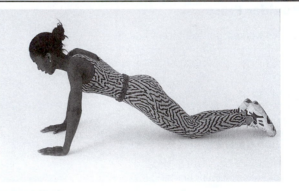

Figure 10.3a

POSITION

Assume the push-up position with your hands on the floor, a little more than shoulder width apart. Extend your legs to the back. Beginners can rest their weight on their knees (Figure 10.3a). If you are more advanced, rest your weight on your toes (Figure 10.3b). In either case, your body should be straight with just a slight lift of the gluteals (buttocks).

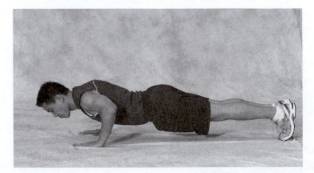

Figure 10.3b

ACTION Bend your elbows to approximately 90 degrees. Then straighten elbows and return to starting position.

VARIATIONS

1. Place your hands farther than shoulder width apart.

2. Place your hands very close together.

3. Place your hands (easier) or feet (harder) on a step (Figure 10.4).

POSITION—BALL

Lie prone on the ball with your hips on top of the ball (beginner) or the lower legs (more advanced) on the

ball. Place your hands shoulder width apart on the floor in front of the ball.

ACTION Bend your arms until your elbows are at a 90-degree bend (Figure 10.5). Keep your body straight (neutral spine) or slightly piked at the hips throughout the exercise.

VARIATION For more difficulty, place the toes on top of the ball.

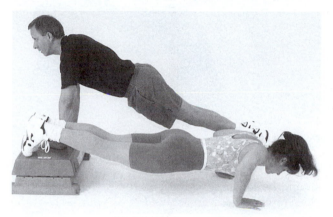

Figure 10.4

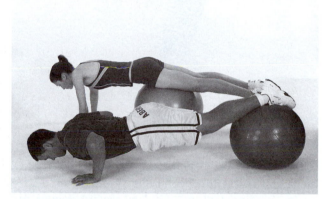

Figure 10.5

Chest Press

Muscles worked: pectorals, deltoids, triceps brachii

Muscle action: shoulder horizontal flexion, elbow extension

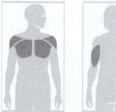
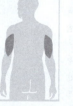

Pectoralis major

Deltoids (anterior)

Triceps brachii

POSITION—BAND

Stand with your knees slightly flexed. Hold one end of the band in each hand with the band running across your shoulder blades and under your arms.

ACTION Extend both arms forward (Figure 10.6a). Slowly flex (relax) your arms.

ACTION Perform the same exercise lying down on a bench with the band or cable running under the bench. Keep your knees bent and your back in a neutral position (Figure 10.6b).

POSITION—WEIGHTS

DUMBBELLS Lie on your back on the floor (or on a bench) with your knees bent and feet flat on the floor (or bench). Hold the weights in your hands, palms facing your knees. Start with your arms fully extended with the dumbbells held directly above the shoulders (Figure 10.7a, back figure). Keep your elbows slightly flexed to prevent locking. Keep the dumbbells parallel to each other.

BARBELL Lie on your back on the step bench in a stable position, with your feet flat on the floor and knees bent. Grasp the bar with a closed pronated grip (palms down, thumb wrapped) slightly more than shoulder width apart. Hold the bar directly over your shoulders with slightly flexed arms (to prevent locking the joint). Wrists should be in line with your forearms (not laid back).

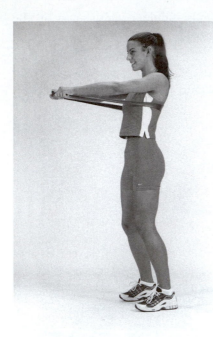

Figure 10.6a

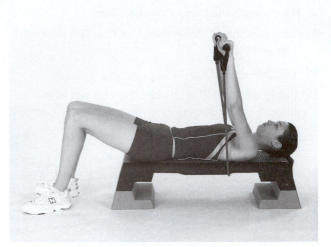

Figure 10.6b

ACTION Lower your arms toward your chest (Figures 10.7a and 10.7b) until your elbows reach a 90-degree angle. The dumbbells will finish near your armpits and should be lowered in unison. The barbell will come close to your chest and should cross your body at the nipple line. Press the weight back up.

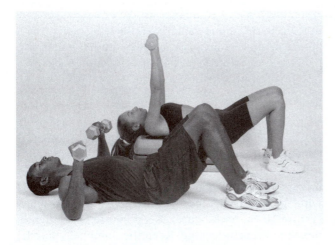

Figure 10.7a

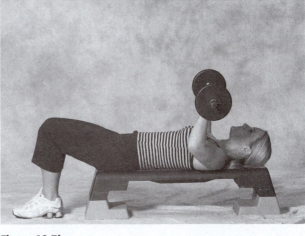

Figure 10.7b

Horizontal Adduction (Imitation Pec Deck)

Muscles worked: pectoralis major, anterior deltoid

Muscle action: chest adduction

POSITION

Stand with your knees slightly bent. Hold your arms out to the side with the upper part of your arms parallel to the floor and the lower part vertical.

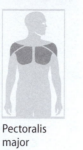

Pectoralis major

Deltoids (anterior)

ACTION Bring your arms forward until your forearms touch (Figure 10.8). Return your arms to the side.

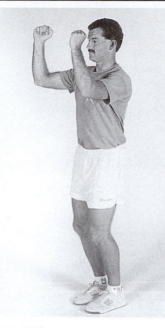

Figure 10.8

Flies

Muscles worked: pectoralis major, anterior deltoid

Muscle action: shoulder horizontal adduction (horizontal flexion)

POSITION

Lie on the floor (or on a bench) with your knees bent and feet flat on the floor. Hold the weights in your hands with palms facing each other and arms extended above your chest. Keep a slight bend in your elbows.

Pectoralis major

Deltoids (anterior)

ACTION Slowly open your arms out to the sides, drawing an arc (Figure 10.9) and lowering your hands until they are even with your shoulders or chest. Keep your wrists in line with your forearms. Maintain a little flexion (bend) in the elbows.

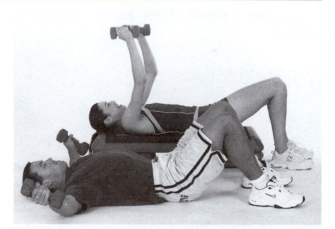

Figure 10.9

Weights should move in unison. Return them to the above-the-chest position.

Row

POSITION—STANDING

Muscles worked: trapezius, posterior deltoid, rhomboids, latissimus dorsi, biceps group

Muscle action: scapular retraction, shoulder extension, elbow flexion

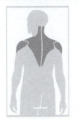 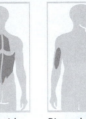

Trapezius
Deltoids

Rhomboids
Latissimus
dorsi

Biceps brachii

Stand with your arms in front of your body parallel to the floor (Figure 10.10a).

ACTION Draw your elbows back, keeping your arms parallel to the floor. Initiate the movement with the muscles in your back. Try to pinch your shoulder blades together (Figure 10.10b). Relax your shoulders and arms.

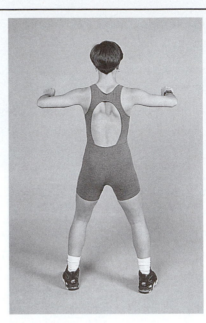

Figure 10.10b

POSITION—SEATED WITH BAND

Sit on the floor with your legs extended forward. (If this position is uncomfortable, bend your knees.) Hold one end of the band with each hand, with the band running across the soles of your shoes.

ACTION Pull both hands back toward the armpits (Figure 10.11). Squeeze your shoulder blades together at the same time. Slowly extend your arms and relax your back.

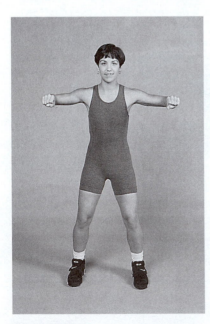

Figure 10.10a

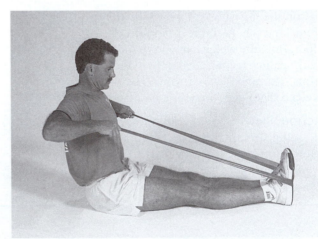

Figure 10.11 Knees can be bent for comfort.

POSITION—UPRIGHT WITH WEIGHTS

Muscles worked: middle deltoid, upper trapezius, biceps brachii

Muscle action: shoulder elevation

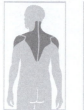 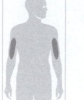

Trapezius
Deltoids

Biceps brachii

DUMBBELLS Stand with your feet shoulder width apart, knees slightly bent. Hold the weights with your arms extended down in front of your body, with your palms facing your legs.

BARBELL Stand with your feet shoulder width apart and your knees slightly flexed. Hold the bar in front of your body with a closed pronated grip (palms down, thumbs wrapped) and your hands slightly narrower than shoulder width. Rest the bar on your thighs. Your elbows should be extended.

ACTION Draw your hands up your torso (Figures 10.12a and 10.12b) toward your chin. Your elbows should point outward and slightly upward at the end of the movement. Slowly extend your arms to return to the starting position.

POSITION—BENT-OVER WITH WEIGHTS

Muscles worked: rhomboids, latissimus dorsi, middle trapezius, posterior deltoid, biceps brachii

Muscle action: scapular retraction (adduction)

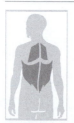 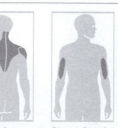

Rhomboids
Latissimus
dorsi

Trapezius
Deltoids

Biceps brachii

DUMBBELLS—ONE ARM Stand in a forward lunge position, bend forward, and place your left hand on your left thigh for support. The fingers of your left hand should face inward. Extend your right arm down toward the ground and slightly forward (near the

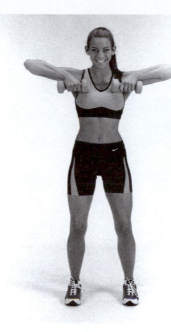

Figure 10.12a

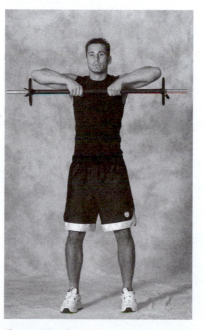

Figure 10.12b

opposite knee). Hold the weight in your right hand with your palm facing in (Figure 10.13a). With a step bench, your front foot can be placed on the bench, or you can place one knee and your support hand on the bench.

BARBELL Stand with your feet shoulder width apart. Using a squatting motion, pick up the bar with a closed pronated grip (palms down, thumbs wrapped), with your hands more than shoulder width apart.

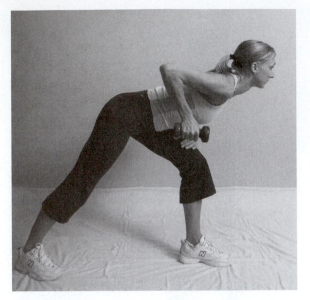

Figure 10.13a

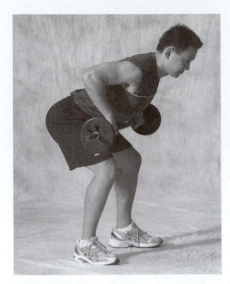

Figure 10.13b

Extend your arms and rest the bar on your thighs. Bend forward at your waist with a straight back until the bar is just above parallel, while simultaneously bending your knees and sitting back with your buttocks. Allow the bar to hang in front of your legs with straight arms. Focus a short distance in front of your feet.

ACTION Using only your shoulder and back muscles, pull your elbow(s) up and back (Figures 10.13a and 10.13b). Make sure your elbow(s) stay close to the side of your body. Maintain the forward body position until all the repetitions are completed. Bring the dumbbells/bar up to your chest, keeping your elbows pointed up. Slowly lower the weight.

Shoulder Shrug

Muscles worked: trapezius

Muscle action: shoulder elevation

POSITION

Stand with good posture.

ACTION Shrug the shoulders up (Figure 10.14), hold for 3 to 5 seconds, and then relax down.

Trapezius

VARIATIONS

1. This exercise can be performed with dumbbells or bar in hands.

2. This exercise also can be performed holding a band/cable in the hands that runs under the feet.

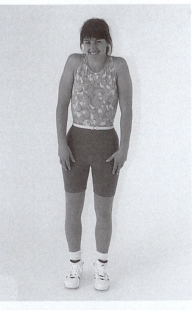

Figure 10.14 Exercise can be done as pictured, but weights can be added to make it more challenging.

Kneeling Back Extension (Back Hypers)

Muscles worked: erector spinae, latissimus dorsi

Muscle action: back extension

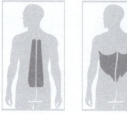
Erector spinae

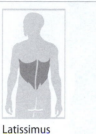
Latissimus dorsi

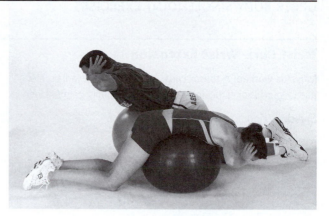
Figure 10.15

POSITION—BALL

Kneel in front of the ball with your trunk on the ball. Rest your hands lightly on the small of your back (beginner), or place your hands up by your ears (advanced).

ACTION Lift your torso off the ball until the back is straight (neutral spine). Do not hyperextend (Figure 10.15).

VARIATION To add difficulty, move from your knees to your toes. This will allow your torso to be farther over the top of the ball. You can also place your arms above your head, with a right-angle bend in your elbows.

Lat Pull-Down

Muscles worked: latissimus dorsi, biceps brachii

Muscle action: arm adduction

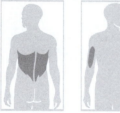
Latissimus dorsi

Biceps brachii

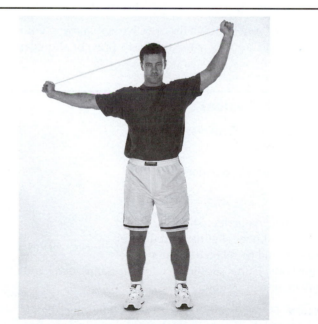
Figure 10.16 Increasing elbow bend will work the biceps.

POSITION—BAND

Stand with your knees slightly bent. Hold the band overhead in both hands, palms forward, with the anchor hand (left) centered above and behind your head and the anchor arm elbow slightly bent.

ACTION Pull the band down and to the side by drawing the working elbow (right) down toward your waist (Figure 10.16). Depending on how you want to work the muscles, you can add more elbow bend as you pull down.

Slowly relax the working arm and allow it to return to its original position. The band may be pulled down in front or behind your head.

UPPER BODY SINGLE-JOINT EXERCISES

Wrist Curl/Wrist Extension

Muscles worked: extensor carpi ulnaris, extensor radialis brevis and longus flexor carpi ulnaris, flexor carpi radialis, palmaris longus

Muscle action: forearm flexion and extension

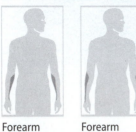

Forearm flexors

Forearm extensors

POSITION

Arms should be straight and may be down, to the sides, in front, or overhead. Hands may be in a fist or open.

ACTION Both wrists can flex, drawing your palm toward your forearm. Both wrists can extend, pulling the back of your hand toward the back of your forearm, or one wrist can flex while one extends (Figure 10.17).

VARIATION Add dumbbells or a barbell. Lower your arms to the front of your thighs to prevent shoulder

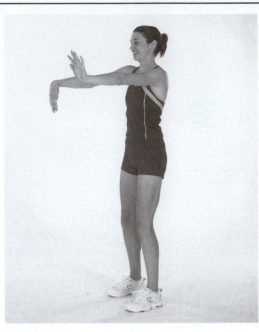

Figure 10.17

fatigue, or sit down on a bench and place your forearms on your thighs with your wrists extending past your knees. Flex and extend both wrists at the same time.

Arm-Curl (Flexion)

Muscles worked: biceps brachii, brachialis, brachioradialis

Muscle action: elbow flexion

Biceps brachii

POSITION

Stand with your feet shoulder width apart and knees slightly flexed. Your arms should be relaxed at the sides of your body. Palms should face forward and your hands may be in fists or open.

ACTION Flex your arms (Figure 10.18). (Pull your palms or fists toward the shoulders.) Relax and extend your arms.

VARIATIONS

1. Hold your arms straight in front of your body, parallel to the floor. Flex, relax, and extend.

2. Hold your arms straight out to the sides, parallel to the floor, palms forward. Flex, relax, and extend.

3. Hold your arms straight out to the sides, parallel to the floor, palms up. Flex, relax, and extend.

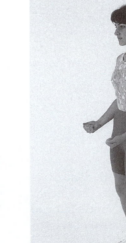

Figure 10.18

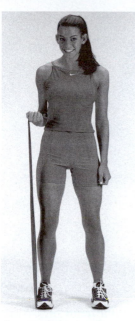

Figure 10.19a

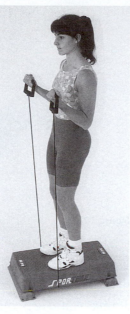

Figure 10.19b

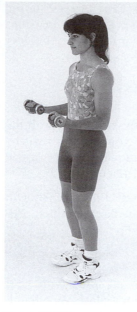

Figure 10.20a

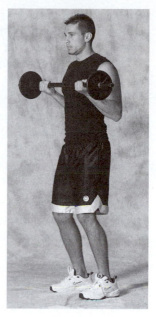

Figure 10.20b

POSITION—BAND/CABLE

Stand with your foot on one end of the band. Grasp or wrap the band around your hand on the same side as the foot you are using to anchor the band (Figure 10.19a). Start with your arm in an extended, relaxed position. Anchor your elbow at your waist. Cables or long bands allow you to work both arms simultaneously. Stand on the cables or place them under a step bench.

ACTION Flex your arm(s), bringing your palm(s) toward your shoulder (Figures 10.19a and 10.19b). Slowly lower your hand(s).

POSITION—WEIGHTS

DUMBBELLS Stand with your feet shoulder width apart and knees slightly flexed. Hold the weights firmly in your hands, with your arms down at your sides and palms facing forward. (Palms may also face inward and rotate forward at the start of the curling action.)

BARBELL Stand with your feet shoulder width apart and knees slightly flexed. Grasp the bar with a closed supinated grip (palms up, thumbs wrapped) with your hands shoulder width apart. Extend your arms and let the bar rest on your thighs.

ACTION Keeping your wrists in line with your forearms, curl the weight up toward your torso until your hands are within 4 to 6 inches of your shoulders (Figures 10.20a and 10.20b). Do not allow any swaying or movement in your torso. Slowly lower the weight until your arms are straight but the elbow joint is not locked.

Arm Extension

Muscles worked: triceps brachii

Muscle action: elbow extension

POSITION—PRESS BACKS

Stand with your knees slightly bent. Lean your trunk forward slightly. Bend your arms with the elbows drawn up and back. Your palms should face back (Figure 10.21).

ACTION Extend your arms (straighten). Relax, allowing your arms to return to the starting position (flexed).

Triceps brachii

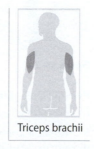

Figure 10.21

VARIATION Rotate your palms 270 degrees to the outside after extending the arm. Rotate your palms back in before lowering your arms. (The shoulder rotator muscles also work in this exercise.)

POSITION—OVERHEAD PRESS

Stand with your knees slightly bent. Extend your arms straight up overhead. Clasp your hands with the palms facing each other. With your elbows right by your ears, flex your arms, allowing your clasped hands to fall behind your head (Figure 10.22).

ACTION Extend your arms until they are straight overhead. Relax and return to the flexed position. This exercise is sometimes called the French curl.

POSITION—DIPS

Assume the crab position, on all fours with your abdomen to the ceiling. You may place your hands on the floor or on a step (Figure 10.23). (If your arms are weak, place your hands and buttocks on the floor.)

ACTION Bend your arms to a 90-degree angle. Extend your arms and then return to starting position.

POSITION—BAND

Stand with your knees slightly bent. Grasp the middle of the band with one hand and hold it against your chest next to the opposite shoulder. Grasp one or both of the ends of the band with your other

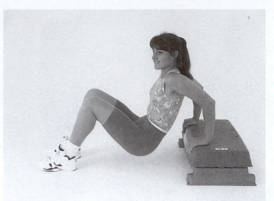

Figure 10.23

hand. The lower hand should be directly below the upper hand.

ACTION Pull down with the bottom hand until your arm is extended (Figure 10.24). Keep your elbow by the body throughout the motion. (You may have to grasp higher on the band with the lower hand to get a full range of motion.) Slowly flex (relax) your arm.

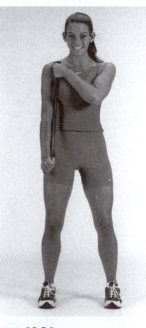

Figure 10.24

POSITION—DUMBBELL KICKBACKS (STANDING)

Stand in a forward lunge position, with your elbow drawn up and back, and your left hand and arm in a support position on your thigh.

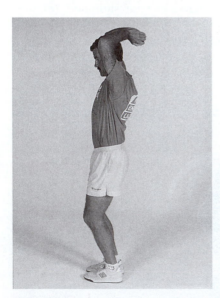

Figure 10.22

ACTION Holding your elbow in position, extend your right arm (Figure 10.25). Slowly bend your arm at the elbow and return to the starting position. This exercise may be combined with the bent-over row (page 125).

POSITION—BARBELL LYING ARM EXTENSION "SKULL CRUSHERS"

Lie on your back on the step bench in a stable position with your legs bent and feet flat on the floor.

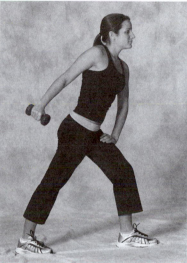

Figure 10.25

Hold the bar over your chest with a closed pronated grip (palms down, thumbs wrapped), hands shoulder width apart. Position the bar directly above your shoulders and extend your arms with a slight elbow bend to prevent locking the joint. Point your elbows toward your knees. Do not allow them to go out to the sides. (**Note:** This exercise can also be done holding the middle of a dumbbell with both hands turned so that it is on end.)

ACTION Slowly lower the bar (Figure 10.26) until it is just above your forehead. Maintain your upper arm position throughout—arms parallel, wrists in line with your forearms, and elbows pointing away from your face. Raise the bar back up.

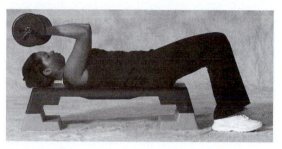

Figure 10.26

Arm Circles

Muscles worked: deltoid

Muscle action: shoulder rotation, flexion, abduction and adduction

POSITION—BAND

Arms extended to the side, elbows straight but not locked (Figure 10.27).

ACTION 1 Move your arms in small or large circles first clockwise and then counterclockwise.

ACTION 2 Raise your arms out to your sides to shoulder height, then lower them down alongside your legs with palms facing in.

VARIATIONS

1. While circling your arms, move them to the front, overhead, down, and to the side again. You can also raise and lower your arms to the front and sides without performing the circular motion.

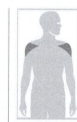

Deltoids

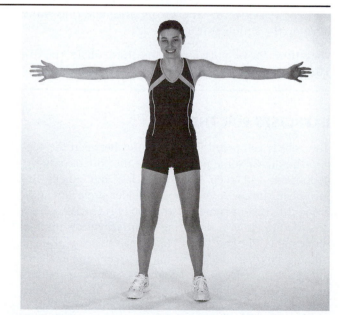

Figure 10.27

2. With your arms to the side, move them forward and back with your palms facing forward, then palms back, palms up, and, finally, palms down.

3. You can perform this exercise while standing or sitting. If you stand, your knees should be slightly bent and your spine should be in a neutral position.

Lateral Arm Raise

Muscles worked: deltoids

Muscle action: arm abduction

POSITION—BAND

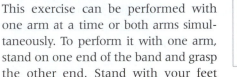

Deltoids

This exercise can be performed with one arm at a time or both arms simultaneously. To perform it with one arm, stand on one end of the band and grasp the other end. Stand with your feet shoulder width apart and with good back alignment. Your knees should be slightly bent. Extend your arm down alongside your leg with your palm facing your leg. There should be a little tension on the band. Move your hand up or down the band to adjust the tension.

ACTION Move your arm outward and upward (Figure 10.28) until it is parallel with the ground (shoulder height). Keep the palm facing downward and wrist firm throughout. Do not take the arms above shoulder height because the joint is more susceptible to injury in that position. To strengthen the shoulders in an overhead position, use the shoulder press exercise. (**Note:** From this position, your arms can also move forward, backward, and across the body to fully develop the shoulder muscles.)

VARIATION Move both arms simultaneously (Figure 10.28). (Make sure that the band or cable is long enough to do this.) Stand with your feet shoulder width apart. Place the center of the band under your feet. Grasp the ends of the band with your hands. Adjust the tension. Move both arms up and out until they are even with your shoulders. Keep your palms facing downward throughout. Lower your arms.

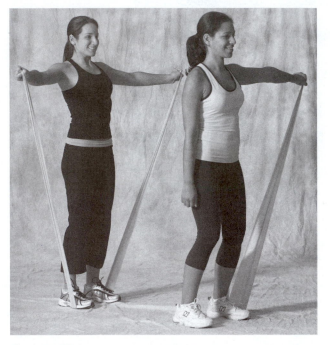

Figure 10.28

EXERCISES FOR THE CORE

The core is composed of the muscles between the hips and shoulders. Some people define the core as only the abdominal and deep spinal muscles, and others also include the buttocks, chest, and shoulder girdle. Strengthening the core, or center, of your body is crucial because it is used in either a stabilizing or an active role in most movements. The core plays a major part in postural alignment (stabilizing and supporting the spine) and in allowing you to optimize sport movements. Some core training exercises are dynamic, such as the curl-up (page 134), whereas others are static, such as the plank (page 139).

These exercises are organized by those that focus on the abdominals, the trunk, and then the hips. Although some core exercises tap a large number of muscles, only the major ones will be identified in the exercises that follow. When you perform core exercises, body position is very important; improper technique can easily lead to an unhealthy load on your back. As you strengthen your core, enjoy the new sense of power and alignment you will feel during both daily and recreational activity. For more discussion about the core, please refer back to pages 54–58 in Chapter 6.

ABDOMINAL EXERCISES

A general understanding of the abdominal muscles and their function will help you select specific exercises for your program. The rectus abdominis is a long muscle that attaches to the pubic bone at one end and the ribs at the other. The whole muscle will contract during any abdominal exercise, but some exercises tend to emphasize the upper two-thirds, whereas others emphasize the lower third. The oblique muscles run from the ribs to the pelvic girdle on an angle. When they contract, they twist (or rotate) the trunk with respect to the pelvic girdle. The transversus abdominis is the deepest of the abdominal muscles. It lies underneath both the rectus abdominis and the obliques. It is often referred to as the transverse abdominal muscle because the fibers run across the body. (Other common names include transversalis and TvA.) Its primary function is postural; practicing good posture by keeping your abdomen lifted and pulled in is one way to keep this muscle toned. It is very important to make sure this muscle is engaged during core exercises because it helps to support the lower spine. If this and other abdominal muscles can't maintain good spinal positioning during exercise, then the exercise is too difficult.

For many years, people have done sit-ups to develop abdominal strength. Sit-ups used to be performed with a relatively straight back and with the hands behind the head. Today, curl-ups are the exercise of choice because they are much easier on the lower back, and they are as or more effective than sit-ups. In a curl-up, your head and shoulders follow a natural curl as you lift. (At one time, people were taught to lift the chin straight up; this is incorrect.) You roll up, initiating the role with your abdominal muscles and engaging the transverse and then the rectus abdominis, until your shoulder blades come off the floor. If you sit all the way up, your abdominals are resting for the last one-half to one-third of the exercise because the pull of gravity lessens in this range. Your hip flexor muscles also come into action in this range, taking work away from the abdominals.

Arm placement can make curl-ups progressively more difficult. With your arms at the sides of your body, your abdominal muscles are lifting only the weight of your trunk and head. When your arms are placed across the chest, the abdominals must lift the weight of your arms, trunk, and head. When you move your arms up toward the head, they represent even more weight. Figure 10.29 demonstrates these three positions. You can use an incline board (or bench) for an assisted curl-up (Figure 10.30).

Placing your hands behind your head can be stressful to the neck; for this reason, many exercise leaders do not use this position. Too often individuals use their arms to pull their body forward, which presses the chin to the chest and stresses the neck. In properly executed curl-ups, the arms remain passive, and the abdominal muscles do all of the pulling.

The position with the arms near or behind the head is included for two reasons. First, some individuals can clearly maintain good technique and handle the weight of the arms in this position. Second, a few individuals experience neck fatigue prior to abdominal fatigue and

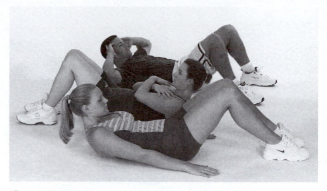

Figure 10.29

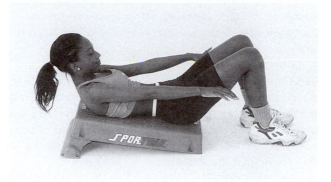

Figure 10.30

like to rest their head in their arms to relieve the neck muscles. However, the majority of individuals will achieve the best results by placing their arms alongside their body or across their chest. Weights can also be held against the chest to make curl-ups more difficult.

To concentrate on the oblique muscles, you have to twist before lifting the torso. (A common error is to lift and then twist.) One way to ensure good twisting action when the hands are behind the head is to leave one elbow flat on the floor while the other lifts across the body.

Strengthening the lower third of the abdomen and not straining the back is a challenge. Eighty percent of all people have back pain sometime during their lives—pain that is often caused by a lack of abdominal strength and leg flexibility. Some exercises seem as though they should increase abdominal strength, but in fact may cause lower back pain. See Figures 10.31, 10.32, and 10.33. Double leg lifts are one such culprit. A double leg lift requires the abdominal muscles to stabilize the spine while about one-half the body's weight is lifted through hip flexion. If the abdominal muscles are too weak, the pelvis is pulled forward by the hip flexors and strain is placed on the low back. The iliopsoas, for example, attaches to the spine in the lower back area. When it contracts, it pulls against the lower spine. If the abdominals are able to stabilize the spine and pelvis, the hips flex raising both legs without

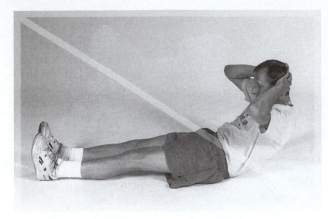

Figure 10.31 Straight-leg sit-ups place stress on the lower back and emphasize hip flexor strengthening, not abdominal strengthening. Placing your hands behind your head and pulling forward puts stress on the cervical vertebrae.

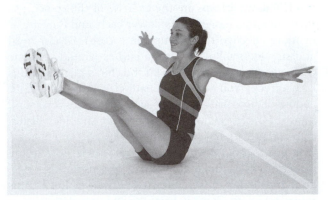

Figure 10.32 The weight of both legs is often more than the abdominals can handle. The result is stress on the lower back area.

incident. However, when the abdominals are unable to stabilize the body, the iliopsoas pulls the lower back up off the floor. This can result in lower back pain. Plus, leg lifts that strengthen the hip flexors (iliopsoas and others) and hurt the back fail to do the one thing you set out to do—strengthen the abdomen.

Only individuals who can keep the back in a neutral position and maintain the natural curves of the spine should lift both legs. Many exercises fall into the "double leg lift" category: straddling the legs 6 inches off the floor, sitting and pushing both legs out, scissoring at a low angle, and others. Exercises that are better for the majority of the population are single leg lifts, bicycling the legs, or reverse curls. Strengthening the abdominals will help support the spine and decrease susceptibility to back pain.

Figure 10.33 The V-seat position is another form of a double leg lift. This may also stress the lower back.

Curl-Up

Muscle worked: rectus abdominis (obliques and transversus abdominis stabilize)

Muscle action: trunk flexion

POSITION

Assume the curl-up position—lie flat on the back with your knees bent, feet flat on the floor and shoulder width apart. Hands may be at your sides, across your chest, or by your head.

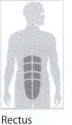

Rectus abdominis

ACTION Lift your upper body up off the floor while pressing your lower back into the floor. Be sure to lift up and "curl" naturally with your body and neck (see Figure 10.29). Roll back down to the floor. Beginners can relax between curl-ups; more advanced

participants should curl down until their shoulder blades touch and then curl up again.

VARIATIONS

1. Lift your feet off the floor, ankles crossed or uncrossed and knees bent. Curl up (Figure 10.34). Roll back down to floor.

2. Bend your left leg and place your left foot on the floor. Place your right ankle on your left knee. Perform curl-ups (Figure 10.35). Curl down to floor.

3. Reach for your toes with your legs extended up in the air (Figure 10.36). Reach with one hand and place the other hand behind your head if you experience neck fatigue. You can also bend your legs during the relaxation phase and extend them during the reaching phase. Curl down to floor.

4. Bench-assisted curl-up. The angle of the bench helps beginners perform a curl-up (see Figure 10.30 on p. 134). Lie down with your back and buttocks on the angled bench and your feet on the floor. (Tall people may have difficulty fitting on a step bench.) Curl up as before.

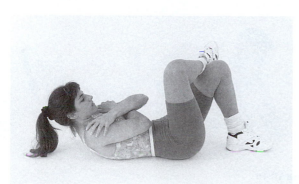

Figure 10.34

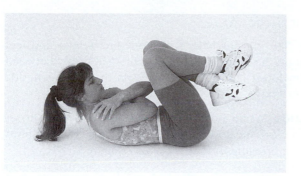

Figure 10.35

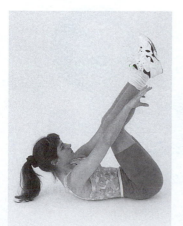

Figure 10.36

POSITION—WEIGHTS

Lie on your back with your knees bent and feet flat on the floor. Hold the weights in your hands and cross your arms flat over your chest.

ACTION Curl up until your shoulder blades come off the floor (Figure 10.37). Slowly lower down.

POSITION—BALL

After taking a seat on top of the ball, roll down the ball until the small of your back is against it. Lean back until your back is in a relatively straight line. Place your hands across your chest (beginner) or up by your ears (more advanced).

ACTION Curl up approximately 30 to 45 degrees (Figure 10.38).

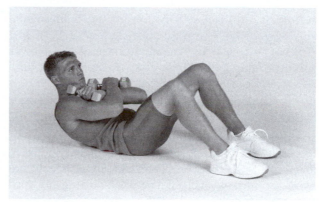

Figure 10.37

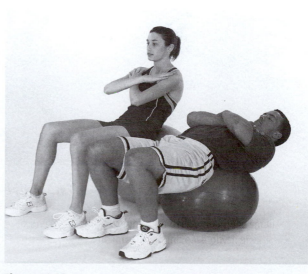

Figure 10.38

VARIATIONS

1. Curls may also be performed lying on the floor with the feet up on the ball.

2. Twisting or oblique curls can be performed by locating the hips on the side of the ball (just off the top) and twisting the torso away from the ball as you curl up.

Reverse Curl-Up

Muscles worked: rectus abdominis (obliques and transversus abdominis stabilize)

Muscle action: trunk flexion

Rectus abdominis

POSITION 1

Lie flat on your back with your legs bent so that your knees are near your chest but your feet are extended upward.

ACTION   Try to lift your hips toward the ceiling while moving your knees toward your chest (Figure 10.39). (Try not to roll or use momentum—make the lower portion of the abdominals work.) Relax hips to floor. This exercise is often called a reverse curl.

POSITION 2

Sit on the floor with your legs extended to the front. Lean back on your elbows. Roll your pelvis under so that your lower back is stabilized. (Some people are more comfortable lying flat and supporting the hips with the hands.)

ACTION   Bicycle your legs (Figure 10.40). If fatigue causes you to arch your lower back, bicycle with just one leg.

(This exercise works a static hold on the abdominals while using the leg and hip muscles to cycle.)

POSITION—BALL

Lie flat on your back with your knees bent and feet flat on the floor. Hold the stability ball firmly between your lower legs. Rest the arms on the floor alongside your body.

ACTION   While holding the ball between your lower legs, curl the lower half of your body toward your chest, bringing the ball with you (Figure 10.41).

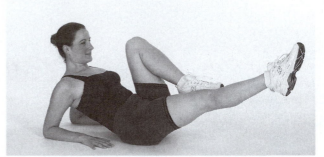

Figure 10.40

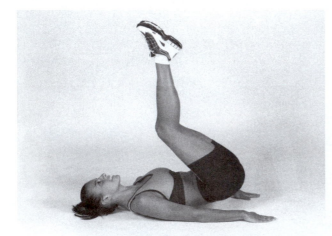

Figure 10.39 Reverse curl.

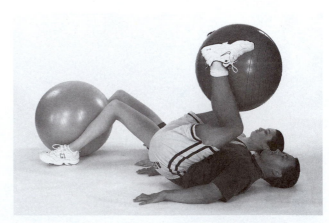

Figure 10.41

Twisting Curl-Up

Muscles worked: obliques, rectus abdominis (transversus abdominis stabilizes)

Muscle action: trunk flexion and rotation

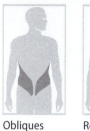
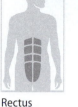

Obliques   Rectus abdominis

POSITION

Assume curl-up position.

ACTION Twist your torso to one side before curling up (Figure 10.42a). If your hands are by your head in a more advanced position, leave one elbow on or near the floor while twisting and lifting with the opposite side of your body (Figure 10.42b). Curl-ups may be performed in a series to one side or alternating sides.

VARIATIONS

1. Alternately extend one leg out and hold it off the floor as you bend your other leg into your chest. As the legs change position, twist and curl, bringing your left elbow to your right leg or your right elbow to your left leg. (Figure 10.43 shows this with an advanced arm position.)

2. Lay your knees over to one side, placing your body in a twisted position. Curl up. (Figure 10.44 shows an advanced arm position.)

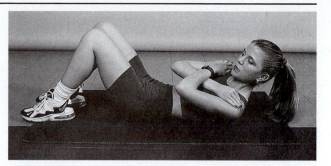

Figure 10.42a

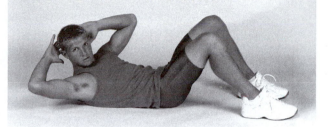

Figure 10.42b Advanced arm position.

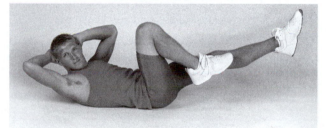

Figure 10.43 Advanced arm position.

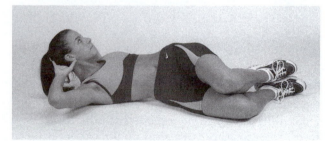

Figure 10.44 Advanced arm position.

Hip and Trunk Curl (Flexion)

Muscles worked: rectus abdominis

Muscle action: hip and trunk flexion

POSITION

Lie on your back, with your knees bent toward your chest. Tie the band around your legs just above your knees. Place your hands inside the band loop, with palms facing your feet.

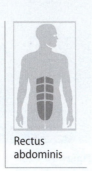

Rectus abdominis

ACTION Curl your knees toward your chest while simultaneously holding the band in position or pushing it away. Your upper body can also be curled toward your knees (Figure 10.45). Slowly uncurl your legs and upper body.

VARIATION You can perform this exercise without the band; curl your shoulders and knees toward each other.

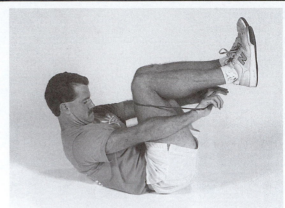

Figure 10.45

(**Note:** This exercise is a curl-up and reverse curl at the same time.)

Lateral Trunk Raise with Ball

Muscles worked: erector spinae, quadratus lumborem (abdominals stabilizing)

Muscle action: lateral lumbar flexion

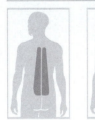 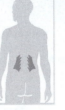

Erector spinae   Quadratus lumborem

POSITION

Lie on your side on the ball. Extend your feet in a forward/backward stride position with the top leg forward. You can place your arms on the ball for balance

purposes or bend your arms with your hands near your ears (advanced).

ACTION Bend at your waist, lifting the trunk up off the ball while maintaining a sideways orientation to the floor (Figure 10.46).

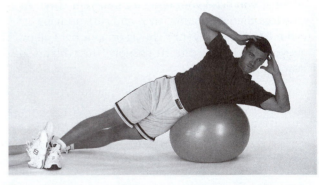

Figure 10.46 A partner is supplying stabilization at the feet. This would not be necessary on a nonslip floor and with practice.

TRUNK EXERCISES

Prone Bridge (Plank)

Muscles worked: abdominals (rectus abdominis, obliques, transversus abdominis), pectorals, triceps, deltoid

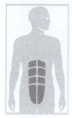

Rectus abdominis	Latissimus dorsi	Transversus abdominis
Pectoralis major	Triceps brachii	Deltoids

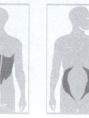

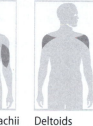

POSITION

From a modified push-up position, drop down onto your forearms. Create a straight line from the knees to the top of your head, with just a slight break (lift) at your hips. Breathe normally. The variations provided make this exercise progressively more difficult.

ACTION Hold the position. Be sure to breathe normally throughout. If you start to shake, take a short break and then resume the position you started with, or if on toes, drop to the kneeling position. Start with short durations (10 to 20 seconds) and build up to longer durations (1 to 2 minutes).

VARIATIONS

1. Curl your toes under and lift your knees off the floor. Create a straight line from your heels to the top of your head, with a slight break (lift) at your hips (Figure 10.47, female).

2. Move up off your forearms to a standard push-up position. Keep the slight lift in your hips and flex your arms slightly to prevent locking the elbow joint.

3. From the standard push-up position described above, lift one leg straight out behind you. Lead with your heel. Do not allow your back to arch or your hip to rotate. After holding the position with one leg up, change legs (Figure 10.47, male).

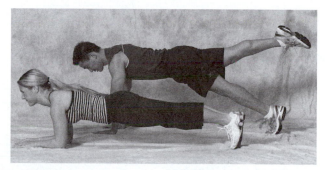

Figure 10.47

Lateral Bridge (Side Plank)

Muscles worked: abdominals (rectus abdominus, obliques, transversus abdominus), latissimus dorsi, deltoid, triceps

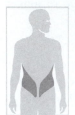
Obliques

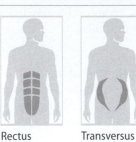
Rectus abdominis

Transversus abdominis

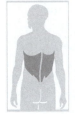
Latissimus dorsi

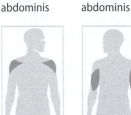
Deltoids

Triceps brachii

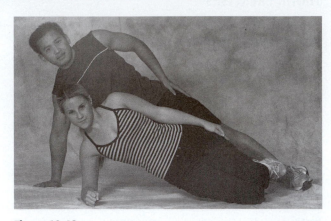

Figure 10.48

POSITION

Sit on the floor on your right hip with your knees bent. Place your right forearm on the floor directly under your right shoulder. Lift your hips off the floor. Create a straight line from your knees through your hips, back, shoulders, and head. Your left arm should lie alongside your torso. Make sure your hips are vertical, one on top of the other (Figure 10.48, female).

ACTION Hold the position described above. Be sure to breathe normally throughout. If you start to shake, take a short break and then resume the position you started with, or if on toes, drop to the kneeling position. Start with short durations (10 to 20 seconds) and build up to longer durations (1 to 2 minutes).

VARIATION To make this exercise more difficult, extend your legs so that your knees are no longer touching the ground. The top foot can be placed on the floor in front of the bottom foot for more stability. The straight line now runs from your feet to the top of your head (Figure 10.48, male).

Overhead Stabilization

Muscles worked: whole body with emphasis on core muscles

POSITION—BAND (WITH PARTNER)

Stand with your feet slightly wider than shoulder width apart and your knees slightly flexed (not locked), or take an athletic stance with one foot in front of the other. If using the latter position, switch the front foot periodically. Hold the band in the middle with both hands (or grasp the handle of a cable band). Extend your arms up overhead. Your partner will stand behind you and take hold of the ends of the band (or the other cable handle). Make sure you are maintaining excellent standing posture.

ACTION Your partner will pull down on the bands while you try to remain steadfast in your posture (Figure 10.49). Your partner should begin gently and increase intensity (pull harder) only when you request it. Partners should use smooth (never jerky) pulling motions. Your partner can pull the band downward toward center and also downward and off

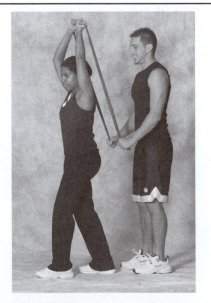

Figure 10.49

to the sides. Partners must be attentive and trustworthy, or else injury can occur.

HIP EXERCISES

Hip and Shoulder Extension (Prone Swim)

Muscles worked: deltoid, gluteus maximus, hamstrings (with assisted abdominal and erector spinae stabilization)

Muscle action: hip extension, shoulder flexion

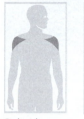
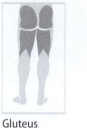

Deltoids

Gluteus
maximus
Hamstrings

POSITION

Lie prone with both arms extended overhead along the floor.

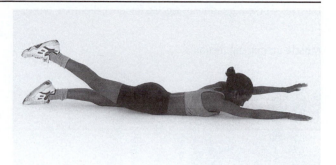

Figure 10.50

ACTION Raise one arm and the opposite leg simultaneously. Keep both your arm and your leg straight. Hold for 5 to 10 seconds and then relax (Figure 10.50). If you experience any pain, discontinue this exercise.

VARIATION Kneel on all fours and raise a leg, an arm, or opposite arm and leg simultaneously. This is often called the quadruped.

Elbow Roll Out with Ball

Muscles worked: rectus abdominis, erector spinae, latissimus dorsi

Muscle action: hip extension

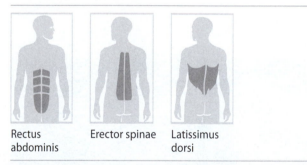

Rectus
abdominis

Erector spinae

Latissimus
dorsi

POSITION—BALL

Kneel in front of the ball. Place your forearms on the near side of the ball with your elbows apart and hands near each other.

ACTION Roll the ball forward using your forearms until your lower body forms a straight line from your knees to your shoulders (Figure 10.51).

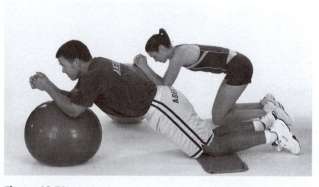

Figure 10.51

Prone Body Tuck with Ball

Muscles worked: quadriceps (rectus femoris), iliopsoas, tensor fasciae latae

Muscle action: hip flexion

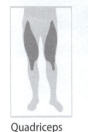
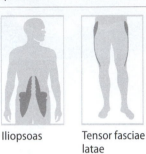

Quadriceps   Iliopsoas   Tensor fasciae latae

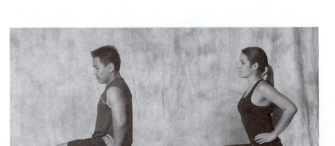

Figure 10.52

POSITION—BALL

Lie prone (face down) on the ball. Position the ball under your hips (beginner) or thighs or lower legs (more advanced). Place your hands shoulder width apart on the floor in front of the ball. Your head and back should maintain a straight line (neutral spine) throughout.

ACTION Bend at your hips, and pull your thighs to your chest. To increase the difficulty, place your legs closer to each other on the ball (Figure 10.52).

VARIATION Perform a knee-tuck press by doing a push-up action when the hips are flexed. This approximates a military press or handstand push-up.

Pelvic Tilts with Ball

Muscles worked: quadratus lumborem, transversus abdominis, rectus abdominis

Muscle action: lumbar spine flexion and extension (hyperextension)

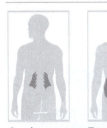
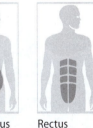

Quadratus lumborem   Transversus abdominis   Rectus abdominis

POSITION—BALL

Sit on the ball with your feet on the floor shoulder width apart. Place your hands on the ball near your hips or on your thighs. Sit up with your spine in a neutral position.

ACTION Tuck your pelvis under by contracting the abdominals and rolling the ball forward. Then roll the ball backward, tilting your pelvis forward and placing your back into slight hyperextension (Figure 10.53).

Figure 10.53

Lateral Hip Tilts with Ball

Muscles worked: quadratus lumborem, obliques

Muscle action: lateral hip and trunk flexion

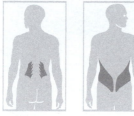

Quadratus
lumborem

Obliques

POSITION—BALL

Sit on the ball with your feet on the floor shoulder width apart. Place your hands on the ball near your hips or on your thighs. Sit with your spine in a neutral position.

ACTION Using the muscles on the side of the trunk, roll the ball first to one side and then the other (Figure 10.54).

VARIATION Perform hip circles.

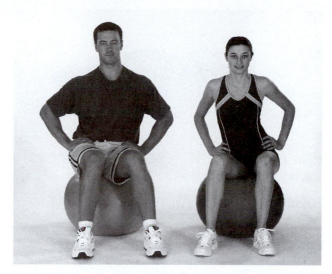

Figure 10.54

EXERCISES FOR THE LOWER BODY

Two basic positions used in leg exercises require special comment. When working on all fours, you can be on your hands and knees (Figure 10.55) or on your forearms and knees (Figure 10.56). In most cases, the latter position is recommended because it allows you to lift your leg higher without causing your back to arch. If you are more comfortable in the first position, lift your leg only until it is parallel with the floor. During exercises in these positions, it is important to use the trunk muscles to stabilize the body.

When you are performing exercises lying on your side, your arm and trunk can be flat along the floor (Figure 10.57), or you can be resting on your forearm (Figure 10.58). Both positions are fine. If you use the latter position, resist the temptation to slouch into your shoulder. Stay pulled up and again concentrate on using the core muscles to maintain good positioning throughout the exercises. Lying flat has the advantage of eliminating undesirable spinal curvature during the exercise.

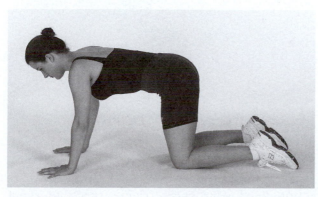

Figure 10.55

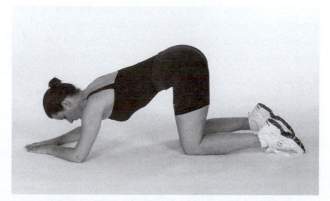

Figure 10.56

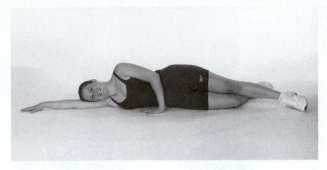

Figure 10.57

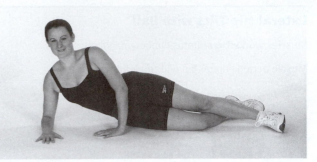

Figure 10.58

LOWER BODY MULTI-JOINT EXERCISES

Squat

Muscles worked: gluteals, hamstrings, quadriceps

Muscle action: hip and leg (knee) extension

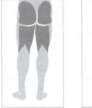

Gluteus maximus

Hamstrings

Quadriceps

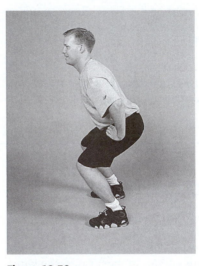

Figure 10.59a

POSITION

Assume the squat position—feet slightly wider than shoulder width apart, heels down, knees bent, trunk on a forward angle. Some back arching is required to maintain balance, but avoid excessive curvature.

ACTION Bend your knees to about 90 degrees. Be sure to retain muscular control throughout the movement (Figure 10.59a). You should sit backward (as though you are sitting on a chair) and keep your head and eyes forward and slightly raised. Straighten legs and relax. Do not perform a full deep knee bend (Figure 10.59b), because this places stress on the knee ligaments.

POSITION—BAND

In a standing position, place the center of the band underneath your feet. Grasp the ends of the band with your hands. When you are standing straight with feet shoulder width apart and arms extended by your sides, the band should have some tension. Move your hands up or down the band (or wrap/unwrap the band around your hand) to adjust the tension. Toes should be pointed slightly outward. Focus is forward and slightly upward. Chest up and out.

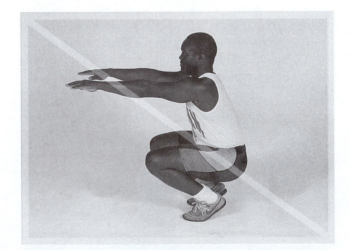

Figure 10.59b Deep knee bends place stress on knee ligaments.

ACTION Bend your knees (Figure 10.60) to about 90 degrees while sitting backward as if sitting down in a chair. Be sure to retain muscular control throughout

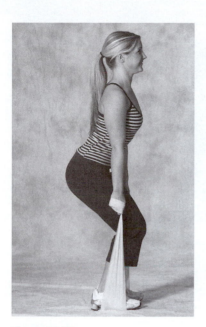

Figure 10.60

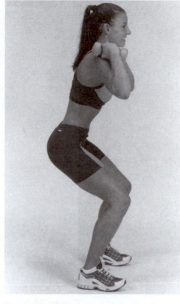

Figure 10.61a

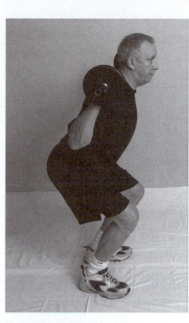

Figure 10.61b

the movement. Keep your head and eyes forward and slightly raised. Straighten your legs slowly against the resistance of the band. Sit down only as far as you can while maintaining control and good back positioning (natural curve). The trunk leans forward slightly as you squat. Flexibility may limit the range of motion.

POSITION—WEIGHTS

DUMBBELLS Stand with your feet slightly wider than shoulder width apart, heels down, toes angled slightly outward, knees bent, trunk on a slightly forward angle. Hold the weights in your hands just above your shoulders (near your ears), palms forward, elbows out.

BARBELL Stand with your feet slightly wider than shoulder width apart, heels down, toes pointing slightly outward, knees bent, trunk on a slightly forward angle. Hold the bar with your hands slightly wider than shoulder-width, with a closed pronated grip (palms down, thumbs wrapped). Balance the bar on your upper back, just above the scapula. Arms should be fully flexed (bent).

ACTION Bend your knees (Figures 10.61a and 10.61b) to about 90 degrees while sitting backward as if sitting down in a chair. Be sure to retain muscular control throughout the movement. Keep your head and eyes forward and slightly raised, chest up and out, shoulder blades down and back. Keep good back alignment, natural curve; avoid excessive arching or rounding of the back. Straighten your legs slowly.

POSITION—BALL (WALL-SLIDE, DOUBLE-LEG)

Place the ball between a flat wall and your back at belt height. Place your feet shoulder width apart and

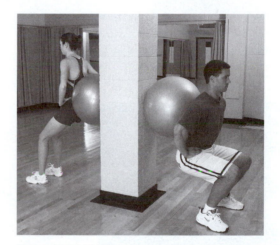

Figure 10.62 This exercise should be performed against a flat wall. A pillar is used here to allow the reader to see both positions simultaneously.

about 12 to 14 inches from the wall (beginner) or place your feet under your hips (more advanced). Place your hands on your hips or extend them in front of your body parallel to the floor.

ACTION While maintaining pressure against the ball, bend your knees until they reach a 90-degree angle (Figure 10.62). Make sure your back stays upright (perpendicular), your hips stay under your shoulders, and your feet stay flat on the floor. Return to a standing position. As you improve, you can narrow your stance, which increases the balance requirement. Your knees should not extend over your toes.

Lunge

Muscles worked: lead leg—gluteus maximus, hamstrings, quadriceps

Muscle action: hip and knee extension

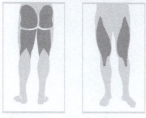

Gluteus maximus   Quadriceps

POSITION

Take a large step forward into a lunge position. Keep the knee on the front leg behind the instep of the front foot. Keep hips square.

ACTION Lower the hips until the front thigh is parallel to the floor. Take another large step forward to a lunge on the other side and repeat (Figure 10.63).

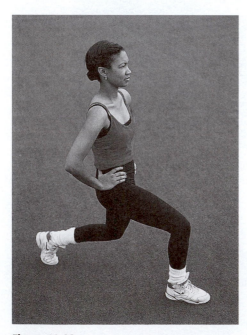

Figure 10.63

POSITION—BAND

Stand in a front lunge position with the center of the band under your front foot. Hold the ends of the bands in your hands with your arms extended down by your sides. Move your hands down the bands or wrap the band around your hands until there is some

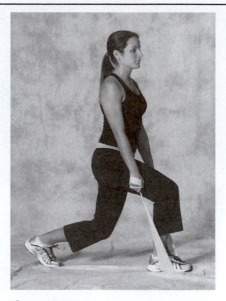

Figure 10.64

tension on the band when your torso is upright. Keep your front knee over your ankle and your hips square. The heel of your back foot should be raised.

ACTION Lower your hips directly down (Figure 10.64) until the thigh of your front leg is parallel to the floor. Raise your hips against the resistance of the band. Repeat 8 to 12 times before switching legs. Make sure the front knee does not move forward; it should stay over the ankle.

POSITION—WEIGHTS

DUMBBELLS Stand with your feet shoulder width apart and arms extended down by your sides (or up by your shoulders). Hold the weights in your hands with your palms facing in.

BARBELL Stand with your feet parallel and shoulder width apart, with your knees slightly bent. Hold the bar with a closed pronated grip (palms down, thumbs wrapped), hands slightly more than shoulder width apart. Place the bar on the base of your neck so that it is balanced by the upper back and shoulder muscles. Lift your elbows to help stabilize the bar. Lift your chest up and out. Look slightly upward. Pull your shoulder blades down and back.

ACTION Take a large step forward with one foot, into a lunge position. Keep the knee of your front leg behind the instep of your front foot. Keep your hips square. Lower your hips (Figures 10.65a and 10.65b) until the thigh of your front leg is parallel to the floor. The heel of your back foot should raise off the floor. Return to the starting position by pushing off the floor with your front leg. (Do not perform this exercise if it causes knee pain.) Flexibility may limit your ability to reach 90-degree flexion.

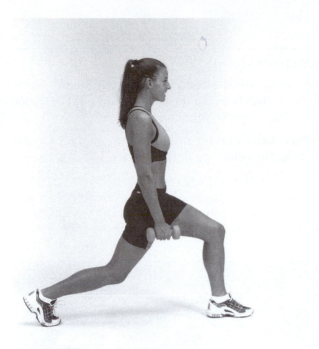

Figure 10.65a

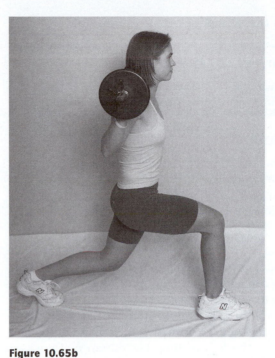

Figure 10.65b

Double-Leg Curls

Muscles worked: hamstrings, quardriceps (rectus femoris)

Muscle action: knee and hip flexion

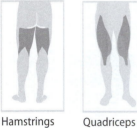

Hamstrings   Quadriceps

POSITION—BALL

Lie on your back on the floor with your ankles and lower legs resting on the ball. Lift your buttocks up until your body forms a straight line between your shoulders and ankles. Arms remain on the floor.

ACTION   Roll the ball toward you by pulling your heels toward you until your knees are flexed to a right angle

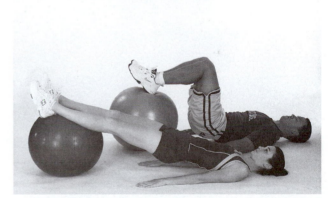

Figure 10.66

(Figure 10.66). To increase the difficulty, place your feet closer together on the ball. If you keep your body straight, bending only your knees, this works primarily hamstrings. If you bend at the hips the quadriceps also become involved.

LOWER BODY SINGLE-JOINT EXERCISES

Leg Curl (Flexion)

Muscles worked: hamstrings

Muscle action: knee flexion

POSITION

Lie prone on the floor. Fold your arms, turn your head to one side, and rest it down on your arms. Place your left ankle over your right ankle.

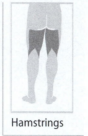

Hamstrings

ACTION Flex your right leg (leg curl) while pushing downward with your left (Figure 10.67). Your left leg should provide enough resistance so that your right leg can only be brought up slowly. Stop when the right leg reaches a 90-degree angle. Be sure that the leg being curled stays in alignment. Do not allow the lower part of your leg to be pushed to the side.

Note: The leg creating the resistance also gets a workout. The quadriceps muscle is slowly lengthening against the push of the curling leg. This creates what is called an eccentric (lengthening) contraction.

POSITION—BAND

Lie prone. Tie the band around both ankles; leave about an inch between the ankles. Hands can be under your chin or under your hips.

ACTION Bend one leg up toward the buttocks while holding the other leg down (Figure 10.68a). Slowly lower your leg.

VARIATION For a more advanced exercise, stand and bend one leg up toward the buttocks (Figure 10.68b). Slowly lower your leg.

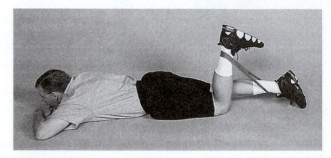

Figure 10.68a

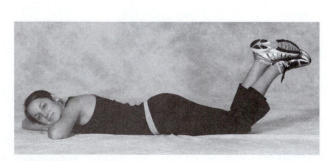

Figure 10.67

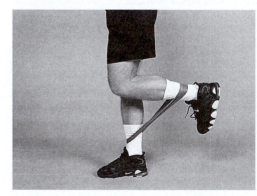

Figure 10.68b

Hip Extension

Muscles worked: gluteus maximus (with hamstring and abdominal stabilization)

Muscle action: hip extension

Note: Hip extension can be performed lying prone on the floor, kneeling, or standing. It can be done in isolation (just hip action) or combined with shoulder action. Two exercises which combine hip and

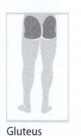

Gluteus maximus

shoulder movement were presented as core exercises earlier in the chapter (see pages 132–143); Figure 10.50 shows you how to lie prone and lift one arm and one leg, and a variation explains how to perform a similar exercise in a kneeling position. The two exercises presented here isolate the hip extension action; using the band adds resistance.

POSITION

Assume an all-fours position. Lift the working leg up off the floor. Flex this leg 90 degrees. Keep your hips flat. Flex your foot (Figure 10.69a).

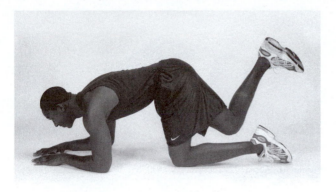

Figure 10.69a

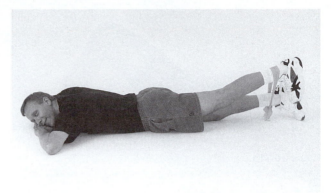

Figure 10.70

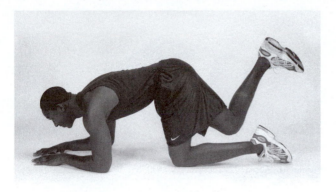

Figure 10.69b Stages of change.

ACTION Keeping your hips flat, lift your leg upward. It probably won't lift very high if you are in a correct position (Figure 10.69b). Lower your leg.

POSITION—BAND

Tie the band around both ankles; leave about an inch between the ankles. Lie prone.

ACTION Keeping your legs straight, lift up one leg with the heel leading. Keep both hips in contact with the floor (Figure 10.70). Slowly lower your leg.

VARIATION A standing hip extension exercise (not shown here) is really an upright version of the prone exercise. Stand on one leg and extend the other straight back with or without a band.

POSITION—PELVIC TILT

Lie on the back with knees bent and feet on the floor about shoulder width apart.

ACTION Press your lower back into the floor by tilting your pelvis. Continue to roll your pelvis under while tightening your buttocks and lift your hips off the floor (Figure 10.71a) until your body creates a straight line. Lifting too high will arch your back. Roll down and release the pelvic tilt or lower your pelvis without touching your buttocks to the floor; repeat the lift. Rolling in and out of the position involves the abdominal muscles to a greater degree.

VARIATIONS

1. Vary the distance between the feet. (Some people feel knee discomfort when the feet are close together. If you feel knee discomfort, don't do this variation.)

2. Cross one leg over the other knee and lift as before (Figure 10.71b), or extend one leg upward and lift as before (Figure 10.71c). When one leg is off the floor, this becomes an advanced exercise, since it requires greater body stabilization.

3. Perform the exercise with the legs resting on a stability ball.

POSITION—WITH LEG FLEXION

Assume the all-fours position (on hands and knees). Lower your shoulders by taking the weight off your hands and putting it onto your forearms. Extend the working leg out to the back. Flex the foot with the heel facing directly up to the ceiling, toes touching the ground (Figure 10.72a).

ACTION 1 Keeping a straight leg, lift the working leg until it is aligned with your back (Figure 10.72b).

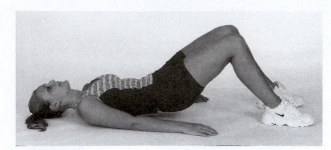

Figure 10.71a

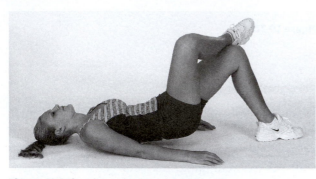

Figure 10.71b Advanced.

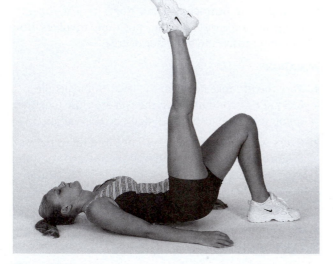

Figure 10.71c Advanced.

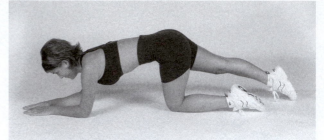

Figure 10.72a

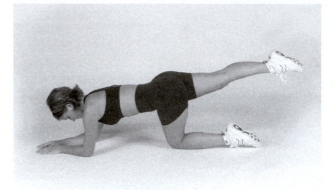

Figure 10.72b

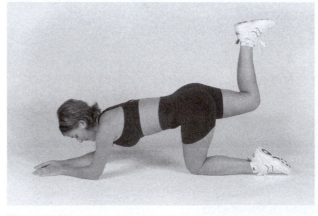

Figure 10.73

Lower and touch your toes to the ground. The gluteals and hamstrings are both active during this exercise.

ACTION 2 Lift the working leg until it is aligned with your back (Figure 10.72b). Maintain the knee position, flex your leg, and bring your heel toward your buttocks (Figure 10.73). Then straighten your leg. In this exercise, the hamstrings are targeted while the gluteals act as stabilizers (along with the trunk and arm muscles).

Note: Muscle action 2 for this position includes both hip extension (Action 1) and leg flexion.

Leg Extension

Muscles worked: quadriceps

Muscle action: knee extension

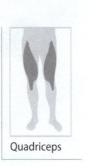

Quadriceps

POSITION—BAND

Tie the band around both ankles; leave about an inch between the ankles. Sit with your knees bent and your feet flat on the floor. Lean back on your forearms. This exercise can also be performed sitting on a step or a stability ball.

ACTION Extend one leg forward (Figure 10.74). Slowly lower the leg.

POSITION—BALL

Sit on the ball with your feet on the floor shoulder width apart. Place your hands on the ball near your hips or on your thighs. Sit with your spine in a neutral position.

ACTION Extend one leg forward and parallel to the floor while maintaining good sitting alignment (Figure 10.75).

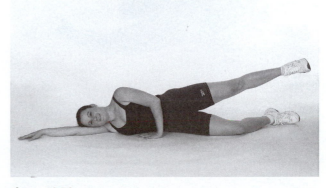

Figure 10.74

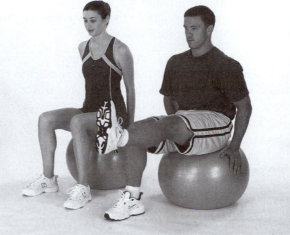

Figure 10.75

Outer Thigh Leg Lift

Muscles worked: gluteus medius, gluteus minimus, tensor fasciae latae

Muscle action: hip abduction

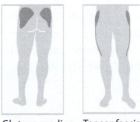

Gluteus medius and minimus   Tensor fasciae latae

POSITION—STRAIGHT LEG

Lie on your right side with your left hip directly above your right hip. Keep your upper body flat along the ground or support raised shoulders with your right

Figure 10.76

forearm flat on the floor. The bottom leg may be bent for balance.

ACTION Lift the top leg straight up, and then lower it down (Figure 10.76). Keep your knee facing directly toward the front. (If the knee rotates to the ceiling, the muscles on the front of the leg, instead of the outer thigh muscles, do the work.)

VARIATIONS

1. Alternately point and flex your toe.

2. Raise the leg only halfway up, and then lower it down (smaller range of motion).

3. Raise the leg all the way up, and then lower it only halfway down.

POSITION—BENT LEG (ACCORDIANS)

Lie on your right side with your upper body positioned as described in the straight leg lift. Bend both knees 90 degrees and flex slightly at your hips for comfort. Adjust the bottom leg for balance.

ACTION Raise the top leg, and then lower it. Keep your knee facing forward and the lower leg parallel to the ground (Figure 10.77). (If the knee points toward the ceiling, the muscles on the front of the thigh will work instead of the outer thigh muscles.) By bending your knees, you will lift less weight than when you keep your legs straight.

Note: This is a modified position, generally less difficult than the straight leg lift.

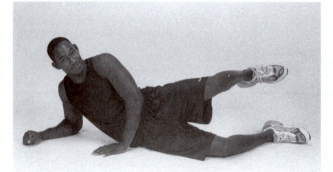

Figure 10.77

POSITION—ALL FOURS (HYDRANTS)

Support your body on all fours. Keep your weight centered. Your elbows should be straight but not locked.

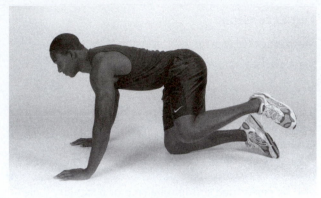

Figure 10.78

Your head should be in line with your back. Turn your body sideways to the instructor so that your head can be turned (rather than lifted) to view the instructor. Place your hands shoulder width apart with fingers facing forward. Pull in your abdomen.

ACTION Keeping your weight centered and leg bent, lift your left leg to the side and then lower it (Figure 10.78). Lift until you feel resistance. Do not lift the working hip. If a yardstick was placed on your back, the yardstick should remain parallel to the floor throughout the exercise. Another test to see if your weight is centered is to raise your right arm when your left leg is working. (If your hip is allowed to rise, some of the back muscles are doing the work.) This exercise requires more core stabilization than the exercises performed lying down.

POSITION—SIDE STEP WITH BAND

Stand with your feet together and knees slightly flexed. Tie and place the band above your knees (beginner), or below your knees (intermediate), or around your ankles (advanced).

ACTION Step to one side, maintaining a slight knee bend. Slowly slide in the opposite foot, bringing your feet back together (Figure 10.79a). The outer thigh can also be worked using a side-lying leg lift (Figure 10.79b).

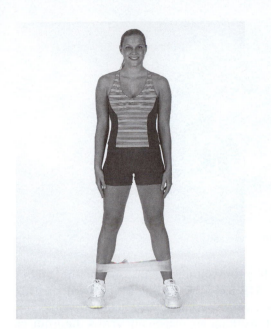

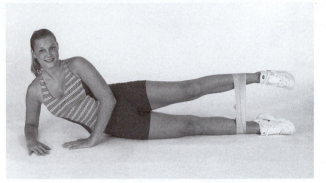

Figure 10.79b

Figure 10.79a

Inner Thigh Leg Lift

Muscles worked: adductors (adductor magnus, adductor longus, adductor brevis, pectineus, gracilis)

Muscle action: hip adduction

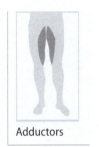

Adductors

POSITION—STRAIGHT LEG

Lie on your right side. Bend your left leg and allow the knee and lower leg to rest on the floor in front of your body (Figure 10.80). Keep your left hip directly above your right hip.

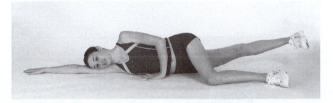

Figure 10.80

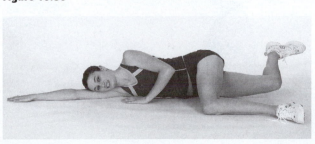

Figure 10.81

ACTION With your inner thigh facing the ceiling, raise and lower your right leg.

VARIATIONS

1. Lift your right leg up and slightly back.

2. Flex and point the toe of your right leg while the leg is held up off the ground. (This involves a static hold of the adductor muscles while flexing the ankles uses the gastrocnemius and soleus muscles.)

3. Circle your right leg forward and then back.

4. Hold your right leg off the ground while bending and straightening your knee (Figure 10.81). (This involves a static hold of the adductor muscles, while flexing the knee uses the hamstring muscles.)

POSITION—STRADDLE

Lie on your back. Extend your legs straight up in the air. Straddle your legs and place your hands or forearms on the inside of your thighs. (Lack of flexibility may make this uncomfortable for some, since it requires the hip flexors and abdominal muscles to hold the legs vertical.)

ACTION Bring your legs together while resisting with your hands (Figure 10.82), then relax. Start with easy resistance and build up. (Arm and shoulder muscles also work in this exercise.) This exercise can also be done with a partner providing resistance.

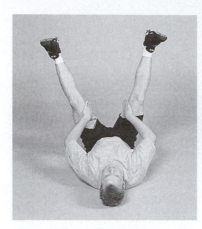

Figure 10.82

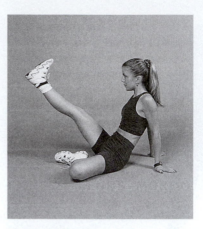

Figure 10.83 Advanced.

POSITION—SEATED (ADVANCED)

This is for people at an advanced fitness level only—it may cause lower back strain. Sit up tall with your legs extended forward along the floor. Place your hands on the floor behind your buttocks. Bend the nonworking leg so that your knee is close to your buttocks. Take the working leg to the side and rotate it at the hip so that your inner thigh is facing the ceiling.

ACTION Raise your leg and then lower it (Figure 10.83).

VARIATION Raise your leg and then lower it as you move it to the front and then back out to the side. (Hip rotator muscles are also worked in this exercise.)

POSITION—BAND

Tie the band around both ankles with about an inch between the ankles. Lie on one side with your top leg bent and the knee placed on the floor in front of the body.

ACTION Lift your bottom leg up toward the ceiling (Figure 10.84). Slowly lower the leg to the floor. This exercise can also be performed in a standing position by pulling the working leg diagonally across the front of your body. You can make this exercise easier by placing the band closer to your knees.

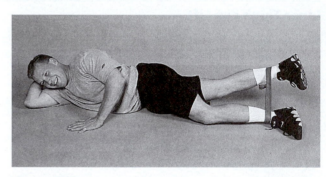

Figure 10.84

LOWER LEG

Ankle Flexion

Muscle worked: tibialis anterior

Muscle action: ankle dorsi flexion

POSITION—BAND

Sit on the floor with your knees bent in front of your body and your hands supporting behind your buttocks. The band, tied snugly around both feet, should run across the top of the arch of your right foot and under the sole of your left foot.

Tibialis anterior

ACTION Flex your right foot—that is, draw your toes toward your shin (Figure 10.85). Slowly point (relax) your foot.

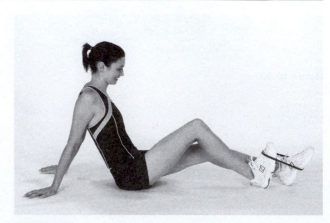

Figure 10.85

Ankle Extension

Muscles worked: gastrocnemius, soleus

Muscle action: ankle extension, point toe

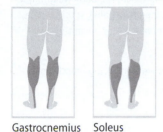

Gastrocnemius   Soleus

POSITION—BAND

Sit on the floor with your legs extended out in front. Hold one end of the band in each hand with the band running across the ball of one or both of your feet. Your foot should be in a flexed position.

ACTION Extend your foot by pointing your toes (Figure 10.86). **Caution:** Do not let the band slide off the foot. Slowly flex (relax) your foot.

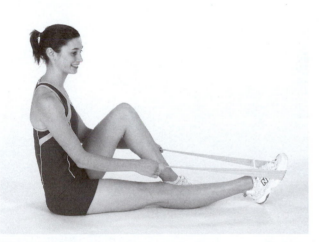

Figure 10.86

POSITION—WEIGHTS

Stand tall with good posture. Hold the weights in your hands down at your sides, palms facing inward.

ACTION Raise up onto the balls of your feet (Figure 10.87). Slowly lower back down until your heels touch. This exercise can be added to the end of a squat to save time.

VARIATION This exercise can also be performed with the balls of your feet on a bench so that your heels can drop below the level of the bench, thus effectively increasing the range of motion in which strength is developed.

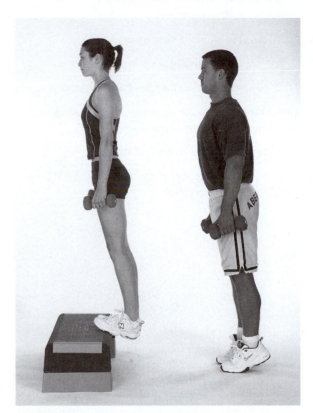

Figure 10.87

SUMMARY

Working muscles correctly will increase your rate of improvement. Be sure to isolate the muscle or muscle group you are trying to train. If your muscles begin to cramp during an exercise, stop and stretch them out. If the instructor and class are doing more of an exercise than you can do, perform one exercise for every two they do. To gain fitness, overload by working until you feel mild discomfort, but never perform an exercise that causes pain. Finally, don't be afraid to modify exercises to make them safer and more comfortable for you.

KNOWLEDGE TIPS

1. The ACSM recommends completing a minimum of 1 set of 8 to 12 repetitions (to near fatigue) of between 8 and 10 exercises that use the major muscle groups on 2 or 3 nonconsecutive days of the week.

2. To progressively overload, increase resistance or perform more sets.

3. You can make an exercise more difficult (intense) by changing position or by adding resistance in the form of weights, bands, balls, or water.

4. Move at a moderate pace and maintain body control throughout resistance exercises.

5. Exercise both muscles of a muscle pair.

6. Use a curling motion during sit-up–type exercises.

7. Avoid exercises that strain the lower back.

8. Protect the lower back during exercises by contracting core muscles and maintaining a neutral spine.

9. If muscle cramping occurs, stop and stretch.

10. Breathe out during the work phase of an exercise and breathe in during the relaxation phase.

THINK ABOUT IT

1. Explain how increasing strength can help increase muscular endurance.

2. Resistance can be created using machines, body weight, free weights (dumbbells, barbells, medicine balls), stability balls, exercise bands, and water. Explain the key advantages to each type of resistance.

3. Identify pairs of exercises that work opposing muscles or muscle groups.

4. Put together a workout with 8 to 10 exercises using the major muscles of the body.

5. What are key technique points for performing resistance exercises? Include body position and proper use of equipment.

6. Stability balls create an unstable environment in which to exercise. Explain why an unstable environment can be an advantage.

7. Explain what proper breathing technique is when using resistance training.

11

The Mind-Body Connection

"Where does the body end and the mind begin?
Where does the mind end and the spirit begin?
They cannot be divided as they are interrelated
and but different aspects of the same all-pervading
divine consciousness."

B. K. S. IYENGAR

- What does a mind-body connection mean?
- How do I develop a mind-body connection?
- How can I get myself to relax? Feel more connected? Less stressed?
- What is the difference between pilates and yoga?

Who hasn't had a nagging thought or an inner voice that just won't go away? Today many of us juggle demands such as coursework, jobs, social events, and family responsibilities; as we run from one activity to the next, we constantly chatter and mutter to ourselves. Sometimes these conversations inside our heads help us solve problems or remember things, but sometimes they can be a nuisance or even hinder us from getting things done. Seldom is the inner voice quieted and thought allowed to shift inward. Those who take the time to tune out the demands of the outer world and focus on the inner one often find an enhanced connection with their bodies and feel physically and mentally renewed. For this reason, over recent years there has been a growing interest in activities such as yoga, pilates, the martial arts, and meditation—activities that encourage a mind-body connection and promote healthy lifestyles.

Before discussing some of the specific methods of achieving a mind-body connection, let's look more closely at what it means to connect the mind and body. Stress, both good (eutress) and bad (distress) and the immune system are at the heart of this idea. That mental stress affects our bodies is pretty intuitive, but how it does so and to what extent is not as obvious. Hans Selye, an astute observer of behavior, recognized in the 1940s that regardless of the type of stress, good or bad, the stress response was similar. For example, the physical stress response of nervousness, sweating, and a pounding heart can occur right before you ask someone out on a date or just before an exam. And a yes for the date provides an adrenaline rush, whereas a failing grade on an exam registers in the pit of our stomach. Interestingly, the stress response will occur whether the cause of the stress is real or perceived. In other words, if you think you are in danger, your body will react the same way as when you are in danger. Furthermore, people's perceptions of the same situation can be quite different. For example, for some people speaking in front of a crowd is frightening, and thus elicits a stress response, whereas others find it enjoyable.

Whatever the cause of stress, once the alarm has been raised you will experience physical reactions that are often described as the "fight-or-flight" response. One of the problems with modern living is that too often we confront stressful situations but do not have the opportunity to vent them physically. The hunter/gatherer who was surprised by a wild animal would run. Today, when presented with an unrealistic deadline, the college student whose blood pressure spikes doesn't usually run—although this might be a very healthy idea—at least initially! As we have become more sedentary, we have lost our physical outlets for stress, and chronic stress with no relief is harmful to our health. Providing a physical outlet can be very positive both physically and mentally. This is when the body can help the mind, and by calming the mind, we help the body.

A Harvard study in the 1970s found physical evidence of the effects of our mental outlook on our immune system. Immune cells were discovered to have receptors for chemicals called neuropeptides. These chemicals are produced by the brain and vary with emotions. In other words, how you are feeling sends out chemicals to your immune system. Negative factors, such as academic difficulties, pessimism, loneliness, and chronic stress, lower the immune system and make us more susceptible to disease, whereas positive factors such as aerobic exercise, social support, laughter, and satisfying relationships, boost the immune system. The study of how our psyche (brain) influences our immune system is called **psychoneuroimmunology.** Negative thoughts, worry, anxiety, nervousness, and panic all work to bring our physical body down. Positive thinking, viewing life as a fun challenge, feeling in control, and good self-esteem can help us stay healthy.

Remember, some stress is good—it pushes us to new heights, allows us to take on challenges, and keeps us engaged in life. The trick is not to eliminate it, but rather to manage it. Blow steam in healthy ways, keep things in perspective, manage time well, and put a good spin on life. This leads to a healthier immune system and better quality of life. Here are a few ways to manage stress. All of the ideas presented here can be found in much more depth in stress management texts, courses, and resources. For more information, contact the psychology department or health center of your institution.

- Engage in physical activity. It can help clear your mind and give you a chance to regroup when you are feeling overwhelmed. Breakthrough thinking often happens during a walk, jog, golf game, dance, or exercise class. It is almost as though taking your mind off a problem allows your mind to solve it. In a grander sense, meditation or yoga can help you reconnect with what is centrally important so that you refocus your energies to what really matters to you.
- Develop supportive relationships. Share your feelings and accept support from those who truly understand your situation.
- Say no to activities and jobs that will put you over your limits. If you feel the need to help, rather than take on the job yourself, help find someone who can.
- Break the "big job" down into smaller, more manageable pieces and then schedule when you will get these done.

- Expect things to change, and allow yourself to adapt. Life seldom stays the same, and people who continue to hang onto what "was" have difficulty enjoying or coping with what "is."
- Take the time to get organized, physically and mentally. Set your priorities and then manage your time so that these things get done first.
- Spend time with positive people. Their attitude wears off on others! There is good evidence that laughter *is* one of the best medicines.
- Eat good foods and get enough rest. Life is much easier to cope with when we take care of our basic needs. You can get a lot more done when you've eaten energizing foods rather than junk foods that make you feel sluggish.
- Do something for someone else. Giving a gift or doing a kind act always makes you feel better.
- Take control of the stressors you can. Identify them and then work to eliminate them. One person who had difficulty getting the equipment she needed asked to be in charge of equipment. Another who hated traffic rearranged his morning routine so he could leave earlier and avoid it.
- Accept your limitations. You can't do it all, and the "I shoulds" will kill you. Maybe this isn't the semester you are going to organize your closets or fix up the car.
- Change your attitude toward stressors you can't change. We can't control everything, but we can control how we react to things. Try reframing. Here is an example. A term paper is due the next day and you cannot possibly finish in time. You can't change the due date. Rather than continue to worry and be unproductive, you can reframe the situation, accept that you will lose a letter grade for being late, take the extra day, and do it well so that even with the penalty you have a good grade.
- Put a positive spin on things. If you're stuck in traffic with children in the car, you have a choice: fret and swear, or spend some quality time with the kids.
- Learn to relax. Try some of the techniques presented in this chapter and create your own way of finding time for yourself.

Pilates, yoga, progressive relaxation, mental imagery, and autogenic training are discussed in this chapter. These activities are often of interest to participants in aerobic dance exercise, and sometimes methods or techniques from one or more of them are incorporated into an aerobic dance (or wellness) class.

PILATES

Pilates is a method of mental and physical conditioning that aims to develop strength balanced with flexibility. To fully appreciate the method and the choices available, here is a little background.

Pilates is the life work of German-born Joseph Pilates. After suffering from rickets, asthma, and rheumatic fever as a boy, Joseph focused his life on finding and honing a method of exercise that promotes strength and good health. He became strong through his dedicated study of exercise, and by age 14 he was modeling for anatomical drawings. By age 32 he had moved to England where he performed in the circus and became a self-defense trainer for English detectives. At the outbreak of World War I, Joseph was interned in England with other German nationals. During this time, he worked in an infirmary and developed a method of exercise he called "contrology," which he taught to others interned with him. He gained recognition when none of his "students" died during the influenza epidemic of 1918. In 1926, Joseph immigrated to the United States. With his wife Clara, he opened a small studio in New York City called Pilates Studio, Inc., to teach his method of exercise. Pilates caught the attention of the dance community, including influential choreographers George Balanchine and Martha Graham, who referred a number of dancers to them. Joseph lived a long, healthy life. When he died in 1967 at the age of 87, his wife continued to operate the studio with the help of one of Balanchine's former dancers, Romana Kryzanowska, who had studied with Joseph many years prior. Romana continues to teach and train instructors today in the original Pilates method, while many other students of Pilates Studio have set up their own classes. Some of them have also trained instructors who, in turn, have gone on to teach contemporized versions of the Pilates method. Although this is discouraged by those who prefer to teach the original method, others recognize the value of embracing more recent research. For example, Moira Stott-Merrithew, the founder of Stotts Pilates, teaches use of a neutral spine position rather than a flat back, because the neutral spine allows for the normal curvatures of the spine and is the position of greatest mechanical advantage.

Instructors who teach contemporized versions of Joseph Pilates' method had to refer to their classes as "like Pilates" or something similar, until the year 2000, when a court decision declared "pilates" a generic term (like yoga and karate) and rescinded the trademarks previously held by Pilates Studio, Inc. This means that now all who teach this type of exercise can use the name and advertise their classes as pilates classes, even if they do not teach the original method.

Joseph Pilates developed more than 500 exercises, most of which are performed lying down. Some are performed using special equipment he designed, and some are done on a mat (hence the pilates term "mat class" for a common type of instruction using no equipment). The equipment, which uses cables and springs to create resistance, adjusts for body size and needs. The most popular pieces of equipment include the reformer, Cadillac or trapeze table, chair, and different sized barrels. Multiple exercises can be performed on each piece of equipment. To see examples of pilates equipment, go online to www.pilates.com.

The Pilates method of body conditioning has six original principles.[1]

1. Concentration: One must pay attention to how the body moves and how each part of the body is interconnected with the rest of the body. The mind must be engaged during every move— the mind and body work as a team.
2. Control: All physical movement must be controlled by the mind.
3. Centering: One's center is the "powerhouse," which consists of the muscles of the abdomen, lower back, and buttocks. These muscles support the spine and internal organs and are important in maintaining good posture. All movement begins at the center and flows out from there.
4. Flowing movement: All movements are to be done smoothly and evenly, not in a rushed or jerky manner.
5. Precision: Control must be used to ensure that all movements are performed correctly each time.
6. Breathing: The bloodstream is purified (oxygenated and eliminated of noxious gases) with proper breathing technique. Breathe in to prepare for a movement, and breathe out as you execute it.

The "core," or basic, exercises of the Pilates method work the core muscles described in Chapter 2. The result is a flatter abdomen, strong lean muscles, and better control and coordination of movements involving the limbs. Pilates also:

- improves core strength and stability (balance)
- balances strength and flexibility (longer, leaner muscles)
- is a nonimpact exercise that is easy on the joints
- improves coordination

1. S. P. Gallagher and R. Kryzanoska. *The Pilates Method of Body Conditioning.* Philadelphia: BainBridgeBooks, 1999.

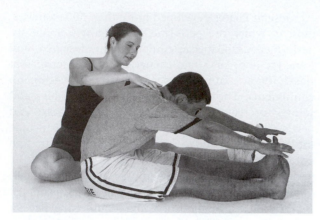

Figure 11.1 The pilates roll-up exercise.

- improves circulation
- improves posture
- heightens body awareness (mind-body connection)
- helps prevent injuries and relieve low-back pain
- improves sports performance
- enhances functional fitness (ability to do daily activities)

Basic exercises include the roll-up, the hundred, the single and double leg stretches, and single leg circles. It is extremely important that these exercises be performed with proper technique and control of the spine. This is achieved by recruiting the deep postural muscles in addition to the more surface abdominal muscles. The roll-up (Figure 11.1) is similar to a straight leg sit-up, which due to the potential for low-back strain is contraindicated for many individuals. However, under proper supervision and with controlled precise rolling of the spine, this can be a safe and effective exercise. The hundred is another example of an exercise in which the back position must be monitored carefully and a progression of positions employed based on the individual's core strength. It is critical that the back remain pressed into the floor (mat) throughout the exercise. (Some instructors refer to this as imprinting the back on the floor.) The easiest body position is lying on the back with the knees bent and feet on the floor. The next position in the progression is with the feet up (Figure 11.2a); shins can be parallel to the floor or higher depending on comfort and strength. The most difficult leg position (Figure 11.2b) is with the legs extended and lowered as far as the individual can go without shaking. This advanced position is, in essence, a double leg lift, which is normally considered an exercise to avoid. It comes off the avoid list when the individual has enough strength to maintain good spinal positioning. The arms extend toward the feet and are held just a few inches off the floor. The upper spine is curled upward lifting the shoulder blades off the floor. To begin the exercise, extend the legs to the desired position while simultaneously curling the upper body. While holding this position, the arms are pumped up and down (a few inches) in coordination with short breaths. The breathing is done in cycles. Each cycle is five short in-breaths and then five short out-breaths. The name of the exercise, the hundred, represents the goal of performing 100 arm pumps with coordinated breathing (10 cycles). The shoulders and neck should remain relaxed throughout. A modification, which leaves the head and shoulders on the floor, can be used as needed. All of the pilates exercises are to be initiated by the center of the body (the powerhouse). To be successful, participants must focus on the deep stabilizing muscles, clearing their minds of everything else.

There are many excellent pilates classes being taught in both traditional and contemporary forms.

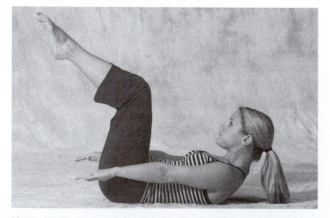

Figure 11.2a Beginner's position for the pilates hundred. This can also be performed with the feet on the floor.

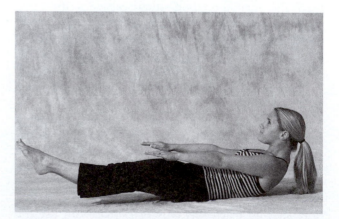

Figure 11.2b Advanced position for the hundred. When the legs are extended, it is critical that the low back remain in contact with the floor or mat.

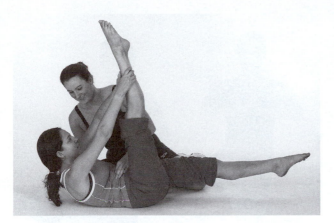

Figure 11.3 An instructor's touch can help a pilates student focus on the right muscles and technique.

Unfortunately, there are also classes being taught by instructors who have minimal training in pilates. Certification programs range from 600 hours of internship to weekend workshops. It is important to select an instructor with both training and experience. Mat classes are the most popular form of pilates because they can be taught in many locations and involve only mats for equipment. They are also more conducive for group instruction. Smaller groups are best because the instructor can better watch and assist participants. An instructor's touch can help a participant mentally and physically locate and focus on muscles and proper technique (Figure 11.3).

Joseph Pilates felt strongly that thought and movement have to emanate from the inside out. He believed that the stabilizing benefits of beginning all movement from the center, accompanied by focused mental practice, will carry over into daily life. He felt that the discipline of focus and the greater body awareness forge a mind-body connection that changes not only how a person moves but also how he or she approaches life. And he is not alone. Pilates exercise is now enjoyed by dancers, theatre groups, professional athletes, rehabilitation clients, and fitness enthusiasts around the world.

YOGA

The practice of **yoga,** an ancient Eastern Indian philosophical tradition dating back 5,000 years, has been growing in popularity in Western countries for a variety of reasons. Some people see it as a way to increase strength, stamina, and flexibility; some use it to reduce stress; others more fully embrace its philosophy and begin the "path to enlightenment." Although it is one of the oldest forms of exercise and has more than 100 years of history in the United States, yoga practice is

one of the top fitness trends in the country. Singing its praises are celebrities, like Oprah Winfrey and Ricky Martin, professional athletes like Kareem Abdul Jabbar and Maria Sharapova, former Supreme Court justice Sandra Day O'Connor, and dancers, physical therapists, and, of course, many of the rest of us. Classes are available at health clubs, yoga centers, dance centers, community centers, hospitals, and rehabilitation clinics, and may be offered at your college or university. Some insurance companies recognize the benefits of yoga and offer their yoga-taking members a discount.

Although in the Western world many people treat yoga as a form of exercise, it is actually a philosophy. Yoga embraces the ideas of living in harmony and achieving an inner peace, and it has as its ultimate goal a journey to *samadhi,* or self-realization. Yoga is accepted by, and influenced by, the Hindu religion. Yet, most people outside the Hindu faith find they can embrace the yoga philosophy and practice it without interference with their religious beliefs. In yoga, there is no distinction between where the mind leaves off and the body begins. The practice of yoga is directed toward realizing this connection between the mind and the body.

Yoga is often described as a tree with deep tangled roots, a big stem, large branches, and many secondary branches. There are six major branches in yoga (although some sources list four pathways, with hatha under raja): hatha yoga, raja yoga, karma yoga, bhakti yoga, jnana yoga, and tantra yoga. Each branch offers a path to the divine. **Hatha yoga** is the physical aspect of yoga; it is what most Americans refer to when they speak simply of yoga.

Hatha yoga is practiced through the use of various poses called *asanas,* through breathing techniques called *pranayama,* and through meditation. The goal of hatha yoga is to transcend the mind-body connection and fuse the mind, body, and soul into one. The asanas are meant to help bring a person away from the awareness of the body toward the consciousness of the soul. In the words of yogi Iyengar:

> The primary aim of yoga is to restore the mind to simplicity and peace and free it from confusion and distress. This sense of calm comes from the practice of yogic asanas and pranayama. Unlike other forms of exercise which strain muscles and bones, yoga gently rejuvenates the body. By restoring the body, yoga frees the mind from the negative feelings caused by the fast pace of modern life. The practice of yoga fills up the reservoirs of hope and optimism within you. It helps you overcome all obstacles on the path to perfect health and spiritual contentment. It is a rebirth.

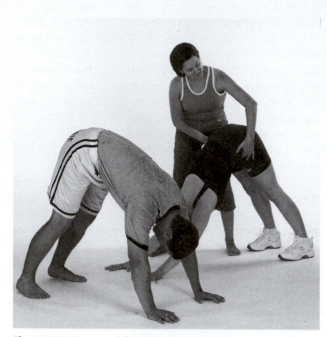

Figure 11.4 Downward facing dog asana.

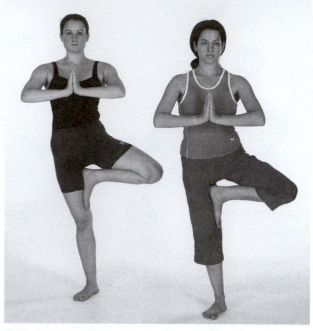

Figure 11.5 Tree asana.

Asanas such as downward facing dog (Figure 11.4) and the tree (Figure 11.5) are used to build strength, flexibility, and endurance. Someone unfamiliar with the tenets of yoga could move through these positions and achieve strength, balance, and flexibility but might miss out on the important philosophy of the mind-body connection.

The practice of pranayama unites the breath with the mind. It is not deep breathing, but rather the gentle, full inhalation and full slow exhalation during which the *prana*, which means energy or life force, is absorbed by the mind and the body. A variety of breathing techniques are used—some to invoke relaxation, others to energize. Respiration is improved through breathing exercises. But more important, breathing is used to focus attention on the body and on the stillness that exists both inside and outside of us.

One of the great beauties of yoga is that a person can focus on the physical, psychological, or spiritual aspects, or combine all three. Yoga is believed to:

- calm/relax and stimulate body and mind
- stimulate organs and glands
- remove toxins
- counteract stress and disease
- produce fitness (strength, flexibility, some cardiorespiratory)
- strengthen bones and muscles
- correct posture
- improve breathing (respiration)

- increase energy
- balance effort and relaxation
- promote healing
- alleviate pain or help in the tolerance of pain
- have a positive effect on hypertension for some
- help control some aspects of asthma and epilepsy
- provide mental clarity
- promote self-understanding
- promote inner peace

One big difference between yoga and other forms of exercise is that it is process oriented versus product oriented. The focus is on how you *feel* during an exercise and is about building an *awareness* of what you are doing rather than counting how many of something you can do. To ensure that a pose feels right, a good instructor will demonstrate modification and encourage you to make the choice that works for you at that moment in time. You should stretch or strengthen in a way that comfortably matches the present condition of your mind and body; this can be different from day to day—even within a day. It is not about straining to achieve a set goal, but rather to enjoy and be fulfilled through the process. Challenging yourself can be part of the process as long as it feels right. Figures 11.6, 11.7, and 11.8 demonstrate how exercises can be modified so that you can choose one that matches your flexibility, balance, and strength. Some yoga positions require extreme flexibility and are contraindicated in

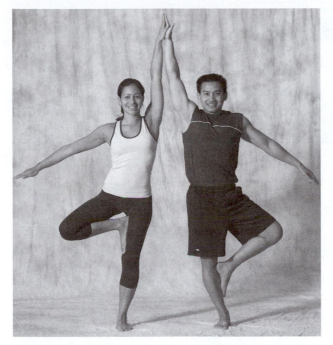

Figure 11.6 A partner is used in this modified tree asana to assist with balance.

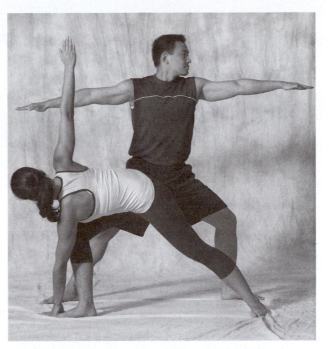

Figure 11.7 As strength improves, the lunge can progress to the warrior (male). The triangle pose can progress to the reverse triangle (female).

traditional exercise programs. In proper yoga practice, a position that is harmful or painful for an individual would never be encouraged. Careful progressions are needed to attain the advanced yoga positions. Although strength can be a by-product, yoga is more endurance oriented than strength oriented. Its goal is to tone muscles, not create size (bulk).

There are a number of styles of hatha yoga, ranging from meditative to highly vigorous. An emphasis may be placed on the release of energy, relaxation, therapy, postural alignment, inner focus, detoxification, strength, balance, or flexibility. In addition, yoga can be challenging or more relaxing, depending on how it is performed. Some styles challenge you by holding poses, whereas other styles link together poses in a single flow, which can be very physically demanding and result in cardiorespiratory benefits. Ashtanga yoga, Bikram's yoga, Iyengar yoga, and Power yoga (based on Ashtanga) are some of the more physically challenging styles. Other types of yoga include Integral, Ananda (more gentle), Kripalu, Kundalini, Sivananda, and Viniyoga. These yogas all share a common lineage back to Patanjali's *Yoga Sutras,* a text written sometime between the second century B.C. and the first century A.D., that outlines the basic philosophy and practices of classical yoga.

Selecting a yoga class and instructor that meet your needs is very important. The styles are quite different, and hybrid styles are continually emerging. The class

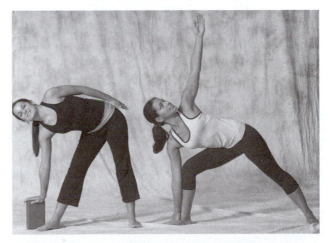

Figure 11.8 During the triangle, the supporting hand can be placed anywhere along the leg, or on a block, to allow for different degrees of flexibility.

should feel comfortable and rewarding (not an obligation), and you can and should modify the movements to meet your energy. Many instructors teach an eclectic style, using methods from more than one traditional approach. It takes considerable training and maturity to be a good yoga instructor. Look for someone with experience, and watch or take a trial class. People are

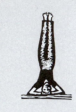

WHO'S WHO IN YOGA

In yoga, there are several terms for those who practice and teach. Here are a few:

• A *yogi* is someone who practices yoga.

• A *yogin* is a male student; a *yogini* is a female student.

• A *guru* is a teacher.

• *Swami* is a title of respect for a spiritual master.

often confused by the terms used to identify those who practice and teach yoga. See the Who's Who in Yoga box for an explanation of some of the names.

A good setting for yoga is one in which the instructor can easily assist you throughout class. If the class is large, you lose important individualization. There are also certain high-risk positions, such as the shoulder stand, that require special attention and will probably need to be modified for safety. Match the style of yoga to your personality, but the style is less important than the relationship between you and your instructor.

The practice of yoga has recently become more interesting to researchers. Many past studies have been dismissed because of a lack of proper controls, but two recent studies provide good preliminary evidence of fitness benefits of yoga. Researchers at University of California, Davis, found significant gains in muscular strength, muscular endurance, flexibility, and aerobic capacity for those who practice yoga. Ball State University researchers found that a yoga program improved the lung capacity of all of its student subjects regardless of whether they were athletes, asthmatics, or smokers. With yoga's increasing popularity, more studies are sure to follow. However, sometimes science need not prove the point. If you participate in yoga and feel better, then keep doing it!

PROGRESSIVE RELAXATION, MENTAL IMAGERY, AND AUTOGENIC TRAINING

PROGRESSIVE RELAXATION

Progressive relaxation is a technique that systematically relaxes your skeletal muscles. Edmond Jacobson developed the technique of progressive relaxation based on his beliefs that relaxing skeletal muscles will also relax nearby organs and involuntary muscles, and that a person cannot be nervous or tense in any body part where muscles are relaxed. The program of progressive relaxation consists of alternately tensing and relaxing muscles in a predetermined order. Purposefully creating tension in your muscles will help you recognize when your body is becoming tense at other times and consciously learn to relax it. Jacobson's full training procedure takes months, with whole sessions dedicated to relaxing a single muscle group. However, it is possible to achieve significant relaxation benefits in less time. A session should begin with muscle tensing, but most of the session should be devoted to achieving full relaxation. In the beginning, it may take a while to achieve muscle relaxation. But with practice (usually several months), you will be able to elicit the relaxation response quickly and counteract stress-induced tension. An example of this classic progressive relaxation technique developed by Jacobson is found in the Progressive Relaxation Exercise box.

MENTAL IMAGERY

Progressive relaxation, a physiological (physical) technique, is often combined with **mental imagery,** a cognitive (thought-based) technique. During mental imagery, you imagine yourself doing something special—often performing a task or athletic move that you want to perfect. You may use external imagery, in which you see yourself going through the movement, or you may use internal imagery, in which you feel yourself going through the movement. Research studies show improved performance when mental imagery is used in conjunction with physical practice.

AUTOGENIC TRAINING

Autogenic training was developed by Johannes H. Schultz as a way to relax the body. It is a psychophysiological technique, which means it is a physiological technique that uses the relationship between physiological processes and thoughts, emotions, and behavior. It uses visual metaphors, such as imagining warmth and heaviness to relax. A variety of mental images can be used, such as imagining your body glowing warm like the sun and sinking into the deepest, downiest cloud to achieve even greater relaxation. To

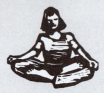

PROGRESSIVE RELAXATION EXERCISE

To begin progressive relaxation, take a comfortable position lying on your back on the floor with your knees straight or bent but not crossed and your arms by your side. Or sit relaxed in a comfortable chair. Spend a few minutes clearing your mind and concentrating on deep breathing. Begin to relax. Now clench your right fist; study the tension in your fist, hand, and forearm as you do so. Relax your fist. Feel the looseness in your hand and arm, and notice the contrast with the tension. Repeat this procedure with your right fist again; always notice as you relax that this is the opposite of tension—feel the difference. Repeat the entire procedure with your left fist, then both fists at once.

Continue this process of clenching and releasing as follows. Always repeat the exercise for each muscle at least once. Flex your biceps (one at a time, then both), scrunch your forehead, squeeze your eyelids closed, bite down with your jaw. Each time you release, notice the sensation of looseness. Really appreciate the contrast between tension and relaxation. Press your tongue against the top of your mouth, purse your lips, press your head back against the floor or back of the chair, then press it forward against your chest, shrug and relax your shoulders.

As your release from each exercise, feel the comfort and heaviness increasing. Breathe in, filling your lungs completely, and hold your breath. Notice the tension. Exhale and let your chest become loose. Repeat several times; notice the tension draining from your body as you exhale. Continue relaxing and breathe freely and gently. Next, tighten your stomach and hold, then arch your back, while keeping the rest of your body as relaxed as possible. Move the clenching and releasing through the rest of your body, one body part at a time: buttocks, thighs, knees, calves, shins, feet, and toes. Feel the relaxation spread deeper and deeper as your focus moves down your body.

Let go more and more until you feel yourself completely relaxed.

---

relax a tense muscle, a person might picture the aching muscle as red and then try to mentally change the color to a cool blue, or imagine the tension as a liquid and let it run out like water. The technique involved is very similar to Jacobson's progressive relaxation method and often begins with muscle-tensing and muscle-relaxing exercises. The full program, a series of six psychophysiological exercises, takes about four months to learn. Audio and video formats and workbooks are available commercially, in addition to course offerings with trained professionals.

SUMMARY

There is strong evidence that the mind and the body are inextricably connected. When either one is out of balance, it affects the other. The basis of pilates is that the focus of the mind helps control and train the body, and the fitness of the body then affects the way we act and think. In yoga, there is no distinction between where the body begins and the mind leaves off. Therefore, the physical training of the body necessarily trains the mind, and similarly the state and discipline of the mind influence the body. They are interrelated and cannot be considered separately. Progressive relaxation, mental imagery, and autogenic training use both the mind and body to help us leave our stressors behind and create a positive internal environment. The belief that the mind and the body are always connected allows us to use both in the healing process of either.

KNOWLEDGE TIPS

1. Many philosophies believe that there is a fundamental connection between the mind and body.

2. Techniques and philosophies such as those used by yoga, pilates, progressive relaxation, mental imagery, and autogenic training promote a mind-body connection and a healthy lifestyle.

3. Aerobic dance instructors sometimes incorporate aspects of mind-body techniques into their classes.

4. Pilates, a practice created by Joseph Pilates, is dedicated to developing a balance between strength and flexibility.

5. Pilates uses exercises on adjustable equipment as well as simple mat exercises to develop the powerhouse, or core muscles of the body: the abdomen, lower back, and buttocks.

6. The six original principles of the Pilates method are concentration, control, centering, flowing movement, precision, and breathing.

7. Yoga is an ancient Eastern Indian philosophical tradition dating back 5,000 years. It consists of physical, psychological, and spiritual aspects to realize the unity of the mind and body.

8. Hatha yoga is the physical aspect of yoga. It is practiced through poses called *asanas,* breathing techniques called *pranayama,* and meditation.

9. Progressive relaxation is a relaxation technique that systematically relaxes your skeletal muscles through tensing and releasing in a specific order.

10. Mental imagery is often used with progressive relaxation. During mental imagery, you imagine yourself doing something.

11. Autogenic training is a psychophysiological technique to induce relaxation through specific mental imagery and muscle-tensing and muscle-relaxing exercises.

THINK ABOUT IT

1. Explain how your mind can influence your body and vice versa. Give an example of a technique that uses the

   - body to influence the mind
   - mind to influence the body

2. If you feel yourself becoming distressed, what can you do to help return yourself to a healthy state of being?

3. What is the philosophical basis behind yoga?

4. What makes pilates different from other forms of strengthening and stretching?

5. Create a mental imagery scenario that will help you handle a stressful situation (i.e., a test).

REFERENCES

Bartholomew, J. B., and B. M. Miller. "Affective Responses to an Aerobic Dance Class: The Impact of Perceived Performance." *Research Quarterly for Exercise and Sport* 73 (No. 3, 2002): 301(9).

Bauman, A. "Is Yoga Enough to Keep You Fit?" *Yoga Journal* 158 (2002): 85–91.

Corliss, R. "The Power of Yoga." *Time,* April 23, 2001, pp. 54–56.

Feuerstein, G., and S. Bodian, with the staff of *Yoga Journal* (editors). *Living Yoga: A Comprehensive Guide for Daily Life.* New York: J. P. Tarcher/Perigee, 1993.

Freedman, F. B., B. Gibbs, D. Hall, E. Kelly, J. Monks, and J. Smith. *Yoga and Pilates for Everyone.* London: Hermes House, 2005.

Friedman, P., and Eisen, G. *The Pilates Method of Physical and Mental Conditioning.* Warner Books, 1982.

Iyengar, B. K. S. *Yoga: The Path to Holistic Health.* New York: Dorling Kindersley, 2001.

Kiecolt-Glaser, J. K., W. Garner, C. E. Speicher, G. Penn, and R. Vlaser. "Psychosocial Modifiers of Immunocompetence in Medical Students." *Psychosomatic Medicine* 46 (1984).

Reddy, P. R., and P. R. Kumar. "A Comparative Study of Yogasanas and Aerobic Dance and Their Effects on Selected Motor Fitness Components in Girl Students. *Research Bi-annual for Movement* 19 (No. 1, 2002): 30–37.

Silvananda Yoga Vedanta Center. *Learn Yoga in a Weekend.* New York: Alfred A. Knopf, 1998.

Stewart, K. *Pilates for Beginners.* Created and produced by Carroll & Brown Publishers, London. First published in the USA by HarperResource, an imprint of Harper-Collins Publishers, New York, 2001.

Stott-Merrithew, M. *Pilates Essential Matwork for Beginners: Stott Pilates with Master Instructor–Trainer Moira Stott-Merrithew.* 2nd ed. Merrithew Corporation, 2001. Videocassette.

Tran, H., J. Lashbrook, and E. A. Amsterdam. "Effects of Hatha Yoga on the Health-Related Aspects of Physical Fitness." *Preventive Cardiology* 4 (2001): 165–170.

12

Nutrition and Weight Control

"Life itself is the proper binge."

JULIA CHILD

- What is a balanced diet?
- What are the best foods to eat?
- Should I drink water or a sports drink?
- How can I best manage my weight?
- How do exercise and diet tie together?

PROPER nutrition and exercise are two of the most valuable tools for developing and maintaining a healthy body. Used together, they are more effective than either one alone. An exercise program without proper nutrition can leave you feeling run-down, depleted of energy, and without the building blocks for muscle and bone development. Similarly, a balanced diet without exercise doesn't result in muscle tone or aerobic efficiency. Put them together, and you not only get the positive effects of each one, you also experience combination benefits. When a weight-loss diet is combined with exercise, more of the weight lost is fat (as opposed to lean body mass) than when dieting is used alone. People are also more successful at maintaining a healthy weight (once they attain it) when exercise is part of the equation. This chapter starts with a review of basic nutritional information, then examines the combined effects of exercise and nutrition on weight control, and finally discredits some popular but false beliefs concerning dieting and weight management.

BASIC NUTRITIONAL INFORMATION

A car needs a variety of fluids to keep it running. You could say its nutritional requirements are gas for fuel; radiator fluid to keep the engine cool; and oil, transmission, and brake fluids to lubricate. If you fail to keep these fluids at appropriate levels, the car either runs poorly or doesn't run at all.

Your body, like a car, requires certain types and quantities of nutrients to function properly. The body's nutrients are chemicals that come from the digestion of food and drink. Your body needs about 50 different nutrients. Organized into six categories, they are referred to as the essential nutrients: carbohydrates, protein, fat, water, vitamins, and minerals.

Collectively, the six essential nutrients provide for the:

- production of energy
- construction and maintenance of cells
- regulation of body processes

Of these six, only three—carbohydrates, fat, and protein—provide energy for the body. When these nutrients are chemically broken down, energy is released. That energy is measured in kilocalories, which the general public calls **calories.** Fat provides almost twice as much energy (9 calories per gram, or g) as carbohydrates and protein (4 calories per g). Although no energy can be obtained from water, vitamins, or minerals, these nutrients play major roles in the many chemical processes of the body, including the processes that result in energy production.

How much of each nutrient do we need? This important question is continually being researched in this country and around the world. Every 5 years in the

United States, this information is reviewed and written into science-based advice (guidelines) on food and physical activity choices for health. The 2005 Dietary Guidelines for Americans is available online at www.health.gov/dietary/guidelines or through the Government Printing Office. Some of the key recommendations are included in this chapter for easy reference.

In addition, the U.S. Food and Nutrition Board of the Institute of Medicine of the National Academies in collaboration with Health Canada released a report in 2002 to provide dietary reference values for the intake of nutrients for healthy Americans and Canadians. The report is titled "Dietary Reference Intakes (DRIs) for Energy, Carbohydrate, Fiber, Fat, Fatty Acids, Cholesterol, Protein and Amino Acids." A summary of some of the key points from this report follows. There will be more on these points in the chapter as the essential nutrients are discussed.

- Adults should get 45 to 65% of their calories from carbohydrates, 20 to 35% from fat, and 10 to 35% from protein.
- Added sugars should comprise not more than 25% of total calories consumed. Added sugars are sugars incorporated into foods and beverages during production, which usually provide insignificant amounts of vitamins, minerals, or other essential nutrients. Major sources include soft drinks, fruit drinks, pastries, candy, and other sweets.
- The recommended daily intake for total fiber for adults 50 years and younger is 38 grams for men and 25 grams for women.
- Using new data, the report reaffirms previously established recommended levels of protein intake, which is 0.8 grams per kilogram of body weight for adults; however, recommended levels for pregnancy are increased.
- The report doesn't set maximum levels for saturated fat, cholesterol, or *trans* fatty acids because increased risk exists at levels above zero; however, the recommendation is to eat as little as possible while consuming a diet adequate in important other essential nutrients.
- To maintain cardiovascular health, regardless of weight, adults and children should achieve a total of at least 1 hour of moderately intense physical activity each day.

You may have already noticed wider ranges on carbohydrates, fats, and proteins. These ranges were expanded to cover a broad spectrum of individual differences and with the goal of minimizing risk of chronic diseases and maximizing the intake of essential nutrients. The recommendations of other health organizations—50 to 60% carbohydrate, less than 30% fat, and 10 to 15% protein—fall within the range of the U.S.-Canada recommendations.

CARBOHYDRATES

Carbohydrates are a major source of energy for the body. They also play a role in the digestion of fat and protein, hence the expression that "fat is burned in a carbohydrate flame," and the concern that low levels of carbohydrates can result in an increased use of protein for energy rather than muscle-building and maintenance.

Carbohydrate foods (sugars and starches) are broken down into the simple sugar **glucose.** Glucose is absorbed into the blood and used by the cells. If it isn't used right away, glucose is stored in the muscles and liver as **glycogen** (long chains of glucose molecules). Glycogen is the preferred fuel for aerobic exercise. There are limits on how much glycogen can be stored. When these limits are reached, additional glucose is converted into fat and stored as adipose tissue.

There are two kinds of carbohydrates: simple and complex. The natural sugars found in fruits and milk and refined sugar are simple carbohydrates. Foods containing high amounts of refined sugars are easily digested and rapidly absorbed into the bloodstream. When enough refined sugar is eaten, it creates a surge in blood sugar. This triggers a release of insulin, which, in reaction to the high concentration of sugar in the blood, sweeps much of the sugar out of the blood. This, in turn, causes a sudden drop in blood sugar that leaves you feeling sluggish, tired, and often hungry. A sugary snack such as a candy bar is not a good way to get quick, lasting energy—that strategy generally backfires!

Foods that are composed of more complex sugars, such as whole-grain cereals and vegetables, are sources of complex carbohydrates. For the most part, these foods take longer to digest, so they are more slowly absorbed into the blood. This prevents quick rises and dips in the level of blood sugar. The resulting steady level of blood sugar helps you maintain your energy level and prevents you from feeling hungry between meals. At least half of all grains should be whole grains. See the accompanying box, Carbohydrates.

Foods can be categorized according to their glycemic index. Foods with a high glycemic index are easily digested and, if eaten alone, result in a surge of sugar in the bloodstream. It may surprise you to learn that some starches have a high glycemic index and can act on blood sugar like simple carbohydrates. These include pasta, white bread, white potatoes, and white rice.

CARBOHYDRATES

KEY RECOMMENDATIONS

- Choose fiber-rich fruits, vegetables, and whole grains often.

- Choose and prepare foods and beverages with little added sugars or caloric sweeteners, in amounts suggested by the USDA Food Guide and the DASH Eating Plan.

- Reduce the incidence of dental caries by practicing good oral hygiene and consuming sugar- and starch-containing foods and beverages less frequently.

Note: DASH stands for Dietary Approaches to Stop Hypertension. The DASH eating plan is available from the National Institutes of Health (NIH). The booklet (also available online) includes two weeks of menus, recipes, and information on weight management.

Good substitutes for these are brown rice and whole-grain breads and pasta.

Nutritionally speaking, it is better to eat complex carbohydrates and natural sugar foods (fruit, milk) than refined sugars because the former contain vitamins, minerals, phytochemicals, and fiber, whereas refined sugars have no nutritional value. Of course, one can't deny that sweets made with those refined sugars have other benefits worth enjoying every now and then! The trick is to consume them in small amounts. As you reach for something sweet, consider also that when it comes to calories (and fat), some choices are better than others. For example, a McDonald's apple pie weighs in at 1,037 calories, a piece of carrot cake rings in at 419, a piece of pumpkin pie at 239, and a brownie or chocolate pudding (4 oz.) at about 150 calories. Of course, if you like to eat four brownies but would eat only one piece of cake, the point is moot.

Fiber (or roughage) is a general term for food substances that the body can't fully digest. Fiber is made up of complex chains of carbohydrates that the human digestive system lacks the enzymes to break. There are two types of dietary fiber: soluble and insoluble. Soluble fiber wraps around fats and promotes their excretion. Insoluble fiber combines with water and gives bulk to the stool. Bulk encourages waste products to move more quickly out of the body, thereby reducing the time that potential cancer-causing substances remain in the colon. Good food sources of fiber include whole (not refined) grains, fruits, and vegetables. Animal foods do not contain fiber. A high-fiber diet:

- helps maintain regularity
- helps fill you up and keeps you from getting hungry so fast
- provides good nutrients because sources of fiber are nutrient dense

- helps prevent constipation, hemorrhoids, and diverticulitis
- reduces cancer risk, especially colon and rectal cancer
- lowers "bad" blood cholesterol (low-density lipoprotein, or LDL)

A coincidental benefit is that high-fiber diets tend to be low in saturated fats and thus help to reduce the risk of cardiovascular disease.

In general, the more a food is processed, the less fiber it contains. See the Fiber: Where It Is . . . Where It Isn't . . . box on page 170 for an example. Women need about 25 grams of fiber per day and men 38 grams—too much or too little can cause difficulties. Add fiber to your diet gradually, and drink plenty of fluids so that you don't experience gastrointestinal distress. Your body needs time to adjust.

PROTEIN

Your body needs **protein** to build and repair body tissues, to make hemoglobin (which carries oxygen), to form antibodies (which fight infection), to produce enzymes and hormones, and, when necessary, to supply energy. When protein foods are digested, they are broken down into amino acids. There are nine amino acids that the body cannot manufacture. These nine are called essential amino acids. Foods that contain all the essential amino acids are called complete proteins; those that contain only some of the essential amino acids are called incomplete proteins. Complete protein sources, such as meat, have all the essential amino acids. If, however, you are a vegetarian or eat very little meat, you need to eat a wide variety of grains, vegetables, and seeds to get all the essential amino acids. In the past, it was believed that two

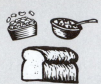

FIBER: WHERE IT IS . . . WHERE IT ISN'T . . .

Fiber is in plant leaves, roots, seeds, and skins. The more plant foods are processed, the less fiber they will contain. Take, for example, an apple:

raw with peel	3.6 g
½ cup applesauce	2.1 g
apple juice	0.2 g

To make sure that you are getting whole grains, read the labels. Do not be fooled by labels with the following ingredients: wheat flour, enriched flour, or degerminated corn meal. Also be careful of 12-grain product labels. Check the ingredient list to see whether any of the 12 grains are whole.

There are many good high-fiber foods. This abbreviated list contains some that students on the go can obtain easily, carry with them, or keep handy in the car. And remember, these foods are excellent fuel sources rich in vitamins, phytochemicals, and minerals.

- salads containing lots of vegetables, tabouli salad
- sandwiches with vegetables: romaine lettuce, peppers, onions, etc.
- pizza with vegetables or fruit: broccoli, green pepper, pineapple, etc.
- apples, pears, and oranges
- pasta sauce with vegetables added
- whole-grain pastas
- whole-grain cereal (for breakfast or eat dry for snack; keeps well in the car)
- seeds or nuts, such as shelled almonds; these make handy "staying" snacks
- baked potato topped with vegetables, such as broccoli (choose instead of fries)
- soups containing whole grains, such as barley
- whole-grain crackers

---

complementary incomplete proteins had to be eaten together at the same meal. Now it is known that as long as they are eaten on the same day, they will offer the benefits of a complete protein. Beans and rice, pasta and peas, and wheat bread and peanut butter are examples of good pairings of incomplete proteins.

It is not necessary to take amino acid pills; it is easy to get all the protein you need in a normal diet. In fact, most Americans eat too much protein. When too much protein is consumed, the extra amino acids are converted to fat and stored. The recommended protein intake for men and women over age 18 is 0.8 grams per kilogram of body weight per day. Research suggests that active individuals, such as endurance and strength-trained athletes require 1.2–1.7 grams per kilogram of body weight per day, and that this amount can generally be obtained through diet alone, without the use of protein supplements. However, even though they require more protein, they also need substantially more carbohydrate and overall calories; therefore, the recommended proportion of protein in the total diet doesn't change significantly.

To determine the protein requirement for a normal healthy adult, you must (1) convert pounds to kilograms, (2) multiply by the recommended amount of protein per kilogram of body weight, and (3) convert grams to calories by multiplying by 4, because protein contains 4 calories per gram. Here is an example using a 143-pound individual:

143 lbs ÷ 2.2 = 60 kg (body weight)

60 kg × 0.8 = 48 g (protein required)

48 × 4 = 192 calories from protein

The 192 calories represents about 10% of a 2000-calorie diet. If you do not want to convert body weight to kilograms, a close approximation can be obtained (for the 0.8 g/kg) by multiplying body weight in pounds by 0.36.

Countries where meat is used more for flavoring and less as a primary food have lower incidents of cardiovascular disease. Although most experts recommend that we consume smaller portions of red meat, remember that it is a good dietary source of iron. Both animal and plant foods contain protein. Some good sources of protein include meat, poultry, eggs, milk products, legumes (beans and peas), whole grains, pastas, rice, and seeds.

FAT

Fat is an essential part of every cell in your body. No fat, no life. The absolute minimum for men is about 3 to 6% of body weight, for women about 8 to 12%. Fats, also known as lipids, have a bad reputation only because most Americans overconsume them. Fat is an excellent source of concentrated energy. It also acts as insulation from the cold and carries the fat-soluble vitamins A, D, E, and K. Fat helps provide energy for prolonged activities performed at low to moderate levels of intensity, but to do so, carbohydrate must also be present.

Dietary fat is 95% triglycerides. Tryglycerides are made up of three fatty acids and one glycerol. Fatty acids come in three varieties: saturated, polyunsaturated, and monounsaturated. Saturated fats in the diet are related to elevated blood cholesterol, stroke, and coronary heart disease. In addition, saturated fats are converted into cholesterol in the liver when the amount of dietary cholesterol is low. Therefore, eating a diet low in saturated fats is as important, if not more important, than eating a low-cholesterol diet. Saturated fats, which are generally but not always solids at room temperature, include animal fats, butter, cheese, chocolate, and coconut and palm oils. (Chocolate, however, does contain some healthful substances—especially dark chocolate.) Unsaturated fats are generally liquids or soft solids at room temperature. Polyunsaturated fats include most of the oils (corn, soybean, cottonseed, safflower, sesame, and sunflower), fish, some nuts (walnuts, pecans, flaxseed), and most margarines. Mono-unsaturated fats include peanut, olive, and canola oils; avocados; olives; and some nuts (peanuts and cashews).

Fat consumption should be between 20 and 35% of energy intake. Unfortunately, the fat content in a typical American diet is 37 to 40%. Extra fat is stored as adipose tissue. You don't have to work hard at getting your required fat, because fat is hidden in so many foods. Red meats, cheese, baked goods, and fried foods are all high in fat. One of the easiest ways to cut down on fat is to switch from whole milk to low-fat or fat-free milk. Nearly half of whole milk's 150 calories per serving come from fat. Reduced-fat milk (2%) derives 38% of its 120 calories from fat, while low-fat milk (1%) drops to 23% of its 100 calories. And the winner, fat-free milk (nonfat or skim), contains no fat in its 80 calories. As you look for the fat content of foods, be aware that many products are labeled by the percentage of *weight* that is fat rather than the percentage of *calories*. Using the milk example above, only 2% of the weight (or 5 g) of reduced-fat milk (2% milk) is fat, but notice that more than a third of its calories come from fat. Many people mistakenly think that only 2%, not 38%, of the *calories* are from fat. To convert grams of fat to calories, you simply multiply the grams by 9. Two-percent milk, for example, contains 5 g of fat, which translates into 45 calories from fat. So, depending on the type of milk you pour in your cup, you can consume as much as 72 or as few as no calories from fat. See the box, Fats, below.

Trans unsaturated fatty acids, often referred to as ***trans* fats,** are fats produced artificially through a heating process that turns liquid (unsaturated) fats into solid fats. Food manufacturers use this process to turn vegetable oil into margarine and shortening. Manufacturers also use oils containing *trans* fats to cook fast foods. Some of the fatty acids that cause fats to become rancid can be removed when creating *trans* fats, which makes *trans* fats commercially attractive because they increase the shelf life of products, especially baked goods. The problem with *trans* fats is that they are linked to higher cholesterol levels (increasing

FATS

KEY RECOMMENDATIONS

- Consume less than 10% of calories from saturated fatty acids and less than 300 mg/day of cholesterol, and keep consumption of *trans* fatty acids as low as possible.

- Keep total fat intake between 20 and 35% of calories, taking most fats from sources of polyunsaturated and monounsaturated fatty acids, such as fish, nuts, and vegetable oils.

- When selecting and preparing meat, poultry, dry beans, and milk or milk products, make choices that are lean, low-fat, or fat-free.

- Limit intake of fats and oils high in saturated and/or *trans* fatty acids, and choose products low in such fats and oils.

low-density lipoprotein, or LDL, and decreasing high-density lipoprotein, or HDL) and an increased risk of coronary heart disease. One difficulty for consumers has been the lack of required labeling of fats on nutrition labels. Manufacturers have been able to make their foods look lower in fat by substituting *trans* fats (not required on the label) for saturated fats, which are required on the label. Some foods containing *trans* fats can also carry labels of "cholesterol free" and "cooked in vegetable oil." Furthermore, fast foods, which are often very high in *trans* fats, do not have to be labeled at all. Many fast foods that are perceived as more healthy because they are cooked in vegetable oil may actually be worse for us. With increasing evidence that *trans* fats are unhealthy, in January 2006 the U.S. Food and Drug Administration (FDA) required that *trans* fats be listed on nutrition labels under the saturated fat line. However, this requirement still does not include fast foods. The good news is that there are already *trans*-free products on the market, and with food labeling more will likely appear. If you are using stick margarine, switching to a softer tub margarine can significantly reduce your *trans* fats as well.

Fats that are health-enhancing include the polyunsaturated fats called omega-3. These are found in fish such as salmon, mackerel, herring, tuna, and sardines and can help reduce cholesterol and inhibit atherosclerosis in the coronary arteries. The American Heart Association recommends eating fish twice a week. Omega-3 fatty acids are also found in walnuts and flaxseeds. Consider little changes, such as adding walnuts to your whole-grain muffin for breakfast or making a tuna fish sandwich for lunch.

Cholesterol is a waxy fatlike substance found in the blood and in body tissues. The body naturally synthesizes it because it is essential in the formation of bile salts, which are used in fat digestion. It is also an essential component of all cell membranes; therefore, it is found in every cell of the body. It is transported through the blood by fat-protein particles called lipoproteins. Lipoproteins are named according to their density. The two major types of lipoproteins are **high-density lipoprotein (HDL)** and **low-density lipoprotein (LDL).** HDL picks up cholesterol from the cells and bloodstream and transports it to the liver, where it is used to make the bile salts. When the bile salts are used for fat digestion, some of them are excreted, thus eliminating cholesterol from the body. HDL is sometimes called the garbage collector of the blood, because it picks up cholesterol and dumps it in the liver. HDL is also referred to as "good cholesterol."

Cholesterol levels can be increased two ways: through our diet (eating cholesterol-rich foods) or through production of cholesterol in the liver. When the body has too much cholesterol, the LDL transporting cholesterol will give up some of its cholesterol to the walls of the arteries. As the fatty deposits (plaque) build up, the arteries become narrow and clogged. This condition, called atherosclerosis, is often accompanied by arteriosclerosis, a hardening of the arteries. Both of these can lead to **coronary heart disease (CHD),** a degenerative heart condition caused by the thickening and hardening of the coronary arteries. To prevent these dangerous diseases, people must control their cholesterol level. This disease does not start only in middle age; plaque has been found in young adults and even in children.

Both the total amount of cholesterol in the blood and the amount of HDL in the blood are good indicators of heart disease risk. A desirable level for **total cholesterol** is below 200 milligrams per deciliter (mg/dl). A low level of HDL cholesterol, 35 mg/dl or lower, is considered a risk factor for coronary artery disease. A high level of HDL cholesterol, 60 mg/dl or higher, is considered protective. If you want to know your cholesterol levels, you can take a simple blood test. A combination of diet and exercise is the best way to control your cholesterol level. Aerobic exercise can increase the amount of HDL cholesterol, and a diet low in cholesterol and low in saturated and *trans* fats can decrease the amount of LDL cholesterol circulating in your bloodstream.

WATER

Water, which constitutes 70% of the body's weight, is the solvent for digestion and waste removal. Water is the major component of blood and of the lubricant found in and around joints and organs. It also acts as a coolant as long as sweat is evaporating. You should consume the equivalent of six to eight 8-ounce (oz.) glasses of fluid daily for normal activity. Most people in the United States do not have a problem staying hydrated. Fluid intake can come from both beverages and foods. Recent research indicates that even caffeinated beverages can assist in hydration.

However, warm environments and exercise can both increase fluid needs. Water losses as little as 2 to 3% of body weight can negatively affect physical performance. You can be this dehydrated and not even be thirsty. Furthermore, thirst can be quenched with small amounts of water, when, in fact, your body may need much more. Be sure to stay well hydrated, and don't trust your thirst as an indicator of dehydration. Water is the best thing to drink for exercise up to an hour. For exercise more than an hour, an electrolyte-replacing sports drink containing less than 8% carbohydrate may help boost energy and aid in endurance activities. For the normal fitness exerciser, water is free, easy to digest, and great for rehydration. Be sure to start class hydrated, and drink again after class. If the environment is very warm, it is a good idea to have a drink in the middle of class. Some students like to keep a water bottle handy.

You want to drink the fluid that will leave your stomach the most quickly and get out to the body where it is needed. Cold drinks (40° to 50°F) leave the stomach more quickly than do warm drinks. They also help cool you off. Even ice-cold water won't hurt you, although you should drink it slowly. Sugars (glucose, fructose, sucrose) in drinks slow down the rate at which the fluid leaves the stomach. If you do use a sport drink and the carbohydrate percentage is higher than recommended (4 to 8%), you can dilute the drink. Soft drinks are not good sources of rapidly absorbed fluid. Fifteen minutes after drinking 12 oz. of a regular soft drink, 95% of it is still in your stomach. In addition, the carbonation can cause stomach bloating and upset. Fifteen minutes after drinking 12 oz. of water, only 30% of it is still in your stomach. Water, under normal conditions, is the most effective drink and also the least expensive.

Don't worry about replacing the electrolytes lost during a regular aerobics class. Sweat is really very diluted. The small amounts of minerals and electrolytes (including sodium [salt], potassium, and magnesium) that are lost through sweat can, under normal conditions, be replaced during your next regular meal. Avoid salt pills during exercise; they create a high salt concentration in the stomach that prevents rapid absorption. They may also cause stomach irritation and nausea.

VITAMINS

Vitamins are organic compounds that are essential for the process of releasing energy from food. As a result, they help to control the growth, maintenance, and repair of body tissues. Vitamins cannot be manufactured by the body and must therefore be obtained through a balanced diet. Research evidence suggests that the lack of vitamins impairs physical performance, but no evidence has proven that large doses enhance performance. Large doses of the fat-soluble vitamins (A, D, E, and K) can accumulate over time and cause serious toxic effects. Excess water-soluble vitamins (B, C, and others) generally wash out of the body daily. However, megadose levels of intake of these vitamins can also result in serious problems. A balanced diet will usually provide all the vitamins you need. Some exceptions include pregnant women, who are usually prescribed vitamins, strict vegetarians, and individuals on low-calorie diets. If you think

that your diet is not sufficiently vitamin rich, you may want to do a diet analysis, consider a nutrition supplement or multivitamin, and consult a registered dietician or other qualified health care provider.

MINERALS

Minerals are inorganic compounds that perform a variety of functions in the body. Some minerals, such as calcium and phosphorus, supply strength and rigidity to body structures like bones and teeth. Adequate calcium intake is important to the prevention of osteoporosis (weakening of the bone). The mineral iron is critical to the formation of hemoglobin, which is the oxygen-carrying pigment in the red blood cell. Lack of iron can cause fatigue. Menstruating and physically active women require more iron than other women, and women in general need more iron than men. Other minerals play a role in the production of hormones, such as zinc with insulin, and still others are involved in the regulatory functions of the body such as muscle contraction, nerve transmission, and blood clotting. A balanced diet will normally provide adequate amounts of all the minerals, although in some cases individuals may benefit from supplementation. Most Americans, especially teenagers, women, and the elderly, do not consume adequate amounts of calcium and iron. Note that some vitamins and minerals, such as calcium and vitamin D, must be taken together to ensure proper absorption and use in the body. Others, such as selenium and vitamin C, should be taken separately. Selenium, which helps reduce the risk of some cancers, can interfere with vitamin absorption. Taking a vitamin C supplement an hour ahead of the selenium supplement solves this problem. Sodium also deserves special mention because many Americans greatly exceed the recommended 2,300 milligrams (mg) a day—the equivalent of one teaspoon of table salt. For sodium-sensitive individuals, high salt intake increases their risk for hypertension. Excess sodium also increases calcium loss through the urine which adds to the risk of losing bone density. See the box, Sodium and Potassium, on the next page.

ANTIOXIDANTS AND PHYTOCHEMICALS

An **antioxidant** is an organic substance that can neutralize particles called free radicals without becoming a free radical itself. Reducing free radicals in the body is believed to prevent or reduce the risk of diseases like cancer, heart disease, and stroke. Vitamins C, E, and A (which is converted from beta-carotene), selenium (a mineral), and phytochemicals are antioxidants. **Phytochemicals** (meaning "plant chemicals") are food components that

SODIUM AND POTASSIUM

KEY RECOMMENDATIONS

- Consume less than 2,300 mg (approximately 1 teaspoon of salt) of sodium per day.

- Choose and prepare foods with little salt. At the same time, consume potassium-rich foods, such as fruits and vegetables.

help ward off cancer, cardiovascular diseases, diabetes, and hypertension. They are found in a wide variety of foods, including colorful fruits and vegetables, grains, legumes, and seeds. Carotenoids (one type of phytochemical), the most common of which is beta-carotene, are the pigments that give many vegetables such as carrots and sweet potatoes their color. Other good sources are green tea, garlic, licorice, and soy.

Free radicals are naturally formed during chemical processes in the cells as well as through exposure to things like solar or cosmic radiation and cigarette smoke. The most damaging source of free radicals in humans comes from oxygen. During oxygen's role of producing energy from carbohydrates and fats, it is usually converted into water and carbon dioxide, but sometimes it loses an extra electron and becomes a free radical. This free radical then steals an electron from another source, which sets up a chain reaction that can result in damage to cell walls, other cellular structures, and the genetic information within the cell. If left unchecked, such damage can become irreversible and lead to disease. When an antioxidant meets and neutralizes a free radical, the chain reaction stops.

Antioxidants are being actively researched. To date, the research is very promising but not conclusive, especially concerning antioxidant supplements. Most of the research has been done using antioxidant-rich foods, so the benefits being documented may be the result of something else in the food, or a combination of the antioxidant with something else in the diet. Furthermore, many studies have been carried out on populations with inadequate dietary intake of antioxidants, thus leaving open the possibility that supplements for individuals with healthy diets may not be necessary or beneficial. Some studies, however, suggest that benefits are derived from antioxidant levels above what can be obtained through diet. Before taking a supplement, consult with your health care provider. To make antioxidants part of your diet, consume lots of fruits, vegetables, and whole grains. Sweet potatoes, carrots, spinach, cantaloupe, and mangoes are all great sources of antioxidants. Research

consistently shows that people with the highest fruit and vegetable intake are the healthiest.

THE FOOD PYRAMID

The Food Guide Pyramid put out by the U.S. Department of Agriculture and the U.S. Department of Health and Human Resources in 1993 got a makeover in 2005. The new design, called *MyPyramid: Steps to a Healthier You*, reflects current scientific evidence and recommendations (Figure 12.1). The pyramid has been tipped on its side so that horizontal lines that once divided the food groups into boxes are now vertical lines. The resulting triangular wedges are designed to emphasize that within each food group there are foods that should be eaten in greater quantities (base foods) and foods that should be eaten more sparingly (peak foods). Base grain foods, for example, include whole-grain breads and cereals, whereas refined sugars, such as table sugar, are at the top. How a food is cooked can affect where it falls in the wedge. Beans are generally at the base of the meat/bean triangle, but if beans are baked in bacon grease, they move dramatically upward. The tip of the pyramid therefore, represents foods that are rich in solid fats and added sugars. The idea is to select the majority of your foods from the base of the pyramid and fewer from the peak. Some wedges are larger than others. This disparity is to represent that more of certain food groups should be consumed than other food groups. This is most obvious when you compare the very slender wedge for oil with the wider wedges for grains, fruits, and vegetables. Finally, the new pyramid includes a human figure walking/running up the steps alongside the pyramid to highlight the importance of combining diet with physical activity.

To accommodate individual differences in gender, age, and activity level, there are actually 12 pyramids. You can access the one that is right for you by going to the website: www.mypyramid.gov. This site also provides you a way to track what you eat, analyze your diet, and find helpful hints on how to eat a

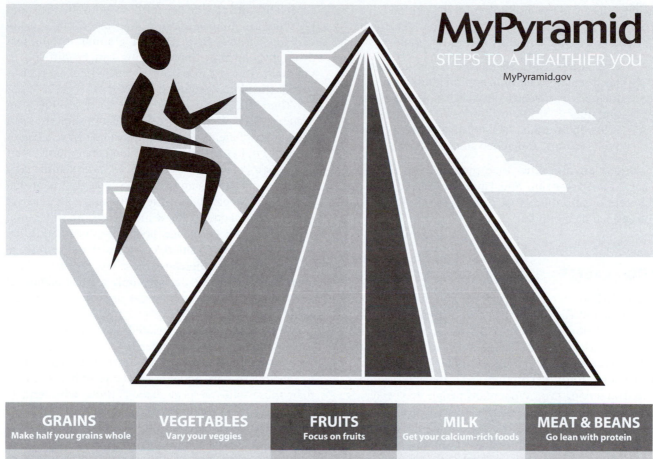

GRAINS	VEGETABLES	FRUITS	MILK	MEAT & BEANS
Make half your grains whole	**Vary your veggies**	**Focus on fruits**	**Get your calcium-rich foods**	**Go lean with protein**
Eat at least 3 oz. of whole-grain cereals, breads, crackers, rice, or pasta every day	Eat more dark-green veggies like broccoli, spinach, and other dark leafy greens	Eat a variety of fruit	Go low-fat or fat-free when you choose milk, yogurt, and other milk products	Choose low-fat or lean meats and poultry
		Choose fresh, frozen, canned, or dried fruit		Bake it, broil it, or grill it
1 oz. is about 1 slice of bread, about 1 cup of breakfast cereal, or ¹/₂ cup of cooked rice, cereal, or pasta	Eat more orange vegetables like carrots and sweet-potatoes	Go easy on fruit juices	If you don't or can't consume milk, choose lactose-free products or other calcium sources such as fortified foods and beverages	Vary your protein routine—choose more fish, beans, peas, nuts, and seeds
	Eat more dry beans and peas like pinto beans, kidney beans, and lentils			

For a 2,000-calorie diet, you need the amounts below from each food group. To find the amounts that are right for you, go to MyPyramid.gov.

| Eat 6 oz. every day | Eat 2¹/₂ cups every day | Eat 2 cups every day | Get 3 cups every day; for kids aged 2 to 8, it's 2 | Eat 5¹/₂ oz. every day |

U.S. Department of Agriculture
Center for Nutrition Policy and Promotion
April 2005
CNPP-15

Figure 12.1 MyPyramid: Steps to a Healthier You.

Source: www.mypyramid.gov.

healthy diet. You can also link from the pyramid to the 2005 Dietary Guidelines for Americans. The Dietary Guidelines describe a healthy diet as one that:

- emphasizes fruits, vegetables, whole grains, and fat-free or low-fat milk and milk products
- includes lean meats, poultry, fish, beans, eggs, and nuts
- is low in saturated fats, *trans* fats, cholesterol, salt (sodium), and added sugars

There are also other food pyramids (for example, Asian, Mediterranean, and Latino) available through different organizations that show how ethnic foods fit into a good dietary plan.

FOOD LABELS

After you know what kinds of foods are good for you and how much of each kind to eat, you need to become a savvy food label reader. The FDA requires food labeling on most packaged foods. Figure 12.2 shows an example of a food label and offers guidelines for interpreting the information contained on the label. Label information is based on serving sizes. What many people don't realize is how much serving sizes, in terms of actual helpings, have increased over the years. The label, however, uses standard sizes that may seem small compared to what is on your plate. To interpret the label correctly, you must know what the label considers a serving. Figure 12.3 on page 178 provides a visual guide to some serving sizes. If you are consuming food in greater quantities, you need to multiply the label information by the number of servings you are consuming. For example, the USDA describes a standard 2-ounce bagel as two servings from the grain group. Many bagels are 6 ounces. This is the equivalent of six servings. Similarly, the label on a single large muffin may state that the package consists of two servings. If the muffin is 250 calories and 10 grams of fat and you eat the whole thing, you have consumed 500 calories and 20 grams of fat. Instead of "biggie-sizing," we should consider "junior-sizing," especially when fats and sugars are involved. One way is to drink a big glass of water and a smaller cup of soda.

WEIGHT CONTROL INFORMATION

To control one's weight at a "desirable" level is one of this nation's most passionate goals. Well-founded weight-loss programs and rip-off fad diets flourish side by side in a society seeking the "beautiful" body. Differentiating fact from fallacy can be difficult at times. But two things are clear: (1) excessive weight, especially fat, can be harmful to your health; and (2) there are no magical diets that take off fat quickly and keep it off. In fact, even gradual weight loss through good nutritional dieting can be difficult to maintain. But it can be done, and when exercise is part of the plan, keeping the weight off is easier.

The extra weight many people carry around is an even heavier burden because of its relationship to disease and quality of life. Overweight individuals have a higher incidence of hypertension, high blood cholesterol, heart disease, stroke, some cancers, diabetes, and arthritis. And this does not even address the psychological pain that overweight people endure due to the unfeeling remarks and attitudes of others. Obese individuals can suffer from depression, poor self-image, poor self-esteem, and even job discrimination. Health risks grow with the percentage of overweightness; therefore, those who are 10 to 15% over their desired weight have only a small additional risk, while the very overweight and obese carry the highest risk.

Body shape is also related to health risk. For reasons not completely understood, individuals with apple-shaped bodies (those who carry extra fat around the abdomen) have a higher incidence of heart disease than those who are pear-shaped (those who tend to store extra fat in the lower body). You can calculate a waist-to-hip ratio to determine if your shape puts you at more risk. Simply measure your waist at your navel, and then your hips at the greatest circumference around the buttocks. Using Worksheet 16, divide the waist measurement by the hip measurement. A waist-to-hip ratio greater than 1.0 for men and 0.8 for women indicates an increased cardiac risk. Some experts believe that waist alone or, even better, in conjunction with BMI, is a better predictor of risk. Women with a waist circumference greater than 35 inches and men with a circumference greater than 40 inches are considered as high risk regardless of their BMI (body mass index, discussed later in this chapter).

Weight control is a complex process involving a number of factors, including genetics, environment, race, gender, economic status, and psychological factors. Why one person stays thin and another doesn't is not as easily answered as one might think. For example, there is good evidence that obesity runs in families. But is this due to a genetic predisposition or to family eating habits and culturally driven food choices? One study using adopted children illustrates the complex, even contradictory evidence often facing weight control researchers. The adopted girls tended to "look" like their biological parents, especially their biological mothers, while the boys did not bear similarities to either biological parent.

The **set point theory** is a genetic-based theory that asserts that the body has a preset level of fat that it

Using the Food Label

The food label carries an easier to use nutrition information guide. It is required on almost all packaged foods (compared to about 60% of products until now). The label below is only an example.

Serving sizes are more consistent across product lines, are stated in both household and metric measures, and reflect the amounts people actually eat (based on consumer surveys).

The **list of nutrients** covers those most important to the health of consumers, most of whom need to worry about getting too *much* of certain items (fat or sodium, for example), rather than too few vitamins or minerals. The numbers next to the nutrients show how much of the nutrient each serving contains.

The label of larger packages must tell the number of calories per gram of the energy-producing nutrients: fat, carbohydrate, and protein.

"Nutrition Facts," signals that the label contains the required information.

Calories from fat are shown on the label to help consumers meet dietary guidelines that recommend people keep total fat intake to between 20 and 35% of calories, with most from unsaturated fats.

% Daily Value shows how much of the recommended amount of a nutrient is in a serving of the food.

Only two vitamins, A and C, and two minerals, calcium and iron, are required on the label. A company may voluntarily list other vitamins and minerals.

Some **Daily Values** are expressed as maximums, as with fat (65 grams or *less*); others are expressed as minimums, as with carbohydrate (300 grams or *more*). The daily values for a 2,000- and 2,500-calorie diet must be listed on the label of larger packages. Individuals must adjust the values to fit their own calorie intake.

Nutrition Facts

Serving Size 1 cup (228g)
Servings Per Container 2

Amount Per Serving

Calories 250   Calories from Fat 110

% Daily Value*

Total Fat 12g	18%
Saturated Fat 3g	15%
Trans Fat 1.5g	
Cholesterol 30mg	10%
Sodium 470mg	20%
Total Carbohydrate 31g	10%
Dietary Fiber 0g	0%
Sugars 5g	
Protein 5g	

Vitamin A	4%	Vitamin C	2%
Calcium	20%	Iron	4%

*Percent Daily Values are based on a 2,000 calorie diet. Your Daily Values may be higher or lower depending on your calorie needs:

	Calories:	2,000	2,500
Total Fat	Less than	65g	80g
Sat Fat	Less than	20g	25g
Cholesterol	Less than	300mg	300mg
Sodium	Less than	2,400mg	2,400mg
Total Carbohydrate		300g	375g
Dietary Fiber		25g	30g

Calories per gram:

Fat 9   Carbohydrate 4   Protein 4

Figure 12.2 Nutrition label.

Source: Food and Drug Administration, 2006.

SERVING SIZE CARD

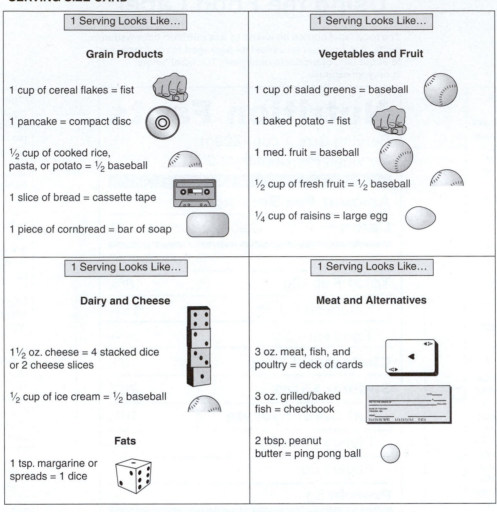

1 Serving Looks Like...	**1 Serving Looks Like...**
Grain Products	**Vegetables and Fruit**
1 cup of cereal flakes = fist	1 cup of salad greens = baseball
1 pancake = compact disc	1 baked potato = fist
½ cup of cooked rice, pasta, or potato = ½ baseball	1 med. fruit = baseball
1 slice of bread = cassette tape	½ cup of fresh fruit = ½ baseball
1 piece of cornbread = bar of soap	¼ cup of raisins = large egg
1 Serving Looks Like...	**1 Serving Looks Like...**
Dairy and Cheese	**Meat and Alternatives**
1½ oz. cheese = 4 stacked dice or 2 cheese slices	3 oz. meat, fish, and poultry = deck of cards
½ cup of ice cream = ½ baseball	3 oz. grilled/baked fish = checkbook
Fats	2 tbsp. peanut butter = ping pong ball
1 tsp. margarine or spreads = 1 dice	

Figure 12.3 Serving size card.

"believes" to be correct and that it will work to ensure. If a person tries to lose weight and drops below the set point, the body encourages weight gain and a return to the set point by conserving fats and increasing appetite. Even when obese individuals (in a controlled setting) are forced to gain weight, they quickly return to their previous weight when allowed to resume their normal eating habits. The biological mechanism at work in set point is still not fully understood. And there are some individuals for whom it doesn't seem to be true: lean people who can eat anything and not gain weight, and a small percentage of obese individuals who can lose weight and keep it off indefinitely. Encouragingly, there is some evidence that aerobic exercise can lower the set point. And a genetic predisposition for something does not mean you will develop it. However, it does signal a need to develop good lifestyle habits in terms of eating well and exercising.

Environment plays the most obvious role in weight control. Environment includes everything from your schedule, to the availability of nutritious food, to cultural influences, to personal choices. It is awfully easy to succumb to high-fat foods when they are quick and convenient. And habits developed in childhood can be very difficult to change. The good news, however, is that personal behaviors, unlike genetics, can be changed. Nutrition awareness exercises can help identify environmental triggers, which can then be avoided or handled with good planning.

Overconsumption explains a lot of overweightness, especially when teamed with a sedentary lifestyle. But it does not account for the fact that many obese individuals eat the same, or less, food than individuals of normal weight and still don't lose weight. There is some evidence that obese individuals burn calories more efficiently and can therefore sustain the same activity level on fewer calories than can a person of normal weight. So again, the equation is not as simple as one would expect. Nor does simple consumption account for the thin person who can eat anything and not gain a pound. Some thin people just seem to "burn calories" sitting still—metabolism no doubt plays a role in this.

Psychological factors such as negative emotions also influence people's eating habits. When dealing with emotions such as rejection, anger, or depression, some people find comfort in eating. This can lead to overeating and/or unhealthy binge behaviors. Feeling "too fat" even though one isn't can also lead to unhealthy habits or eating disorders.

One has to wonder what socioeconomic and gender influences are at work when people under the poverty line are fatter than those at the top of the socioeconomic ladder, especially women. The research on weight control is many-faceted and is not always conclusive, but each study brings us a little closer to understanding the puzzle of weight control and management.

OVERWEIGHT, OVERFAT, OBESE

The word "overweight" comes from the idea that there is an ideal weight for each of us, and if you weigh more than that, you are overweight. In the past, if you wanted to see if you were overweight you checked a height/weight chart. One well-known chart was produced by Metropolitan Life, an insurance company that was interested in body weight as a predictor of life expectancy. One problem is that there are a number of charts with various weight ranges for the same height. Today, the phrase "ideal weight" has been replaced with "healthy weight," and in place of the traditional height/weight chart, many professionals recommend calculating **body mass index (BMI).** BMI is easy to calculate and provides a fairly good estimate of healthy weight when the more accurate methods of measuring body fat are not available. (See the section on body composition later in this chapter.) BMI is calculated by dividing your weight in kilograms by the square of your height in meters. The higher your BMI category, the greater your risk for health problems. To calculate your BMI and determine your weight category (healthy weight, overweight, or obese), turn to Worksheet 16. For both a quick estimate of BMI and to see what category you are in at your height and weight, see Figure 12.4 on page 180. Healthy or normal weights, based on BMI, are believed to be protective. However, recent research suggests that a normal weight as determined by BMI may not be sufficient by itself to lower disease risk; it may be that normal weight must be coupled with cardiorespiratory fitness.

This bolsters the argument that diet and exercise should happen together.

BMI is not without limitations. It may surprise you, for example, to learn that athletes and other highly muscular individuals weigh more than normal and may be incorrectly categorized as overweight. And BMI doesn't take into account where extra fat is stored. Remember that abdominal fat is associated with a higher risk of disease than fat stored in the lower body. Nor can BMI tell you how many of your pounds are fat rather than lean body mass (muscle, water, organs, etc.). In fact, no distinction can be made between a round, soft person and a lean, muscular person as long as they are the same height, weight, and gender. Using a waist circumference measure together with BMI does help establish risk level.

If instead of thinking in terms of being **overweight,** you think in terms of being overfat, the distinction can be made. **Overfat** is a condition in which the percentage of body weight that is fat weight is too high. A person can be a little or very much overfat. Using fatness as the measure, the muscular "overweight" person can be differentiated from the overfat "overweight" person. **Obese** is a medical term that refers to the storage of excess body fat. It is generally agreed that men with more than 25% stored fat and women with more than 30% stored fat are considered obese. How much of your body is fat weight and how to measure it is discussed in the next section.

BODY COMPOSITION

Imagine the look of confusion you would receive if you walked up to the counter at a delicatessen and asked for 10 pounds. The store clerk would probably look annoyed and ask, "Ten pounds of what? Ham? Salami? Cheese?" Yet every day, people say they are going to lose (or gain) 10 pounds. And who thinks to ask the same critical question: 10 pounds of what? Would a person claiming to be 10 pounds overweight be satisfied if she or he lost 10 pounds of muscle? Would a person trying to gain weight want to gain 10 pounds of fat? Probably not. It is helpful, then, to differentiate between weight and fat weight.

The body's weight can be broken into two components: fat weight (FW) and lean body mass (LBM). Fat weight is made up of two kinds of fat: subcutaneous fat, which is stored between the skin and the muscles, and intramuscular fat, which is stored between muscle fibers. By pinching yourself, you can feel the subcutaneous fat. To picture intramuscular fat, think of how a prime piece of steak (cow's muscle) is marbled with fat. **Lean body mass (LBM)** is derived from the weight of the skeleton, muscles, water, organs, and connective tissue.

ARE YOU A HEALTHY WEIGHT?

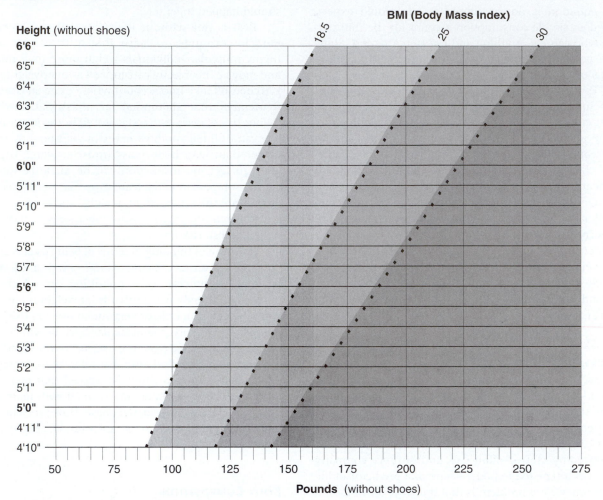

BMI measures weight in relation to height. The BMI ranges shown above are for adults. They are not exact ranges of healthy and unhealthy weights. However, they show that health risk increases at higher levels of overweight and obesity. Even within the healthy BMI range, weight gains can carry health risks for adults.

Directions: Find your weight on the bottom of the graph. Go straight up from that point until you come to the line that matches your height. Then look to find your weight group.

Healthy Weight BMI from 18.5 up to 25 refers to healthy weight.

Overweight BMI from 25 up to 30 refers to overweight.

Obese BMI 30 or higher refers to obesity. Obese persons are also overweight.

Figure 12.4 Are you a healthy weight? BMI chart.

Source: Report of the Dietary Guidelines Advisory Committee on the Dietary Guidelines for Americans, 2000, page 3.

It is possible to estimate how much of your body is fat weight and how much is lean body mass. This is called assessing your body composition.

Body composition is usually measured and discussed as the percentage of weight that is fat weight. For example, an individual might be said to be 18% fat.

Guidelines for healthy percentages of fat for both men and women are shown in Table 12.1. Note that healthy women have higher levels of fat than healthy men do.

To illustrate the importance of examining body composition, consider the following two women. Both are 5'4" and 120 lb and have a small frame size. Both

Table 12.1 Standards for Fatness (Percent Body Fat)

PERCENT BODY FAT

CLASSIFICATION	MEN	WOMEN
Essential fat	no less than 5%	no less than 8%
Desirable fatness for good performance	5–13%	12–22 %
Desirable fatness for good health	10–25%	18–30%
Overfatness (Obesity)	> 25%	> 30%

Source: Adaptation of Table 1, "Standards—Percent Body Fat" from "Body Composition: A Round Table" by J. H. Wilmore, et al., from *The Physician and Sportsmedicine*, p. 152, 1986; 14(3): 144–162. Copyright © 1986 by The McGraw-Hill Companies. All rights reserved. Reprinted with permission.

would be considered at an ideal weight according to a height/weight chart.

PERSON A		**PERSON B**	
Total weight:	120 lb	Total weight:	120 lb
Fat weight:	24 lb	Fat weight:	38 lb
LBM weight:	96 lb	LBM weight:	82 lb
Percent fat:	20%	Percent fat:	32%
Rating:	**healthy**	Rating:	**obese**

Until groups such as the military, commercial airlines, and cheerleaders realized the difference between overweight and overfat, they were denying valuable, highly fit individuals entry to their programs. Unfortunately, some programs still expect individuals to be at certain weight levels to participate. When a trim, toned individual goes on a crash diet to reach this level, it usually means losing water and muscle to do so. Not only is this highly undesirable, it is also dangerous. People should not be expected to reduce weight levels, they should be expected to attain appropriate body compositions.

The most accurate way to determine the amount of fat a person has is to measure it directly, but unless you are willing to be a cadaver, an indirect and slightly less accurate method is the way to go. There are four common ways to assess body composition. One of the more accurate indirect measures is taken using **hydrostatic** or **underwater weighing.** With this method, a person sits on a platform that is attached to a scale. The platform is lowered into the water until the person is totally submerged. After the person exhales as much air as possible, a weight measurement is taken. Because fat floats, a fatter person will weigh less under water than a lean person. The underwater weight is adjusted to account for any air left in the lungs after full exhalation and any gas trapped in the

gastrointestinal tract. Finally, an estimate of fat is computed.

This process is fairly costly in both time and facilities. It requires expensive equipment and well-trained technicians. Although you do not have to be a swimmer to participate, this procedure does not work well with individuals who are uncomfortable under water. If you are comfortable in water and wish to be underwater weighed, check with the physical education department at a university or college or with a local sports medicine center. Most places charge a fee for this service. Sometimes when people are being trained in the procedure, volunteers are weighed at no cost. Be prepared for the process to take at least an hour.

A less expensive, quicker, and more convenient method of assessing body fat is the **skin-fold technique.** It is a little less accurate than underwater weighing, but it still provides a good useful estimate. A caliper is used to measure the thickness of the subcutaneous fat at several sites. The technician uses one hand to pull the skin and subcutaneous fat away from the muscle with his or her thumb and forefinger. With the other hand, she or he uses the caliper to measure the width of the pinched fat (Figure 12.5). The measurements from the different sites are added, and this sum is put into a formula. Some formulas use only one site, some three, and some six or more. Scientists use the multiple-site formulas for accuracy and then recommend the most predictive sites for general use. Some of the most commonly used sites

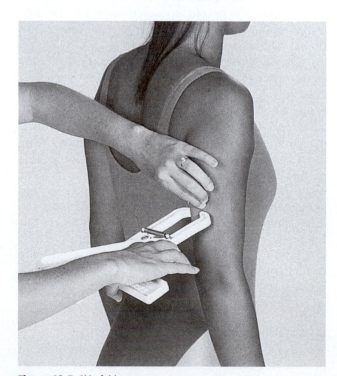

Figure 12.5 Skin-fold measurement.

are the back of the arm, just above the hip, the abdomen, just below the shoulder blade, and the front of the thigh. It is easier to train technicians to measure skin folds than to perform underwater weighing. In addition, skin-fold equipment is easily brought to the exercise site. When a fee is charged for this service, it is usually quite small and the test takes only a few minutes.

Another method of analyzing body composition uses what is called a body analyzer or impedance machine. This machine sends a small, harmless electrical impulse through the body. The computer records both the time the impulse takes to travel through the body and the amount of resistance the impulse encounters. The impulse travels quickly and with little resistance through water, which makes up a good portion of muscle. It meets more resistance and travels more slowly through fat, since fat is a poor electrical conductor. The computer uses this data to compute your percentage of body fat. Because this method depends on total body water values, it is important to be at an appropriate level of hydration each time you are tested. Working out before the test or retaining water due to menstruation can throw off the accuracy of this test. Some universities, hospitals, and health clubs have these machines available but usually charge a fee for their use. The test only takes a few minutes and may be accompanied by a computer printout that includes your percentage of fat, recommended weight, and how to attain your recommended weight. Some professionals still question the accuracy of this test, while others believe it to be as accurate as the skin-fold technique when subsequent tests are performed at a similar hydration level.

The newest method for determining body composition uses air displacement and pressure-volume relationships. In this method, a person sits inside an egg-shaped fiberglass chamber commercially called the Bod Pod. The air inside the unit is measured before and after the person enters. The difference represents the person's body volume. This is then used to calculate body density and percent body fat. One big advantage to this method is that people are much more comfortable sitting in an air-filled chamber than being dunked underwater for hydrostatic weighing. The air displacement plethysmography method has shown some encouraging results, but is in need of additional research testing. It is also a more expensive test at this time.

DETERMINING YOUR "HEALTHY" WEIGHT

While we do not know for sure what constitutes a healthy weight, we do know enough to make educated guesses. How healthy your weight is depends on how much of it is fat, where on your body extra fat is located, and whether or not you have weight-related medical problems or a high risk of weight-related disease. There are several ways to determine your healthy weight. You can consult a height/weight chart or use BMI to identify a healthy weight, as described in the previous section. The most accurate way is to calculate your healthy weight using your present percentage of body fat. You will need to have your percentage of body fat estimated using one of the techniques described in the body composition section. Using Table 12.1 on page 181 to guide you, determine the body fat percentage you would like to have. The range for good health is 10 to 25% fat for men and 18 to 30% fat for women. (If you are interested in competitive athletics, you may want to select a percentage of fat from the performance range.) Turn to Worksheet 16 and subtract your desired percentage of fat from your actual percentage of fat. If the result is a positive number, multiply your present weight by it and subtract the answer from your present weight; if it is a negative number, drop the negative sign, multiply your present weight by it, and then add it to your present weight. Here is an example of the calculation for a woman weighing 160 lbs with 32% body fat who wants to drop to 25% body fat. (Remember to convert the percentage to decimal form before multiplying. For example, 6% = 6/100 = 0.06.)

32% − 25% = 7% = 0.07

160 lbs × 0.07 = 11.2 (rounded down to 11)

160 − 11 = 149 lbs (healthy weight)

Use your "healthy weight" to determine how much weight you need to lose or gain.

WEIGHT MANAGEMENT

The goal of weight management is to achieve a healthy weight and then maintain it. Diet and exercise can be used to maintain, gain, or lose weight. When the number of calories you consume matches the number of calories you expend, you are in **energy balance.** When you consume more calories than you expend, you create a positive energy balance, and you gain weight. When you consume fewer calories than you expend, you create a negative energy balance and lose weight. To change your energy balance, you can change the number of calories you eat, change the number of calories you burn, or, best of all, combine the effects of both. The next three sections discuss how exercise and diet can be used to achieve a desired weight loss, a healthy weight gain, and weight maintenance. See also the accompanying box, Weight Management.

WEIGHT LOSS

Weight loss should be gradual, about 1 lb a week. This gradual weight loss will keep you off the dieting roller coaster and give you the chance to change your lifestyle so that the weight stays off. One pound of fat contains 3,500 calories; to lose it in 1 week you have three choices. You can eat 3,500 fewer calories per week, which is 500 fewer calories per day; you can eat your same diet and exercise off the 500 calories every day; or you can eat 200 fewer calories and exercise off the other 300. The latter is the easiest approach and meets the health recommendation of expending 300 to 500 calories through exercise.

During the first week of a proper diet, you may experience a rapid weight loss. After this initial weight loss, work for a steady 1 lb loss per week, and don't feel discouraged if your weight remains constant from time to time.

It is a good idea to limit caloric decreases to 500 calories per day or 1,000 calories per day if your diet is above 3,000 calories. Also, women should be sure to consume a minimum of 1,200 calories a day and men a minimum of 1,500 calories a day to maintain the basic nutritional needs of the body. Diets that contain fewer calories should be performed only under the care of a physician.

The following is a short list of helpful hints if you are trying to eat fewer calories.

1. Eat planned meals evenly spaced throughout the day to help keep your level of blood sugar steady.
2. Eat fiber-rich foods, which are bulky and will help make you feel full.
3. Eat baked, broiled, or poached meats and steamed vegetables. Avoid fried or sautéd foods.
4. Eat more slowly so that the meal lasts longer even though you are eating less.
5. Switch to skim milk and low-fat dairy products.

6. Eat low-fat meats whenever possible. Poultry (except duck and goose), especially white meat, and fish are good low-fat choices. Red meat is generally high in fat.
7. Limit the number of times you eat out. This will keep you from eating foods you ordinarily wouldn't cook. And remember, restaurants cook with lots of butter, salt, and fattening sauces.
8. Plan your meals. It's easy to end up eating fat-laden fast foods when you are hungry and there is nothing to eat in the house.
9. Write down everything you eat. Awareness is half the battle.
10. Keep fattening foods out of the house. This helps eliminate temptation.
11. Allow yourself a few sweets during the week, or daily if necessary, so that you aren't tempted to binge on them.
12. Pick one or two areas to improve in at one time. Gradual changes in lifestyle are easier to accept than radically new ones. In other words, don't try to break two favorite habits at the same time, such as drinking too much soda and overeating sweets; take them one at a time.

WEIGHT LOSS AND EXERCISE

The key to weight loss with exercise is high frequency (exercising most days of the week) and building up to substantial durations (60 to 90 minutes). See the Physical Activity box on the next page. Shorter, more intense workouts may also be effective after a sufficient fitness level is achieved. If you have not been exercising, you may need to start with fewer days a week, shorter exercise sessions, or both. Consult a fitness professional. People with excess weight may also need to begin with non-weight-bearing activities, such as cycling or aquatic exercises. As weight diminishes, weight-bearing activities such as aerobic dance exercise can be added to the program. With a high-frequency program for weight loss (exercise 5 to 6 times a week), it would probably be best to limit your participation in

---

WEIGHT MANAGEMENT

KEY RECOMMENDATIONS

- To maintain body weight in a healthy range, balance calories consumed with calories expended.

- To prevent gradual weight gain over time, make small decreases in caloric intake and increase physical activity.

PHYSICAL ACTIVITY

KEY RECOMMENDATIONS

- Engage in regular physical activity and reduce sedentary activities to promote health, psychological well-being, and a healthy body weight.

- To reduce the risk of chronic disease in adulthood: Engage in at least 30 minutes of moderate-intensity physical activity, above usual activity, at work or home on most days of the week.

- For most people, greater health benefits can be obtained by engaging in physical activity of more vigorous intensity or longer duration.

- To help manage body weight and prevent gradual, unhealthy body weight gain in adulthood: Engage in

approximately 60 minutes of moderate- to vigorous-intensity activity on most days of the week while not exceeding caloric intake requirements.

- To sustain weight loss in adulthood: Participate in at least 60 to 90 minutes of daily moderate-intensity physical activity while not exceeding caloric intake requirements. Some people may need to consult with a health care provider before participating in this level of activity.

- Achieve physical fitness by performing cardiovascular conditioning, stretching exercises for flexibility, and resistance exercises or calisthenics for muscle strength and endurance.

aerobic dance exercise to 3 or 4 days a week and use a non-weight-bearing or low-impact activity for the other days.

FUELING YOUR WORKOUT

Fat, carbohydrate, and protein can all be used to fuel movement. The amount of each that is used depends on the intensity and duration of the activity, a person's fitness level, and diet. Fat and carbohydrate are the main sources for movement energy. Protein only contributes about 2% of the fuel for less than an hour of exercise, slightly higher for intense prolonged exercise.[1] At rest, almost all of the body's energy is provided by fat metabolism, but because little energy is being expended, not much fat is burned. Moving at low intensities (less than 30% of VO_2max), energy is still predominantly supplied by fat with carbohydrate supplying the balance. Consider then what happens when the intensity or duration of activity increases.

- If a person increases activity or exercise to a higher intensity (above 30% VO_2max), the percentage of fat burning will decrease and that of carbohydrate increase. The point where carbohydrate exceeds fat is called the "crossover point." As intensity continues to increase the reliance on carbohydrates will grow.

- If a person stays at a relatively low intensity, one where the percentage of fat to carbohydrate is fairly equal, and is active for a prolonged amount of time (more than 30 minutes), the percentage of fat being burned will slowly increase and the percentage of carbohydrate slowly decrease. In other words, prolonged low intensity exercise results in a higher percentage of fat burning.

These discoveries have led individuals to believe that because exercising longer at low intensities burns more fat, it is the preferable way to approach weight management. This is, however, only partially true. If the individual trying to lose fat is at a low fitness level and low-intensity activity is the healthiest choice, then exercising at a low intensity for longer (building up to 60–90 minutes) is the way to go. If, however, the individual is able to exercise at a higher intensity, shorter duration exercise can actually burn as many or more calories from fat. Less time, more fat burned? How can this be if higher intensity activity favors carbohydrates? The answer has to do with how many calories are being burned. The more vigorous the exercise, the more calories burned. As exercise intensity goes up, the *percentage* of fat being burned goes down, but the actual *number* of fat calories burned will increase because the total number of calories used increases.

Imagine that you are eating at a slow pace. You consume 12 food items: 50% are carrots, 50% are avocado slices. Eating at a faster pace, you consume

1. S. K. Powers and E.T. Howley. *Exercise Physiology: Theory and Application to Fitness and Performance*. 6th ed. New York: McGraw-Hill, 2006, 62–9.

24 items: 66.6% are carrots, and 33.3% are avocado slices. Notice that in the first case you ate 6 avocado slices (50% of 12), while in the second case you consumed 8 avocado slices (33.3% of 24). The percentage drops (50% to 33.3%), but the actual number of avocado slices increases.

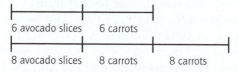

Now turn it around and think of the avocado as fat being burned. Moderate exercise burns more fat calories than low-intensity exercise if the two are performed for the same amount of time. (*Note:* The percentages used in the avocado/carrot example do not represent the real percentages of fat being burned.)

Increasing the amount of time you exercise at low intensity can offset this difference. Very high intensities burn a lot of calories per minute, but most people find it difficult and uncomfortable to sustain high-intensity exercise. The risk of injury also increases, and mainly carbohydrate is burned. Regardless of how much fat or carbohydrate you are burning at any given time, the key is to burn more calories than you take in over the day.

Fitness professionals recommend that a person expend 300 to 500 calories per exercise session. Individuals at a low fitness level may have to begin with a 200-calorie expenditure, but with gradual overload, they can safely reach a 300-calorie expenditure in about 8 to 12 weeks.

A heavy person will burn more calories than a lighter person doing the same activity because the former must move more weight. Corbin and Lindsey in *Fitness for Life* estimate the following numbers of calories per hour for dance exercise for the body weights listed:

POUNDS	CALORIES/HOUR	CALORIES/MINUTE
100	315	5.25
120	357	5.95
150	420	7.00
180	483	8.05
200	525	8.75

To estimate the number of calories you burn in your class, perform the following easy calculation: Multiply the calories/minute for your weight by the number of minutes in your class.

A 150-pound person would burn 7 calories per minute (420 ÷ 60). In a 50-minute class, this person would burn 350 calories (50 × 7). This class would fulfill the 300- to 500-calorie expenditure requirement for those trying to lose weight. Keep in mind that these are averages (calories/minute). If you are performing an intense version of aerobics, the calorie burn may be higher.

Besides the obvious calorie-burning effect, exercise also provides hidden benefits. Your basal metabolic rate is the rate at which your body uses energy to sustain vital functions when you are at rest. When you exercise, your metabolism increases; therefore, you burn more calories. What you may not be aware of is that your metabolic rate remains raised for a period of time following exercise. In addition, every pound of muscle gained through exercise burns an additional 50 calories as compared to a pound of fat. This means you are burning more calories without even trying.

A final advantage for adding regular exercise to your diet regimen is that fit people start to burn fat more quickly during exercise than unfit people do. It may seem unfair, but fit people have a definite advantage when it comes to weight control. If it is possible, have your percentage of body fat estimated in about 8-week intervals to see how you are doing. You can also take body measurements to see whether you are slimming down. Inches may come off even when pounds don't. Muscle-weight additions may be counteracting fat-weight losses. You can actually lose fat, gain weight, and look better all at the same time!

UNBALANCED DIETS, FADS, AND GIMMICKS

Some of the best nonfiction sellers are diet books. An amazing amount of money is spent on diet books, counseling, and products. Many good diet books and diet plans are available, but a tremendous number also violate the most fundamental rules of good nutrition. They are called fad diets because someone makes a lot of money on them when they first come out, and then they pass into anonymity when dieters find out they don't work. Weight-loss fad diets are easy to spot. They promise quick weight losses and advocate unbalanced diets. They depend on your not caring what kind of weight you lose. When you lose more than 1 to 2 lbs a week, you will lose beneficial muscle and water weight to do it. For example, you can wrap yourself in plastic and sweat off pounds of water, pop diet pills that cause food to race through your system without being digested, or drink protein drinks and avoid carbohydrates so that you lose substantial amounts of lean tissue and water. If it is fat you are trying to lose, don't get drawn into a fad diet.

A fad diet that stresses one type of food does so by limiting or excluding intake from one or more of the other food groups. When you don't eat adequate amounts from each food group, you don't obtain all of the essential nutrients. This lack of necessary nutrients can leave you fatigued, depressed, and irritable. Even top athletes who manipulate their diet to carbohydrate load (a process of lowering and raising carbohydrate intake to "trick" the body into storing more glycogen for big events) will tell you that irritability and discomfort often accompany the periods of low carbohydrate consumption.

High-protein diets translate into low-carbohydrate and, often, high-fat diets. When your body does not have sufficient quantities of carbohydrates and fats, it uses protein for energy. Nitrogen is a by-product of the protein energy cycle. Too much nitrogen can be toxic. In an effort to clear the body of excess nitrogen, the kidneys combine it with water to make ammonia. The ammonia is excreted in the urine. (It can also be sweated out in small amounts.) When a lot of protein is consumed, the body has to work very hard to clear the nitrogen. Large quantities of water are needed for this process. High-protein diet plans usually tell you to drink an additional 6 to 8 glasses of water per day. Try drinking 16 glasses of water a day; few people can, and so too often the result is dehydration. If the diet is continued, dehydration can become severe, which can lead to kidney failure and death. Even if you don't dehydrate, the low level of carbohydrates will probably make you feel irritable, sick, and fatigued. High-protein diets often encourage high consumption of meats and dairy foods, which can lead to an unhealthy diet full of saturated fats.

Near-starvation diets, crash diets, and prolonged fasting send signals to your body that food is not available and that your life may be threatened. Sensing starvation, the body conserves the energy it has available. In fact, your body may even begin storing the energy as fat to compensate. Your body actually adjusts itself to survive on fewer calories. Activating this survival instinct makes it more difficult for you to lose fat or, eventually, any form of weight. In fact, some people who are overfat actually eat fewer calories than individuals of normal weight. When you've been on the crash-diet roller coaster, your body needs some time to readjust to a steady caloric diet.

You have already learned how important it is to stay well hydrated. It doesn't make sense, then, to purposely try to lose water. Keeping this in mind, you can avoid some of the diet gimmicks that promise you weight loss and deliver by causing a water-weight loss. For example, rubber suits and plastic wrappings trap in heat so that you sweat out pounds of water. Saunas and whirlpools also sweat out water weight. Some of the diet pills are diuretics that cause you to lose water through frequent urination. Waist and thigh belts temporarily push and sweat water out of targeted areas so that measurements taken immediately after the belt is removed show lost inches. In a couple of hours, the inches are back. Any program that depends on excessive water loss for weight reduction is dangerous and ineffective. You want to lose fat, not water.

Also watch out for "all you can eat" approaches to dieting. If you eat more calories than you expend, you will gain weight. The origin of the calories doesn't matter; if there are too many, they will be stored as fat. Moreover, if all the calories come from a restricted list of foods, you may miss some essential nutrients.

Perhaps one of the all-time biggest diet and exercise myths is **spot reducing.** You cannot choose where the fat will come off your body. In general, it will come off gradually all over. If fat tends to accumulate in one place on your body, you can speculate with some certainty that where it went on first, it will come off last. Don't fall into the trap of thinking that because you use your legs to run, you will get rid of the fat on your thighs more quickly. Running on your hands could be just as effective in removing leg fat. Of course, running on your legs will tone up the leg muscles underneath the fat, and running on your hands would certainly help tone your arms.

EATING DISORDERS

Some individuals start to diet and then can't stop. They look in the mirror and continue to see a fat person. One such disease, **anorexia nervosa,** is widespread among women. Men can also suffer from it, but the estimated cases of men with anorexia nervosa are thought to be relatively few (about one in ten) at this time. Anorexia nervosa is often associated with life-threatening weight losses and denial of weight loss by the dieter. This disease requires both psychological and medical assistance. If you know anyone suffering from anorexia, do everything possible to get him or her to professional help. Otherwise, your friend may literally starve himself or herself to death.

Bulimia, another eating disorder, is characterized by eating regular-sized or large meals and then intentionally emptying the food out of the stomach by self-induced vomiting or the use of laxatives. The lining of the throat and esophagus can become damaged from repeated contact with stomach acids during regurgitation. People suffering from bulimia look healthy, especially since they try to hide their binge-and-purge behavior. Like people who exhibit anorexia, those who suffer from bulimia need immediate psychological and medical attention.

Binge-eating disorder is characterized by episodes of uncontrolled excessive and rapid overeating. Because there is no purging, theses individuals tend to be overweight or obese. Often ashamed of their eating habits, they dine alone. The cause is not known, but this disorder may be accompanied by feelings of anger, sadness, boredom, or depression. Both women and men suffer from this disorder, approximately two men for every three women. Eating disorder conditions are completely reversible if caught early enough. Help is as close as the health and counseling centers on campus.

WEIGHT GAIN

At first it's hard to imagine that anyone would want to gain weight, but there are actually quite a number of people who need weight-gain diets. Certainly, undernourished individuals and people recovering from illnesses and accidents fall into this category. On a brighter note, so do athletes and body builders who are trying to put on lean body mass and a few, such as sumo wrestlers, who are actually trying to put on fat as well. Of course, pregnant women must be on weight-gain diets.

To gain lean body weight, you increase your calorie consumption so that it exceeds your calorie expenditure and continue to exercise. If you only increase what you eat and don't exercise, you store the extra calories as fat. (Pregnant women are the exception to this rule.) As mentioned previously, you should add the calories in a way that maintains the recommended percentages of carbohydrates, protein, and fat. A common mistake is to increase protein intake without making a corresponding increase in carbohydrate intake. The body ends up with an excess of protein and too few carbohydrates to fuel the exercise workout.

Muscle (lean body mass) is most effectively increased through progressive resistance exercises such as weight training. Participants in aerobic dance exercise may be able to gain some lean body mass through endurance exercises, depending on their initial strength and whether they use step aerobics, exercise bands, or hand and wrist weights. Aerobic exercise usually reduces fat and maintains lean tissue.

A pregnant woman's weight gain is a little different, but it still involves eating more calories than daily activity expends. The extra calories are used to sustain the higher metabolic rate of the mother and for the growth and development of the baby. Roughly speaking, a pregnant woman needs to consume an extra 300 calories per day. If a woman begins an exercise program after getting pregnant, she needs to eat enough extra calories to support the activity as well. Pregnancy weight gains and exercise programs during and after pregnancy should always be done in consultation with a physician.

WEIGHT MAINTENANCE

Maintaining a healthy weight is like standing on your hands. Watch gymnasts carefully and you will see them make slight adjustments with their fingertips and wrists the whole time they are upside down. Balance is dynamic, not static. To keep your weight and body composition in balance, you constantly need to be aware of your body's needs and activity level and adjust your intake accordingly. The first lesson in this adjustment usually occurs in the late teens when you hear yourself remarking, "I haven't changed my diet at all, and suddenly I'm gaining weight." This is probably because you are done growing and don't need as many calories. It may also reflect a change in lifestyle. Whenever you become more or less physically active, whether the activity is job or exercise related, you need to adjust your diet accordingly. Imagine the different caloric needs of a teenager, a nursing mother, a construction worker, a business executive, and an elderly person. Some of the critical adjustment periods occur during and after pregnancy, around middle age, and at retirement. Listening to your body, adjusting your dietary intake, and maintaining a regular exercise regimen can keep you in balance throughout your life.

COMMONLY ASKED QUESTIONS

Will exercise increase my appetite?

Some people worry that exercise will make them hungrier and that they will eat as many or more calories than they exercised off. This does not seem to be the case. Most people who exercise at a moderate intensity eat the same or just slightly more calories—not enough to overtake their increased expenditure. Lean individuals will generally increase their caloric intake to maintain their weight. Moderate exercise one to two hours before a meal may actually decrease appetite, but there is some evidence that hunger returns several hours later. You can take advantage of this if you plan a low-calorie snack for later.

Is yo-yo dieting dangerous to my health?

Yo-yo dieting, losing and gaining back weight repeatedly, was initially reported to be harmful and connected to an increased risk of some diseases. More research on this has not been able to conclusively link yo-yo dieting with greater health risk, other than perhaps depression and loss of self-esteem as a result of repeated failures. Professionals recommend that people who are obese or substantially overweight should try to lose weight even if they tend to put it back on, because any weight loss at this level can have significant health benefits.

Someone who is not substantially overweight and who does not have other medical reasons or disease risk factors should aim for maintenance. Just a 10% weight loss greatly reduces disease risk and may improve blood pressure, lipids, and blood glucose.

Should I eat more when I exercise?

If you are trying to maintain or gain weight, yes. If you are trying to lose weight, no. You should, however, maintain at least a 1,200-calorie diet if you are a woman, and 1,500 calories per day if you are a man. Pregnant women who exercise should eat enough additional calories to offset the exercise plus the recommended extra 300 calories a day.

How do I get rid of cellulite?

Cellulite is ordinary fat stored under the skin where it is separated into little compartments by connective fibers. It gets its dimplelike appearance when the fat cells increase in size and bulge out between the connective fibers. The extent to which you develop cellulite is dependent on the amount of fat you store, the strength of the connective fibers, and the thickness of your skin. In women, as compared with men, the fibers tend to be more taut and the skin thinner so that the dimpling is more apparent. Pills, teas, creams, and rolling it under grandmother's rolling pin will not rid you of this fat. Like all fat, it responds to exercise and a balanced low-fat diet. If you have attained a healthy percentage of fat and still have some cellulite, you may have to call a truce.

When should I drink water?

You should stay hydrated at all times. This means that you should drink water about half an hour before class and be sure to replenish your liquids after exercising. Drinking water during class is also a healthy habit. If the class is only an hour long, you probably don't need to stop and get a drink. But if you are thirsty, by all means get one. If you are involved in prolonged exercise, you should drink about half a cup of fluids every half-hour. It is even more critical to drink water on hot days. Thirst is not a good indicator of your need for water during exercise. Drink before you get thirsty.

Will a candy bar before class give me quick energy?

It will give you a short burst of energy and then actually drop your blood sugar. Whenever the blood glucose level gets too high, the pancreas excretes insulin, which acts to lower the blood sugar. When a lot of sugar is introduced to the system quickly, the pancreas puts out a lot of insulin. That much insulin ends up dropping the blood sugar below the level it was at prior to the candy. Halfway through class, you may suddenly feel very hungry or even sluggish from low blood sugar. Some people are affected more than others. You would be better off eating a few crackers or a piece of fruit before class.

Do I really need to eat breakfast before a morning aerobics class?

Not necessarily. The important thing is that you eat a balanced diet over the course of the day. Many early-morning exercisers eat breakfast after they exercise. However, it would probably be a good idea to hydrate yourself by drinking water or juice before exercising. Other people find they need to eat breakfast to boost their blood sugar before exercising.

Does caffeine improve exercise performance?

Research has shown that caffeine can improve long-distance running performance, but ingesting caffeine has two drawbacks. One is that you end up needing to go to the bathroom in the middle of the race. The other is that since caffeine is a diuretic, you will dehydrate more quickly. There doesn't appear to be any advantage in having caffeine before aerobic dance exercise. In fact, in terms of your health, you are better off limiting your caffeine intake, especially if you have high blood pressure.

Can I eat just fruits instead of fruits and vegetables?

A variety of just fruits can provide you with about the same compliment of vitamins and minerals as vegetables but will not provide you with the same richness of phytochemicals and carotenoids needed to help fight heart disease and cancer. There is also still much to understand about how different foods interact. So the healthiest path today is to provide your body with a wide variety of both fruits and vegetables.

Should I change my diet if I start an exercise program?

That depends on what your current diet is and whether you are trying to maintain, lose, or gain weight. If you are eating a healthy, well-balanced diet and are content with your present body composition, you will need to consume more calories to replace the calories you will expend during exercise. For more information, refer to page 185.

If I stop exercising, will my muscle turn to fat?

Not exactly. The muscle does not magically turn into fat. However, when you stop exercising, you will likely lose lean body mass (muscle) from disuse, and, if you do not alter your diet, the calories once expended during exercise will be stored as fat. This is the problem many athletes experience when they graduate and decrease their high levels of training. The key is to keep moving and adjust diet and exercise to your ever-changing life needs.

Are there good carbohydrates and bad carbohydrates?

Yes, there are nutrient-dense and nutrient-empty carbohydrates. See page 168.

Are there good fats and bad fats?

Saturated fats increase the risk of some diseases, whereas unsaturated fats are either neutral or help decrease cholesterol and disease risk. Some, such as omega-3 fatty acids, promote health. See page 171.

Do I need more protein if I am resistance training? Endurance training?

You may need more than the recommended 0.8 g/kg per day, but you will also need more calories overall to sustain your diet. The percentage of protein compared to carbohydrates and fats will not change significantly, but the total amount of calories will. Most individuals already consume more protein than they need, even for active exercising regimens.

How can I eat healthy when I'm so busy?

There are a lot of healthy foods that are easy to carry with you. Consider stocking up on these and keeping them handy where you live and in your car if you are a commuter. At first this will take some effort (for example, reading food labels), but when you've become used to doing so, you'll find that it's pretty easy. For example, when you find yourself hungry, avoid the temptation to go for fast food. Instead, eat a handful of nuts. They are better for you and will hold you until you can get to a healthier meal.

SUMMARY

Each nutrient plays a special role in your health and well-being, which makes it vital to eat a balanced diet. Being aware of what you are putting in your mouth is the key to eating a balanced, nutritious diet. As an awareness project, record what you eat on a weekday and a weekend day using Worksheets 17 and 18 and answer the questions. You may be surprised at what you discover.

The bottom line of weight control is that there are no known quick and easy ways to lose fat. You put it on gradually; it must come off gradually. Exercise makes the process a little easier and a lot more fun.

KNOWLEDGE TIPS

1. The diet should consist of 45 to 65% carbohydrates, 10 to 35% protein, and 20 to 35% fat.

2. Carbohydrate is the primary source of energy for the body. Fat is used for energy when prolonged periods of activity demand it. Protein is used for energy when there is a shortage of available carbohydrate.

3. Dietary fat from unsaturated fats is healthier than saturated or *trans* fat.

4. A balanced diet should depend primarily on foods from the base of the food pyramid: fruits, vegetables, whole-grain breads, cereals, rice, pasta, low-fat milk, yogurt, and cheese, and meats, poultry, fish, dry beans, eggs, and nuts.

5. Vitamins play an essential role in the release of energy from foods.

6. Minerals are inorganic compounds that supply strength and rigidity to body structures and play an important role in the regulation of body processes.

7. Eat fruits and vegetables high in antioxidants and phytochemicals to help reduce risk of cancer and heart disease.

8. Proper hydration is critical to physical health and performance.

9. Plain cool water is the best source of hydration/rehydration for fitness exercisers exercising for one hour or less. Water is absorbed into the body more quickly than sugared drinks.

10. Healthy body composition is characterized by a relatively low percentage of body fat and a relatively high percentage of lean body mass. Healthy women require a higher percentage of fat than do healthy men.

11. During energy balance, caloric intake is equal to caloric expenditure. Weight is gained when intake surpasses expenditure. Weight is lost when expenditure surpasses intake.

12. Genetics, environment, socioeconomic status, gender, and psychological factors all play a role in weight control.

13. High-intensity activity burns more calories per minute than low-intensity activity. Yet, most people are more successful using longer durations at lower intensities than shorter durations at higher intensities to burn the same number of calories.

14. High-intensity work primarily burns carbohydrate. Moderate-intensity work burns carbohydrate and fat.

15. Aerobic exercise most days of the week, for 60 to 90 minutes at a low to moderate intensity, is recommended for weight loss.

16. Anorexia nervosa, bulimia, and binge-eating are eating disorders that require immediate medical and psychological attention.

17. Unbalanced and rapid weight-loss diets can be dangerous, even life-threatening.

18. Most weight-loss experts recommend losing about 1 lb per week.

THINK ABOUT IT

1. Identify the six essential nutrients and explain their key roles.

2. Why do some foods give you more nutrition than others? Give examples.

3. What is the difference between simple and complex carbohydrates?

4. What are "good" fat and "bad" fat?

5. Identify good food sources of fiber.

6. Explain the concept of energy balance and the role exercise can play in it.

7. Describe the role and quantity of protein needed for muscle building.

8. Why is it better to measure body composition than weight?

9. What are some techniques for measuring body composition?

10. What are some good strategies for managing weight?

11. Explain how fat and carbohydrate burning are affected by exercise intensity and duration.

12. What kinds of substitution changes can you make to eat healthier (such as switching to skim milk from whole milk)?

13. How can your diet affect your mood? How can your mood affect your diet?

REFERENCES

Ahrens, J. N., L. K. Lloyd, S. H. Crixell, and J. L. Walker. "The Effects of Caffeine in Women During Aerobic-Dance Bench Stepping." *International Journal of Sport Nutrition and Exercise Metabolism* 17 (No. 1, 2007): 27–34.

American College of Sports Medicine. "Appropriate Intervention Strategies for Weight Loss and Prevention of Weight Regain for Adults." *Medicine and Science in Sports and Exercise* 33 (No. 12, 2001): 2145–56.

American College of Sports Medicine and American Dietetic Association. "Joint Position Statement on Nutrition and Athletic Performance." *Medicine and Science in Sports and Exercise* 41 (No. 3, 2009): 709–31.

American Dietetic Association. "Position Statement on Nutrition and Physical Fitness." *Journal of the American Dietetic Association* 76 (1980): 437–43.

——. "Position of the American Dietetic Association: Nutrition Intervention in the Treatment of Anorexia Nervosa, Bulimia Nervosa, and Binge Eating." *Journal of the American Dietetic Association* 94 (No. 8, 1994): 902–7.

——. "Position of the American Dietetic Association: Vegetarian Diets." *Journal of the American Dietetic Association* 97 (No. 11, 1997): 1317–21.

Food and Nutrition Information Center. *Dietary Guidelines for Americans: A Historical Overview*. Beltsville, MD: National Agricultural Library USDA, 2008.

Foster, C., D. L. Costill, and W. J. Fink. "Effects of Preexercise Feedings on Endurance Performance." *Medicine and Science in Sports* 11 (No. 1, 1979): 1–5.

Kirk, E. P., J. E. Donnelly, B. K. Smith, J. Honas, J. D. Lecheminant, B. W. Bailey, D. J. Jacobsen, and R. A. Washburn. "Minimal Resistance Training Improves Daily Energy Expenditure and Fat Oxidation." *Medicine and Science in Sports and Exercise* 41 (No. 5, 2009): 1122–9.

Lee, C. D., A. S. Jackson, and S. N. Blair. "U.S. Weight Guidelines: Is It Also Important to Consider Cardiorespiratory Fitness?" *International Journal of Obesity* 22 (1998, Suppl 2): S2–S7.

National Dairy Council. "The New Food Guidance System." *Dairy Council Digest* 76 (No. 4, 2005): 19–24.

National Research Council, National Academy of Sciences. *Diet and Health: Implications for Reducing Chronic Disease Risk*. Washington, DC, 1989.

Powers, S. K., and E. T. Howley. *Exercise Physiology: Theory and Application to Fitness and Performance*. 6th ed. New York: McGraw-Hill, 2006, 62–9.

Rixon, K. P., P. R. Rehor, and M. G. Bemben. "Analysis of the Assessment of Caloric Expenditure in Four Modes of Aerobic Dance." *Journal of Strength and Conditioning Research* 20 (No. 3, 2006): 593–6.

The USDA Food Guide in "Preparing Foods and Planning Menus Using the Dietary Guidelines." *HG*, 232–8, 1989.

U.S. Department of Health and Human Services and U.S. Department of Agriculture. *Dietary Guidelines for Americans*. 6th ed. Washington, DC: U.S. Government Printing Office, January 2005.

13

Prevention and Care

Pain to gain . . . you'll wind up lame! No pain, gradual gain . . . win the health fitness game.

- It seems like every time I start exercising I get hurt. How can I avoid this?
- What are the most common injuries in aerobic dance exercise?
- How can I prevent and/or treat shinsplints? Knee pain? Back pain?
- What should I do if I get injured?

IF you are in pursuit of health and fitness, there is no reason to beat your body into the ground. Leave the pain and agony to the professionals who are paid handsomely to put their bodies at risk. Some soreness at the beginning of a program is normal, but if you are hurt, exhausted, and run-down after a workout, something is wrong. You should feel temporarily tired and then actually get a lift of energy from the workout.

Aerobic dance exercise is a safe, fun way to exercise, yet injuries do occur. Most of the injuries that occur in aerobic dance exercise can be prevented.

A quick look at the research on aerobic dance injuries can lead you to the wrong conclusions. About 75% of instructors and 45% of students reported having injuries; this percentage might make one think that aerobic dance exercise is a high-risk activity. Examining the research more carefully, however, shows that most of the injuries were not debilitating, did not require medical treatment, and could be remedied without requiring the person to stop exercising. Instructors most likely report more injuries because they spend more time doing the activity. Instructors are often guilty of exceeding the recommended frequency of 3 to 5 times per week and duration of 20 to 30 minutes. This makes them more susceptible to overuse injuries. Participants who get hooked on aerobic dance exercise sometimes become overzealous. It is a good idea to take at least one day off a week

and/or use non-weight-bearing aerobic activities such as swimming or bicycling to supplement your aerobic dance exercise. This relieves some of the stress on the lower legs. Not surprisingly, more than half of the reported injuries were below the knee. The most common injuries were shinsplints and tendinitis. In most cases, these are overuse injuries that can be prevented by altering the frequency, intensity, and duration of activity. Other injury prevention strategies are working out on a shock-absorbing floor; wearing supportive, shock-absorbing shoes; using equipment properly; and practicing the proper techniques, positions, and alignments for each exercise. If you do experience problems, be sure to check with your health care provider. One big mistake is to continue to exercise "through pain." Injured body parts need rest and time to heal. At the same time, the exercise program and the participant's exercise technique may need to be adjusted to prevent reinjury. When returning to exercise after an injury, participants need to start slowly and be careful not to overload their "weakest link," the injured part. For example, after a sprained ankle, you should add weights back to a lunge or squat exercise only when you can perform a regular lunge or squat without pain.

When the cause of injury can be identified, the program or facility can be modified to eliminate or minimize the risk of future injury. For example, one major cause of shinsplints in aerobic dance exercise is impact stress. Modifications that have been made to minimize shinsplints include the production of better-designed aerobic shoes, the installation and use of better floors, and the introduction of low-impact aerobics.

Participants can also protect themselves against injury by increasing their strength and flexibility. Back pain, for example, can often be prevented or relieved by adopting a good stretching and strengthening program. More group fitness classes are offering ways to increase resistance during muscle-toning exercises. The addition of equipment such as barbells, dumbbells, bands, and stability balls can increase the risk of injury. However, when exercises are done properly and with qualified supervision, the result is a stronger body with a greater resistance to injury. Using the appropriate overloads and good technique is what makes the difference. Ask your instructor to check your alignment, especially on exercises such as squats and lunges, where proper back, hip, and knee alignment is critical.

People who are beginning a program and those with a history of orthopedic problems run a slightly higher risk of injury. To reduce this elevated risk, they should seek advice from their physician, start slowly, overload gradually, and avoid exercises that hurt.

Unfortunately, there will always be unforeseeable accidents. When an accident occurs, the best thing to do is to have a qualified person administer prompt, proper first aid. Make sure the facility where you exercise is prepared to handle injury and emergency situations.

In the following pages, you will see **RICE** listed as a treatment for some of the injuries. RICE stands for **rest, ice, compression, and elevation.** This is a standard first-aid treatment for injuries such as a muscle strain or sprain. If done soon after the injury, RICE can help cut down on inflammation and swelling and decrease the recovery time. "Rest" means to immediately stop using the injured part. "Ice" means to apply something cold to the injured part. You can use crushed ice in a bag, a cold pack, or, in a pinch, something like a cold drink can until you can find a better source of cold. Ice is usually administered in cycles of 20 minutes on and then 20 minutes off. "Compression" means to apply pressure. This is usually accomplished with an ace bandage. (If there is bleeding, pressure points and more bandaging may be required.) Wetting the bandage on a sprain or strain will help transmit the cold from the ice more effectively. Finally, "elevation" means to put the injured part above the heart. This helps keep the swelling down.

Too often, people who have pulled a muscle or twisted an ankle use heat instead of cold. Heat is therapeutic when the time is right. Check with a health care professional before switching from cold to heat.

Another mistake is to avoid performing RICE because you are embarrassed or don't wish to be fussed over. Doing these simple things while the injury is new can make a significant difference to your recovery.

Learn how to put prevention in your program. Listed below are some of the injuries that can occur during aerobic dance exercise. The common causes, preventive actions, and proper first aid for each injury are described.

FOOT INJURIES

BLISTER

DEFINITION Inflammation of the skin that results in a collection of fluid below the skin.

SYMPTOMS Hot and red skin.

CAUSE Friction of the skin against something else.

PREVENTION Wear shoes that fit properly; wear socks. Put bandages or skin tape or rub petroleum jelly over the heel and other high-risk locations before breaking in new shoes or doing a prolonged physical activity.

TREATMENT Apply ice, rest, and put a felt or moleskin donut around the blister so that no further rubbing will occur. If the blister opens, wash with soap and water, dry, apply antibiotic ointment, and cover the area. Do not intentionally pop a blister. If it is in a very uncomfortable location and must be drained, use a sterilized needle to make a small hole in the lower side, drain, use antibiotic ointment, and cover. Do not remove the skin. If the blister develops red streaks or looks infected, see a physician immediately.

BUNION

DEFINITION Irritation of the toe joint (usually the big toe) resulting in a fluid build-up in the capsule surrounding the joint. Toe may turn inward.

SYMPTOMS Burning, tenderness, swelling, redness, pain, and misalignment of toe.

CAUSES Wearing shoes that are too narrow or too short. Individuals with flat feet or who have feet that pronate are more susceptible since their big toe is rolled down and inward which can result in friction.

PREVENTION Wear shoes that fit well and have a sufficient toe box. Orthotics may be needed to correct pronation, flat feet.

TREATMENT Reduce friction by using a felt donut and wearing new shoes with a large enough toe box. Soak your feet in cool water. See a physician. Surgical correction may be necessary.

METATARSALGIA

DEFINITION Irritation of the nerves that lie between the metatarsal bones. (Metatarsals are the bones between the toes and the arch.)

SYMPTOMS Pain under the ball of the foot.

CAUSES Shifting forward of the protective fat pad under the ball of the foot from excessively landing on it; overuse.

PREVENTION An aerobic shoe with good metatarsal (forefoot) padding, good jump-landing technique, and resilient floor. Avoid overuse.

TREATMENT Ice, rest, and cushioned foot pads. If the pain persists, see a physician. You may need metatarsal lifts or orthotics.

PLANTAR FASCIITIS

DEFINITION Strain to the broad sheet of connective tissue that runs from the heel to the metatarsals, which supports the longitudinal arch. When weight is shifted to the ball of the foot, the tension held by this connective tissue equals twice the body's weight. Microtears may occur where the fascia attaches to the heel bone.

SYMPTOMS Pain just in front of the heel where the connective tissue connects to the heel bone. Heel may feel bruised. Pain may also radiate along the arch.

CAUSES A rapid increase in activity that requires pushing off the ball of the foot, particularly on a hard surface; wearing unsupportive shoes.

PREVENTION Work into a new program gradually. Wear shoes that support the arches. Develop calf flexibility. Strengthen the muscles in the foot and ankle.

TREATMENT Rest, soak your feet in cool water, buy new shoes or arch supports. If pain persists, see a physician; you may need orthotics or anti-inflammatory drugs, or surgery.

MORTON'S NEUROMA

DEFINITION Localized swelling of the sensory nerve that lies between the metatarsals (bones in the ball of the foot) and innervates the toes.

SYMPTOMS Pain radiating up between the third and fourth toes.

CAUSES Overuse, too much running on the ball of the foot.

PREVENTION Well-cushioned aerobic shoes. Avoid overuse by doing a practical exercise program. Use a metatarsal arch pad (a felt pad that fits under the ball of the foot).

TREATMENT See a physician.

SHIN INJURIES

SHINSPLINTS

DEFINITION This is a general term for pain on the front or side of the lower leg. Some believe the pain comes from minute tearing of the muscle sheath from the shin bone membrane. Others believe the pain comes from damage caused by excessive vibration of the bone.

SYMPTOMS Pain and aching in the shin area after and sometimes during exercise. May be specific areas of tenderness or swelling over the bone.

CAUSES Impact stress from a hard floor, poorly cushioned shoes, too much jumping, poor foot mechanics, poor posture, fallen arches, insufficient warm-up, fatigue, training too fast or too soon, poor exercise technique.

PREVENTION Dance on a resilient floor with good arch-supporting shoes and use proper footwork. Strengthen the foot muscles and muscles that surround the shin, especially the anterior tibialis. Stretch calves well before and after working out. Also keep shins warm before and during class. Warm-up socks are helpful for this.

TREATMENT Ice shins for 20 to 30 minutes following exercise. You may want to freeze water in a paper cup and use it to massage your shins. Just peel down the cup as the ice melts.

If any bruising, swelling, or specific point tenderness occurs, stop exercising and rest your legs. If pain persists or worsens, consult a physician. You may need to take an anti-inflammatory drug or be fitted for orthotics.

Some individuals get relief from having their arches, shins, or both taped—consult an athletic trainer or podiatrist. Some people also get relief by running backward.

If your shins start to bother you during a class, try modifying the movements to a low-impact style. At some facilities (i.e., a health club), you can leave the floor during the standing aerobics to bicycle, row, or do stairs, and then rejoin the class for muscle-toning exercises.

STRESS FRACTURE

DEFINITION Very thin, undisplaced hairline break in a bone.

SYMPTOMS Pain along the lower leg bones. If you have a stress fracture in the lower leg, it will hurt before, during, and after class and even when you get off your feet. Painful when you touch it, especially in one area.

CAUSES Same as shinsplints.

PREVENTION Wear cushioned, supportive shoes, avoid overuse and nonresilient surfaces.

TREATMENT See a physician. Stress fractures are difficult to diagnose because they don't show up on X-ray images until calcium deposits are made during the healing process. When a stress fracture is diagnosed, activity is restricted and the fractured part of the leg may be immobilized in a cast.

KNEE INJURIES

CHONDROMALACIA PATELLAE

DEFINITION Roughening or softening of the joint surface of the knee cap (patella).

SYMPTOMS Pain when patella is pressed on, maybe creaking and popping noises. May hurt when climbing stairs or kneeling. Knee pain while exercising.

CAUSES Knee cap may be sliding out of alignment and causing irritation. Cartilage may be inflamed or degenerating. May be caused by deep knee bends or other exercises that stress the knee.

PREVENTION Perform a good warm-up. Avoid deep knee bends and knee hyperextension positions. Strengthen the muscles that surround and support the knee, using straight-leg exercises if you already have some knee irritation. Stretch leg muscles, especially the hamstrings and calves.

TREATMENT Ice the knee. See a physician. Strengthen supporting muscles. Avoid kneeling versions of exercises.

MENISCAL INJURIES

DEFINITION Strains or tears of the cartilage that stabilizes the knee joint.

SYMPTOMS Acute pain, popping noise, swelling, knee may "give out" or lock.

CAUSES Rotation or twisting of the knee joint beyond normal limitations. Foot remaining planted when the body turns so that the knee is forced to accept the rotational force. A floor with too much cushion allows the foot to sink into it and remain planted. Sticky floors or treaded shoes on nonslip surfaces may also cause the foot to remain planted. Injury can also be caused by working the knee joint with too much weight.

PREVENTION Select the appropriate shoe for the surface. Select the best possible surface. Use workout routines that don't require sudden pivots or turns, particularly on soft floors. Work with reasonable amounts of weight during leg exercises. Overload gradually and strengthen the supporting muscles.

TREATMENT Support the back of the knee and pack the knee in ice. Move the person only if the knee is supported. Keep injured person warm and call a doctor. Joint may have to be aspirated (excess fluid removed from the joint).

MULTIPLE SITE INJURIES

STRAIN

DEFINITION A **strain** is an injury to a muscle or a tendon. (**Tendons** connect muscles to bone; e.g., the Achilles tendon connects the calf muscle to the heel.)

SYMPTOMS There are three degrees of injury. First-degree symptoms: local pain and tenderness, usually accompanied by swelling and pain. Exercise may be continued when pain and swelling are absent and range of motion is complete. Second-degree symptoms: pain with muscle movement, muscle spasm, increased swelling, and tearing of tissue. Do not continue exercise. Third-degree symptoms: severe pain and disability, severe muscle spasms, and complete tearing of tissue. Do not continue exercise.

CAUSES Pushing a muscle or tendon beyond its normal range, often by a ballistic movement before the body is fully warmed up. May also occur from overuse or flinging the arms, especially when arm weights are used. Older persons are more prone to injury.

PREVENTION Warm up and stretch well before working out. Strengthen both agonists and antagonists.

TREATMENT Rest, ice, compress, and elevate (RICE) the injured muscle or tendon. If pain is acute or persists, see a physician. Do not move anyone who has a third-degree strain. Call a doctor; surgery may be necessary.

SPRAIN

DEFINITION A **sprain** is an injury to a ligament. (**Ligaments** attach bones to bones.)

SYMPTOMS First-degree symptoms: twinge of discomfort, slight skin discoloration from internal bleeding, some ligament fiber damage. Exercise may be continued when pain and swelling are absent and range of motion is complete. Second-degree symptoms: pain, swelling, loss of function for several minutes, tender to the touch, loss of strength, definite tear of fibers. Do not continue exercise. Third-degree symptoms: severe pain and swelling, discoloration of skin, complete tear of the ligament, loss of function. Do not continue exercise.

CAUSES Any movement that pulls two connected bones apart more than a normal amount.

PREVENTION Warm up and stretch before working out. Exercise regularly so that ligaments are strengthened. Overload gradually and remember that ligament strength gains are usually slower than cardiorespiratory gains. When your heart says keep going, check in with the rest of your body. Strengthen muscles that surround joints so that they can minimize the stress put on the ligaments. Avoid exercises that put pressure on ligaments, and do exercises that strengthen muscles. For example, squats and lunges strengthen the legs as long as you don't bend the knee too much; deep knee bends stress the ligaments, and because the muscles are in a weak mechanical position, they can't help the ligaments.

TREATMENT Rest, ice, compress, and elevate (RICE) the injured part. If pain is acute or persists, consult a physician. If it is a third-degree sprain, do not move the person. Keep the person warm and call a doctor. Surgical repair may be necessary.

TENDINITIS

DEFINITION Chronic inflammation or irritation of a tendon. Microscopic tears in the tendon tissue may be the cause of the inflammation. In aerobics, the most commonly injured tendons are the Achilles, shoulder, and elbow.

SYMPTOMS Area may be painful to the touch, warm, and swollen. Skin may be red.

CAUSES Repeated excessive stretching of a tendon; excessive running or jumping, especially on hard surfaces; flinging of arms, particularly when wrist weights are used.

PREVENTION Use careful, deliberate movements rather than flinging movements. Gradually overload. Warm up and stretch out prior to vigorous activity.

TREATMENT Ice and rest the tendon. If pain is acute or chronic, see a physician. May require anti-inflammatory drugs or surgery.

BURSITIS

DEFINITION Inflammation or irritation of a bursa. Bursas are fluid-filled sacks found around the body at sites where friction might occur, such as where muscle tendons and sheaths cross over bones.

SYMPTOMS Localized inflammation, pain, swelling, and heat.

CAUSES Overstretching of the Achilles tendon, direct blow to the elbow or knee, pressure on an area such as the knee, or overuse of a joint, such as the deltoid at the shoulder through unaccustomed overhead arm activity.

PREVENTION Avoid overuse of muscles and joints. Avoid kneeling on a hard floor. Use gradual overloads, especially when adding resistance through weights or exercise bands. Use good exercise technique.

TREATMENT Ice and compress the area. If pain, swelling, or loss of motion persists, consult a physician.

MUSCLE CRAMP

DEFINITION Painful muscle contraction that will not voluntarily release.

SYMPTOMS Acute pain.

CAUSES Fatigue or heat. (Also common among pregnant women, possibly due to chemical changes.)

PREVENTION Warm up well before vigorous exercise. Stretch a muscle following strength and aerobic workouts. Stretch whenever even slight muscle cramping occurs. Wear comfortable, lightweight clothing to prevent heat buildup. Hydrate with water prior to exercise and if cramps develop.

TREATMENT Stretch and massage the muscle. (You can also ice the opposing muscle because its contraction will cause the other muscle to stretch.)

LOW BACK PAIN

Low back pain is actually a symptom and may be the result of a number of underlying causes. For this reason, if you experience back pain you should consult your health care provider. Some of the causes of low back pain include:

- muscle strains or sprains
- disc herniation
- genetic abnormalities
- bony abnormalities
- pregnancy or premenstrual/menstrual symptoms

A normal healthy person may help prevent low back pain by:

1. exercising with good technique and alignment
2. exercising with gradual overloads
3. avoiding positions that put strain on the low back area
4. strengthening and stretching the muscles, especially the core muscles
5. using good postural positions throughout daily life
6. engaging the abdominal muscles when lifting
7. modifying exercises that are too advanced for one's present fitness

Please also refer to Chapter 6 for a discussion on back care and prevention of low back pain.

HEAT-RELATED INJURIES

HEAT CRAMP

See Muscle Cramp.

HEAT EXHAUSTION

DEFINITION Overheating of the body.

SYMPTOMS Muscle spasms or cramping, cold and clammy skin, chills, nausea, dizziness, and profuse sweating.

CAUSES Inability to dissipate heat because the air is too hot or humid for the level of activity. Sometimes aerobic studios are not properly ventilated, or the cooling systems are insufficient. Situations can also arise when the exercise room shares air from a pool.

PREVENTION Exercise in a well-ventilated, controlled-temperature environment, or adjust the exercise level so that it is safe for the environment. Keep yourself well hydrated and wear comfortable, lightweight clothing.

TREATMENT Drink water and cool the body by going to a cooler place or using ice. Rest.

HEAT STROKE

DEFINITION Inability of the body to handle heat stress. This is a medical emergency. The core temperature is rising, and brain damage and death can result.

SYMPTOMS Dry and hot skin, pale or flushed skin, nausea, dizziness, faintness, weakness, or exhaustion. Skin may be still sweating if exercise has just stopped.

CAUSES Overexposure to a hot or a hot and humid environment.

PREVENTION Keep yourself well hydrated. Do not exercise in very hot weather or when the heat and humidity combine to cause a hazardous condition. Although these conditions do not occur often in most places, a wise participant will not continue to take a class if the air conditioner fails (or if he or she is attending a class outdoors) on a very hot day. Such a day may be good for water aerobics.

TREATMENT Immediately cool the body. Put person in a cold shower or dump cold water all over him or her. Call an ambulance immediately.

COMMONLY ASKED QUESTIONS

Should I exercise when I'm sick?
No, exercise is a stressor. When your body is trying to fight off infection, it needs rest, not stress.

How can I tell if I am overtraining?
One way to tell is to monitor your resting heart rate first thing in the morning. If it starts to increase, give yourself a day off. Another sign of overtraining is loss of strength. Strength gains are made only when the muscle has enough time to rebuild between exercise bouts. Chronic injury, lethargy, lack of motivation, overuse injuries, and chronic fatigue are all signs of overuse.

Why do I get muscle cramps during class?
Most cramps occur when a muscle is fatigued. If you experience cramping, stretch out better before class, lower your exercise intensity, and stretch the muscle more often during class. Sometimes poor choreography overworks one set of muscles. This can make you stiff and sore or make you cramp. The best choreography works both muscles in a muscle pair. If you know that you worked one muscle harder than another, do a set of exercises to balance the workout.

Other causes for cramping include overheated muscles, dehydration, and electrolyte imbalance. Drinking water prevents heat cramps. Taking salt pills to prevent heat cramps is not a good idea. The salt can upset your stomach during exercise; furthermore, most American diets contain more salt than is recommended. Only in rare cases is a salt supplement required. Some people find that eating a banana (a good source of potassium) and calcium-rich foods helps prevent cramping. Consult your physician if cramping is persistent.

Sometimes I feel dizzy during class. Can I prevent that?

Dizziness can be caused by a number of things. It may be brought on by low blood sugar. This is often the case when people take a morning class without eating anything for breakfast or skip lunch and take a late afternoon class. Another cause can be heat stress. Wear loose, comfortable clothing and drink water. Dizziness may also be a sign of illness. Medications, both over-the-counter and prescription, can also be the reason. If dizziness occurs, stop exercising and walk around. If you feel as though you are going to faint, lie down and elevate your feet. If dizziness persists, check with a doctor.

I get a side ache (stitch) when I exercise. Why does this happen, and what should I do?

A side-stitch, a pain just under the ribs, can be caused by a poorly conditioned diaphragm muscle, a food allergy (usually to milk), gas, or exercising too soon after eating. To relieve a side-stitch brought on by gas, try stretching up with the arm on the side giving distress. If it continues, slow down your activity and try doing some side and waist stretches.

The diaphragm is a muscle that separates the chest and abdomen. It moves down when you inhale and up when you exhale. When you exercise more, or faster than usual, this muscle can cramp. Try starting more slowly and performing a more gradual overload. Belly breathing (allowing the abdominal muscles to relax and push out as you inhale and contract slightly when you exhale) may help. Belly breathing in combination with exhalations through pursed lips may also help. Strengthening the abdominal muscles by performing curl-ups may help prevent side stitches.

SUMMARY

Many injuries are preventable. Avoid the kinds of exercises that cause injury; you must take responsibility for keeping yourself injury free. If an unforeseen accident does occur, seek proper first aid and then consult a doctor. When you return to class after recovering from an injury, be sure to start out slowly to prevent reinjury.

Much of the fitness information available today is very easy to understand; some of it is very complex; much of it can be misunderstood. Like dieting, exercise information is regularly abused in an attempt to sell quick-fix equipment and programs. The best way to avoid being misinformed is to read exercise literature written by qualified professionals and to ask questions of the experts you have available. Ask your instructors questions—they will welcome the opportunity to enhance your knowledge.

KNOWLEDGE TIPS

1. You can prevent injuries by wearing good shoes, exercising on a resilient surface, using good exercise technique, maintaining proper alignment throughout the class, and modifying exercises to suit your ability.

2. Most of the injuries that occur during aerobic dance exercise are the result of overuse.

3. Only a very small percentage of aerobic dance exercise injuries require the person to stop exercising until the body can heal. Most injuries can be cared for by cutting back overuse activity and using proper shoes and technique.

4. Instructors receive more injuries than do students, probably because instructors spend more time doing aerobics and strength-training classes and are therefore more susceptible to overuse injuries.

5. The immediate first aid for a sprain or strain is RICE: rest, ice, compression, and elevation.

6. Aerobic dance exercise is one of the safest activities available.

THINK ABOUT IT

1. What are the most common injuries in aerobic dance exercise?

2. What is the first aid for injuries? (*Hint:* RICE)

3. What are some strategies for preventing injury?

4. If you are experiencing pain during an exercise, what should you do?

5. What are some specific strategies you can use to prevent shinsplints?

6. What are the symptoms of heat exhaustion? heat stroke?

7. What is the difference between a muscle sprain and a muscle strain?

8. How are the shoes you wear related to injury prevention?

REFERENCES

Belt, C. R. "Injuries Associated with Aerobic Dance." *American Family Physician* 41 (June 1990): 1769–72.

Bishop, J. G., and D. Booth. "Injury Prevention and Care of Aerobic Dance-Exercise Injuries." *National Aerobics Training Association Manual.* Mesa, AZ: National Aerobics Training Association, 1986.

Burkett, L. "Causative Factors in Hamstring Strains." *Medicine and Science in Sports* 2 (1970): 39–42.

Clement, D. B., W. Ammann, J. E. Taunton, R. Lloyd-Smith, D. Jesperson, H. McKay, J. Goldring, and G. O. Matteson. "Exercise-Induced Stress Injuries to the Femur." *International Journal of Sports Medicine* 14 (No. 6, 1993): 347–52.

Clippinger, K. S. *Dance Anatomy and Kinesiology.* Champaign, IL: Human Kinetics, 2007.

du Toit, V., and R. Smith. "Survey of the Effects of Aerobic Dance on the Lower Extremity in Aerobic Instructors." *Journal of the American Podiatric Medical Association* 91 (No. 10, 2001): 528–32.

Fardy, P. S. "Isometric Exercise and the Cardiovascular System." *The Physician and Sportsmedicine* 9 (No. 9, 1981): 42.

Garrick, J. G., D. M. Gillien, and P. Whiteside. "The Epidemiology of Aerobic Dance Injuries." *The American Journal of Sports Medicine* 14 (1986): 67–72.

Hickey, M., and C. A. Hager. "Aerobic Dance Injuries." *Orthopedic Nursing Journal* 13 (No. 5, Sept.–Oct. 1994): 9–12.

Janis, L. R. "Aerobic Dance Survey. A Study of High-Impact Versus Low-Impact Injuries." *Journal of the American Podiatric Medical Association* 80 (No. 8, August 1990): 419–23.

Liemohn, W. "Factors Related to Hamstring Strains." *American Journal of Sports Medicine* 18 (1978): 71–6.

Martin, K. "Soft Aerobics: Gain Without Pain?" *Ms* 14 (May 1986): 52, 54, 113.

Michaud, T. J., J. Rodrigues-Zayas, C. Armstrong, and M. Hartnig. "Ground Reaction Forces in High Impact and Low Impact Aerobic Dance." *Journal of Sports Medicine and Physical Fitness* 33 (No. 4, 1993); 359–66.

Pollock, M. L., L. Gettman, C. Mileses, M. Bah, J. Durstine, and R. Johnson. "Effects of Frequency and Duration of Training on Attrition and Incidence of Injury." *Medicine and Science in Sports* 9 (No. 1, 1977): 31–6.

Richie, D. H., S. F. Kelso, and P. A. Bellucci. "Aerobic Dance Injuries: A Retrospective Study of Instructors and Participants." *The Physician and Sportsmedicine* 13 (No. 2, 1985): 134–5.

Vetter, W. L., D. L. Helfet, K. Spear, and L. S. Matthews. "Aerobic Dance Injuries." *The Physician and Sportsmedicine* 13 (No. 2, 1985): 114–20.

14

A Lifetime of Aerobics . . .

"Light tomorrow with today."

ELIZABETH BARRETT BROWNING

- How do I find a good place to work out during vacation or after I graduate?
- I find health clubs intimidating. Are there alternatives? Or, how do I get past this feeling?
- What should I expect when I visit an exercise facility?
- What questions should I ask before joining a program?

HEALTH-RELATED physical fitness is a lifetime endeavor. It is relatively easy to exercise in a collegiate setting since you are surrounded by other exercisers, recreational facilities, and qualified instructors. After you leave school, your surroundings will change; hopefully your exercise habits will not. To help you take the first step toward continuing your commitment to a lifetime of aerobic conditioning, this chapter offers a few suggestions on how to find aerobic dance exercise and/or group fitness classes outside the college setting.

SELECTING A FACILITY

Exercise programs are offered at a variety of places ranging from town recreation offerings to health clubs. If you are only interested in an aerobic dance exercise class, a health club may be an unnecessary expense. Quality aerobics instructors can be found teaching in places such as churches, town halls, schools, hospitals, and town recreation facilities. Some programs let you pay as you go; others will ask you to sign up and pay for a period of weeks. The fees for programs will vary depending on their overhead costs. The three most important things to investigate concerning these classes are the quality of instruction, the type of floor on which you will be exercising, and how convenient the time and location are for you.

If you are looking for more, such as a weight room, aerobic machines, a pool, or a nursery, check out your local health clubs, employee (corporate wellness) programs, YMCA/YWCA, town recreation programs, and large churches. Knowing some of the characteristics of good programs can help you formulate questions and make decisions as you look at the possibilities in your area.

When you visit a fitness facility, you should receive a full tour and a thorough explanation of the classes that are offered, available equipment, daily hours, and fee structure. Take time to really look around. Bring a friend along if you can so that you feel more relaxed during the tour and can take in more information. Compare notes when you leave. It is easy to feel intimidated when you first visit a facility. A trial membership (2 to 4 weeks) is often available. This gives you a chance to try out equipment, take classes, and see whether you like the instructors. After a few classes and as the staff and other members begin to know you, you should feel more comfortable. Surveying the new scene from a cardio-machine or from a mat where you can stretch are a couple of other ways you can ease yourself into life at a club. Over time, you will become more aware of what a program/facility offers . . . or lacks. Attending the facility during the time you plan to use it gives you a chance to see how crowded it is, the level of cleanliness, staff availability, and the type of classes offered. If after several visits you don't feel positive when you walk in the door, keep looking. It has to be a good match, or you won't go. When you join a fitness program, you should receive an orientation to the facility and

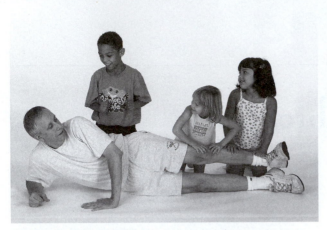

Figure 14.1 A lifetime of fitness. Resistance and encouragement come in many forms!

programs. This orientation should include an introduction to the facility and equipment, a medical history, a fitness evaluation, and exercise prescription. A member of the staff should show you the entire facility and teach you how to use available equipment. A good program will always have someone to help you with exercise questions, equipment, and fitness testing. Sometimes this person is the aerobics instructor, sometimes an additional staff person.

The medical history you complete allows the instructor to work in an informed environment, to decide whether certain exercises should be modified. Find out if the instructor reviews your medical questionnaire or whether it is just filed away.

The fitness evaluation provides baseline data about your personal fitness level. Based on this information, goals and a plan of action can and should be formulated. The program should offer periodic testing to measure improvement, provide motivation, and evaluate the effectiveness of your exercise program. The fitness evaluation should offer measures of cardiorespiratory endurance, muscular strength and endurance, body composition, and flexibility. The person conducting these tests should be knowledgeable and, preferably, have a college degree and/or certification in fitness testing and exercise prescription.

Watch the group fitness class you want to join from beginning to end. If it is an aerobics class, see if it includes a warm-up, 20 to 30 minutes of aerobics, a standing cool-down, resistance exercises (time permitting), and a cool-down stretch. Listen for heart rate or other intensity checks during the class. Check the starting and finishing times for promptness. Make sure you like the instructor's style, and check to see if there is room for you in the class. Check to see if enrollment is limited and if it guarantees you space on the floor. If the class runs on a first-come, first-served basis, be sure you will have enough time to arrive early.

Program variety allows you to select a class that most closely fits your fitness goals and interests. Many programs now offer a variety of workout levels. Check with the instructor to find out what constitutes a beginning, intermediate, and advanced class. Different programs use different criteria for establishing class levels.

As a guideline, beginning aerobic dance exercise classes usually have a 15- to 20-minute standing aerobics section, work at near-threshold intensities, and include shorter sections of resistance exercises. Intermediate classes work aerobically for a minimum of 20 minutes and include fairly demanding resistance exercises, possibly using weights, bands, or balls. Advanced classes work at high intensities and may include workouts with more difficult regimens of weights, bands, or balls. The aerobic section may be 20 to 30 minutes or longer.

Low-impact and step classes are offered in both low and high intensities. Find out when each kind meets and whether equipment like weights and bands are used and supplied. Many clubs also offer group fitness resistance training. If this interests you, see whether there is a convenient class that matches your fitness level.

Special classes may be taught for children, elderly persons, pregnant women (pre/postnatal), people with disabilities, and people who are overweight (overfat). Each class should use music and techniques appropriate to the people involved. Instructors should be qualified to teach these specialty classes.

Select a program that can meet your needs now and in the future. For instance, if you are very active now and are considering becoming pregnant, select a program that has both an advanced class and a pre/postnatal class. That makes it easy to switch from one to the other at the appropriate time. If you can attend only one time of day and one class, look for an instructor who has experience working at different intensities of classes and who is capable of effectively handling people of different fitness levels within one class.

Although major injuries are rare in group fitness classes, it is always comforting to know that the program or facility has an emergency procedure. Check for easy exits, sprinklers, and an available telephone. In addition, the instructors and staff should be educated and certified in cardiopulmonary resuscitation (CPR) and standard first aid. Ice should be readily available in the event of a strain or sprain.

The following is a quick checklist of items to look for as you select an exercise facility. The perfect facility is difficult to find and may be expensive to join, so decide which items are most important to you.

1. The facility should be in a convenient location near home or work.
2. The building should be well ventilated and the temperature set at a comfortable exercise temperature.
3. The lighting should be good quality and nonglare.
4. The whole facility, including locker rooms, should be clean and well supplied even at peak hours.
5. The water in pools and whirlpools should be clear and clean.
6. Mirrors should be strategically placed so that you can check your alignment during exercise.
7. The best aerobics floor is a wooden floor with air space underneath it so that it "gives." Carpet over cement is very hard on shins. Heavy padding can have a tendency to grab your shoe and make changes of direction hazardous.
8. There should be 25 square feet (sft) of space available for each person on the aerobics floor. (The absolute minimum is 9 sft.)
9. The stereo equipment and facility acoustics should project music with a quality sound. The instructor should also be easily heard—many now wear wireless microphones.
10. For larger classes, the instructor should stand on a platform for easy visibility. Mirrors also enhance visibility for both the instructor and the participant.

Selecting a facility is similar to buying a car. Shop around and visit last the place you think you'll like the most. Many clubs offer a first visit (or initial visit) discount. If you have shopped the competition and like what you see, you'll be able to take advantage of the discount. However, the initial visit discount should not pressure you into buying. Clubs often offer a membership plan on your second visit that is similar to the offer on your first visit.

When you enter into a contract with a health club, it is good to know your consumer rights. Start by checking to see if the club is listed with the Better Business Bureau and then check with your state's Consumer Protection Agency to find out what regulations health clubs must meet. Don't feel pressured to sign a contract; take it home and read it over carefully. Make sure that it includes all the services you want and that all the promises made to you verbally are written in the contract. Look for cancellation policies including the ability to cancel penalty-free within 3 days of signing and cancellation terms if you move a distance away from the club and/or the club goes out of business. In the case of the latter,

check the state regulations for terminating the contract. If your club is bought out by another and you want to continue to attend, see if you have the right to continue your original contract, as it may have better rates and services than a contract with the new owner. If you opt for direct deposit payments, be sure to cancel them if the club goes out of business as the club may continue to collect from you. Long-term memberships are often less expensive, but before choosing this option check the track record of the club for longevity and ask for monthly payments instead of a one time up-front payment.

Many clubs will not disclose their membership costs over the telephone. Most recreation, school, or church groups will tell you the cost of the program, if any, over the telephone.

In all cases, the facility should be well staffed with friendly, qualified people. Some locations include a juice bar, weights, a pool, a sauna, a hairdresser, a nursery, and other amenities. Determine what is important to you before you look, so that you won't be distracted by things you don't need and won't use. Find the best facility for you at the most affordable price.

SELECTING AN INSTRUCTOR

As you move away from the college or university setting where aerobic dance exercise and fitness/wellness classes are offered by physical fitness educators, it is helpful to know how to select a qualified instructor in a club, dance studio, or recreational setting. Some program directors and club owners carefully screen their fitness instructors and only hire qualified individuals; some unfortunately are not as careful. The private sector also has to handle staffing demands for trends that gain popularity quickly. It can be difficult to find enough qualified instructors for what is often part-time work.

To help you be a good consumer, here are some ways you can determine the qualifications and traits of a good instructor:

- *Meet the instructor.* Ask the person how he or she feels about lifetime fitness and how he or she can help you toward your goals.
- *Watch and listen to the instructor in action.* Qualified instructors will constantly demonstrate different levels of intensity, offer tips on positioning and alignment, provide safety guidelines, and move around the room to assist individuals as needed.
- *Check the instructor's training and experience.* Find out if the instructor has a fitness education or is certified by a reputable fitness certification program. There are a number of groups that certify aerobic instructors and still more that

offer certifications for personal training and fitness education. Some training programs are more comprehensive than others. The strongest preparation is through a higher education program (such as an exercise science, physical education, or health promotion major in college) or through a specific course of study through a trade school. Other programs offer training ranging from a weekend up to several weeks. There are no rules governing certification of an aerobics instructor, so the quality of the programs varies. In the United States the two most recognized certifying bodies for aerobic instructors are the American Council for Exercise (ACE) and the Aerobics and Fitness Association of America (AFAA). Other, broader certifications include, but are not limited to, ones through the American College of Sports Medicine (ACSM), the National Academy of Sports Medicine (NASM), and the National Strength and Conditioning Association (NSCA). There are also a number of regional certification programs, and the quality of these programs depends on the expertise of the individuals doing the training and the rigor of the certification testing.

At this time, there are no national or state mandates for certification or strict controls over what such a program offers. Therefore, certification alone does not ensure a good instructor, but it does demonstrate a certain commitment toward learning and attaining basic knowledge. In addition to his or her training, find out how much experience the instructor has teaching a particular type and level of course.

- *Determine whether the instructor is up-to-date.* Information changes, and instructors need to stay updated. Find out how the instructor is staying current. You may want to ask a question about something you've read recently to see if the instructor can speak about current issues in fitness and wellness.
- *Find out the procedure for new people joining a class.* When new people join an exercise class, they should have to fill out a medical form, and the instructor should speak with them concerning their exercise background, level of fitness, and how to monitor their exercise intensity.
- *Determine whether the instructor is "onstage" or focused on participants.* Look for an instructor who is clearly watching the class and adjusting the pace and exercises to match the class's needs.
- *Check the instructor's attendance record.* Instructor consistency means that the instructor has a chance to get to know you, identify your needs, and guide your progression. When you keep getting different instructors (substitutes) you lose this personalization.
- *Talk to other members or previous members of the class.* Participants can give you a sense of whether the instructor is prepared for class, personable, and motivating.

FITNESS TRENDS—MORE OPTIONS

Fitness opportunities have expanded, and cross-training (using a variety of fitness modes) is a great way to keep things interesting. You may want to try one or more of the following.

- Dancing is getting some wonderful television press and dance studios and dance clubs are growing in popularity, offering lessons in hip-hop, Latin dancing, line dancing, ballroom, and other styles.
- Some boxing clubs now offer a wider variety of programs including some group fitness classes.
- You can join a walking or running club or take friends or family on a town- or state-managed trail.
- Par courses are located in many parks; these are trails with embedded exercise stations.
- You can hire a personal trainer or join a group training for a charity event.
- In winter climates, consider snowshoeing or cross-country skiing.
- In summer (or indoors), experiment with water aerobics, water polo, canoeing/kayaking, or a nice long swim.

Health clubs are offering more specialized classes so that you can take one just for an aerobic workout or just for muscle fitness. Some have 30-minute classes back to back so you can combine two if you wish. More programs are offering functional fitness—building your fitness in a way that helps you meet daily activity. Balance and coordination and core training are often at the center of these workouts. Other approaches use these ideas (and more) with the intent of building sport-specific fitness and skill. Wellness centers, hospitals, and universities offer programs that combine healthy habits, good nutrition, and physical activity. If you are seeking the mind-body connection, there are studios and clubs and recreation departments offering yoga, pilates, and the martial arts. Or perhaps you'd enjoy tapping into technology using a pedometer or a heart-rate monitor, tune into a workout via your ear buds, or pop in a DVD or use a game console and exercise at home. The options are many and new ideas develop everyday—all you have to do is put on your exercise clothes and jump into activity.

SUMMARY

Make finding a place to continue your aerobic dance exercise (or other exercise program) a priority. In addition to staying fit, going to exercise class is a great way to meet other people who, like you, enjoy an active, healthy lifestyle.

KNOWLEDGE TIPS

1. Before looking for a fitness facility, make a prioritized list of features to look for.

2. Visit a facility at the time of day you will be most likely to use it.

3. Look for a fitness facility that will take you on a complete tour, have you complete a medical/health questionnaire, give you a fitness evaluation, explain how to use the equipment, help you get started in an exercise program, and have someone available for consultation on an ongoing basis.

4. Look over the whole facility. Check for cleanliness, ventilation, good lighting, sound acoustics, well-maintained equipment, and a good aerobics floor.

5. Find out how qualified the instructor is in terms of education, certification, and experience.

6. Check the instructors' educational backgrounds to see if they are certified in CPR, first aid, aerobic dance exercise, or another group fitness specialty.

7. A quality instructor is a good role model, knowledgeable, experienced, up to date, well prepared, places students' needs first, can individualize the lesson, has regular attendance, and is personable and motivating.

8. Observe, from start to finish, the classes you want to join.

9. Consider the financial commitment carefully. Be sure to ask about all the plans.

10. Join and have fun!

THINK ABOUT IT

1. Where are exercise programs available?

2. What types of services do clubs offer?

3. What are desirable qualifications for an instructor?

4. Identify the qualities of a facility/program (i.e., location, cost, etc.) that are most likely to keep you coming back long term.

5. What time of day are you most likely to exercise and what implications does the time of day you are most likely to exercise have on selecting a program and facility?

6. What are some ways that you can find out if the instructor and program you are interested in are of good quality?

7. Where can you obtain consumer information on health clubs?

REFERENCES

American Council on Exercise. *Aerobics Instructor Manual: ACE's Guide for Fitness Professionals.* San Diego, CA: American Council on Exercise, 2000.

Champion, N., and G. Hurst. *Aerobics Instructor's Handbook.* Sydney: Kangaroo Press, 2000.

Kernodle, R. G. "Space: The Unexplored Frontier of Aerobic Dance." *Journal of Physical Education, Recreation, and Dance* 63 (May–June 1992): 65–9.

Muscles of the Body

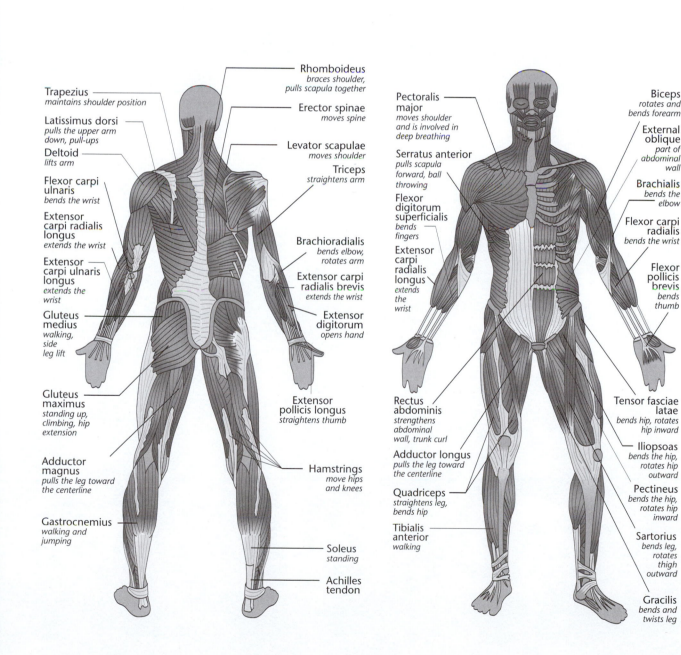

Trapezius
maintains shoulder position

Latissimus dorsi
pulls the upper arm down, pull-ups

Deltoid
lifts arm

Flexor carpi ulnaris
bends the wrist

Extensor carpi radialis longus
extends the wrist

Extensor carpi ulnaris longus
extends the wrist

Gluteus medius
walking, side leg lift

Gluteus maximus
standing up, climbing, hip extension

Adductor magnus
pulls the leg toward the centerline

Gastrocnemius
walking and jumping

Rhomboideus
braces shoulder, pulls scapula together

Erector spinae
moves spine

Levator scapulae
moves shoulder

Triceps
straightens arm

Brachioradialis
bends elbow, rotates arm

Extensor carpi radialis brevis
extends the wrist

Extensor digitorum
opens hand

Extensor pollicis longus
straightens thumb

Hamstrings
move hips and knees

Soleus
standing

Achilles tendon

Pectoralis major
moves shoulder and is involved in deep breathing

Serratus anterior
pulls scapula forward, ball throwing

Flexor digitorum superficialis
bends fingers

Extensor carpi radialis longus
extends the wrist

Rectus abdominis
strengthens abdominal wall, trunk curl

Adductor longus
pulls the leg toward the centerline

Quadriceps
straightens leg, bends hip

Tibialis anterior
walking

Biceps
rotates and bends forearm

External oblique
part of abdominal wall

Brachialis
bends the elbow

Flexor carpi radialis
bends the wrist

Flexor pollicis brevis
bends thumb

Tensor fasciae latae
bends hip, rotates hip inward

Iliopsoas
bends the hip, rotates hip outward

Pectineus
bends the hip, rotates hip inward

Sartorius
bends leg, rotates thigh outward

Gracilis
bends and twists leg

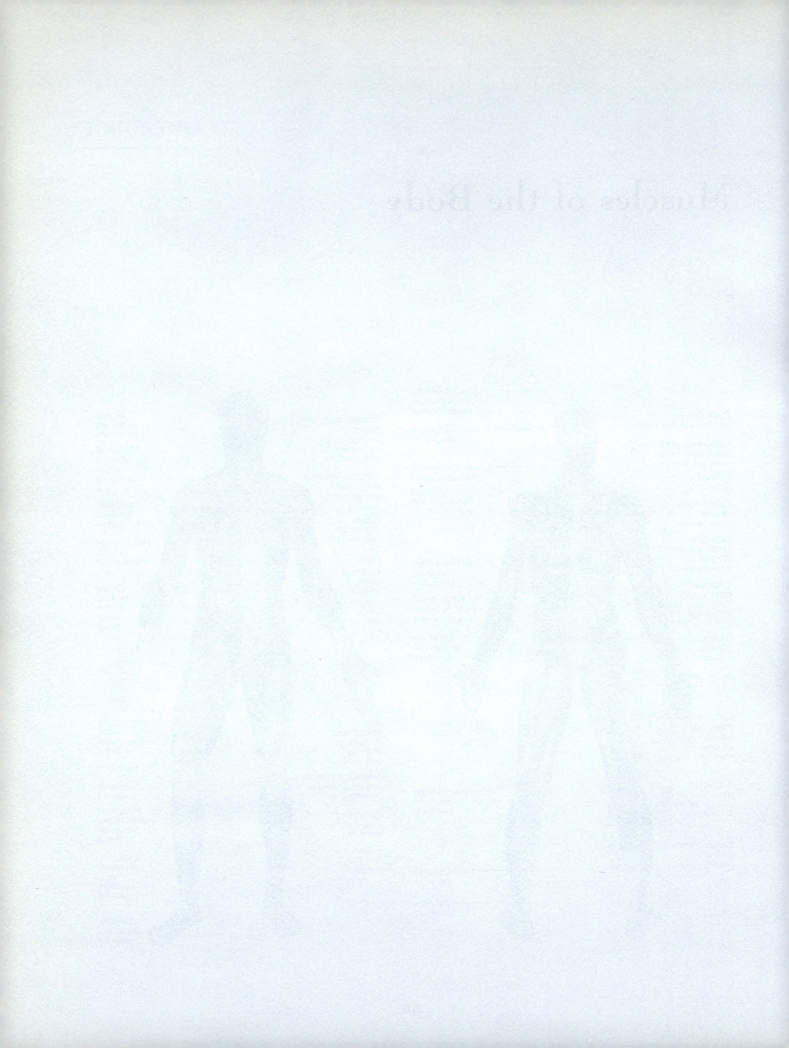

The Aerobics Look: Clothing and Equipment

ALTHOUGH aerobic dance exercise has introduced a style of dress all its own, to get started all you really need are shoes that provide good support, flexibility, and cushioning, and clothes that allow you to move, breathe, and sweat freely.

Avoid materials such as nylon that trap heat and moisture. Stick with cotton, which absorbs moisture, or one of the newer materials that wick away moisture. Loose clothing allows for freedom of movement, but a baggy outfit can make it difficult for an instructor to see your body alignment and can keep you from getting the most out of your exercises. Wear layers if you are in a cooler environment so that you can strip off outer garments as you warm up. A sweatband or rolled and tied bandanna can be worn around your forehead to absorb perspiration and keep it out of your eyes. Wrist sweatbands can be worn as well to absorb arm sweat or to wipe your brow.

SHOES

Put your money where the stress is: Invest in good shoes! Each time you jump, your feet absorb the impact of 3 to 6 times your body weight. The impact vibrations (shock) that cannot be absorbed by your arches are transmitted up your ankles, shins, knees, thighbones, hips, and spine and are eventually dissipated in the soft viscera (organs) in your trunk. With normal, routine activity, this system works beautifully, but when you add repetitive high-impact jumping, your body's shock-dissipating system needs help. Shoes with good support and cushioning help absorb impact shock and prevent chronic stress injuries. In addition to handling impact stress, shearing forces can be decreased if you wear the correct shoes and socks.

Athletic and dance shoes are designed to meet the needs of specific physical activities. The best shoes are those designed for the specific activity. Specialized aerobic shoes, cross-trainers, and fitness trainers are preferable because they are designed for multidirectional activity.

Aerobic/fitness shoes are designed to be lightweight, flexible, and shock absorbing. If you are a big person bringing a lot of weight down on the shoe, a slightly heavier, sturdier shoe may be better than a light shoe. Some very lightweight shoes are on the market today for use in resistance training and for cycling. These do not have enough shock absorption for an aerobic dance exercise class. When purchasing shoes, let the shoe salesperson know all of the types of activities (cardio-machines, kickboxing, court games, step aerobics, high- or low-impact aerobics, etc.) in which you plan to engage. See the box, Shoe Features and Functions.

The main difference between high- and low-impact shoes is the amount of shock absorption you need. If you are doing a high-impact or mixed class, it is worth the extra money to get superior cushioning. Ideally, a shoe for step aerobics has good forefoot padding and good flexibility, because you are repeatedly stepping down on a flexed foot.

The most common mistake beginning students make is to wear a running shoe. Here are some good reasons not to do that:

- You want smooth tread for easy pivoting on floors and rugs, NOT the heavy tread of a running shoe made for road and track use.

SHOE FEATURES AND FUNCTIONS

OUTERSOLE

- Traction—match grid to surface and movement (pivots, etc.).

- Durability—less toughness is needed for indoor sports. Save your soles by wearing your shoes only for class.

- Flexibility—aerobic dance requires a fair amount of this. Look for outersole grooves and flex points.

INSOLE

- Arch support—the arch cookie (bump in the insole) supports the arch.

- Cushioning—the insole provides some, but most comes from the midsole; can supplement with upgraded insoles.

MIDSOLE

- Cushioning—needed to offset impact stress; more cushioning is needed for high-impact exercise than for low-impact exercise.

- Flexibility—needed for stepping off steps, landing on ball of foot, etc.

- Motion control and support—needed to keep foot in control during lateral and twisting movements as well as forward and back motions.

UPPER

- Motion control and support—strong, well-designed lateral straps, heel support, etc., prevent pronation or supination of the feet.

- Durability—not as big an issue; usually cushioning wears out first.

- Fit—should be snug and comfortable.

- Heat dissipation—shoes need ventilation, especially if your feet sweat a lot.

- You want an outersole with pivot points that allow you to turn easily, NOT a running shoe with a tread pattern designed for forward motion only that will cause you to come to sudden stops (because of its gripping power) when doing aerobic steps.
- You want a moderate cut-out in the arch with midfoot lateral support, NOT a high arch cut-out that makes running shoes lighter and more flexible but less stable during side-to-side motions.
- You want a well-padded, shock-absorbing forefoot so you can do the many steps in aerobics that require you to land on the balls of your feet, NOT a running shoe designed with a wide flared heel to prevent heel strike. (Both shoes will offer some shock absorption throughout the shoe, but an aerobic shoe will offer more in the forefoot than other shoes.)
- You want the lateral support of an outersole that wraps up on the sides as well as the front, NOT an outersole that just wraps up on the front.
- You want a shoe with a wider, more stable base (sole) to prevent ankle injuries during

multidirectional movement, NOT one with a narrower base that allows slippage during lateral movements.

FEATURES

Most aerobics shoes have similar features. The bottom of the shoe is called the outersole. Select tread to coincide with the surface on which you will be exercising. Smoother treads help you pivot more easily on wooden floors and carpeted surfaces. The outersole may be cut away under the arch to save on materials and weight, and many of the new shoes also have a shank made up of supportive material running across the midfoot section of the outersole to provide lateral stability. Most companies also groove the outersole to promote flexibility. Look on the bottom of the shoe for these grooves. The outersole should also have flex points so that the shoe bends easily. Test the flex point locations by standing on the balls of your feet; see if the bend of the shoe agrees with the bend in your foot.

The midsole rests on top of the outersole and supplies most of the shock absorption. Many aerobic dance exercise steps involve landing on the ball of the foot first; therefore, forefoot padding is crucial. A good shoe

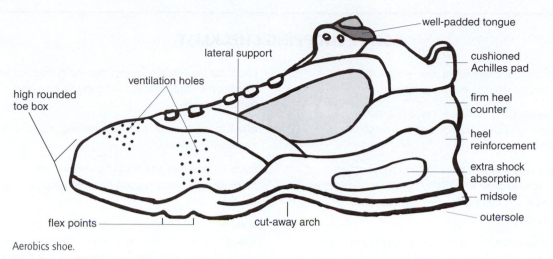

high rounded toe box

ventilation holes

lateral support

well-padded tongue

cushioned Achilles pad

firm heel counter

heel reinforcement

extra shock absorption

midsole

outersole

flex points

cut-away arch

Aerobics shoe.

Source: "Aerobics Shoe" by Melissa Galen Benine. Reprinted by permission.

will have shock absorption under both the ball of the foot and the heel. Manufacturers are using three shock-absorbing materials for midsole construction: EVA (ethyl vinyl acetate), compressed molded EVA, and polyurethane. The compressed molded EVA is an improved version of EVA and is therefore preferable. Polyurethane provides the best shock absorption but is slightly heavier and is thus not used or used only sparingly. In addition to these effective synthetic foams, manufacturers have designed unique shock-absorption systems. For example, Avia uses a cantilever system, Nike an encapsulated air system, Asic an encapsulated gel, Ryka encapsulated nitrogen, and Reebok a honeycombed inset called Hexalite. All of them are effective. Check for midsole flexibility by performing toe raises while wearing the shoes. Check for shock absorbency by jumping up and down and performing aerobic steps. See the box, Shoe Shopping Checklist.

Your feet rest on insoles inside the shoe; along with the midsoles, insoles provide arch support and cushioning. Look for insoles that pull out so they can be aired between classes and replaced when worn out. You can purchase insoles made of compressed molded EVA, polyurethane, or neoprene at stores that sell athletic shoes. If you plan on using one of these insoles, try on the shoe with the insole. You may need a half-size larger shoe. Regularly washing the insoles will allow them to breathe better and keep your feet cooler. You will be unclogging their pores, so to speak.

Materials that provide lateral support help stabilize your foot during side-to-side movements and keep it from twisting when you place your weight on the ball of your foot. The previously mentioned midfoot shank, as well as reinforcement in the heel cup and, in some cases, thermoplastic urethane supports in the

midsole, help stabilize the foot. Leather straps that run from the midsole up to the lacing provide lateral support; some lacing systems run on the sides of shoes to add support. Other sources of lateral support include outersoles that wrap up the sides of the shoe and insoles and midsoles that curve up on the inside edges of the shoe to cradle the foot. Beware of cosmetic stitching that looks like lateral reinforcement. You can purchase aerobic shoes, cross-trainers, and fitness shoes in low- and mid-cut models. The mid-cut or three-quarter-cut shoes provide additional ankle support.

To prevent side-to-side slippage in the heel, the shoe should have a firm, reinforced heel counter. The sole beneath the heel should extend out a little wider than the upper but should not have the flare of a running shoe. The heel should also be well padded and notched to support but not irritate the Achilles tendon during jumping and stepping.

Both leather and synthetic leather are good materials. Firm leather provides support, and soft leather stretches out and allows the feet to roll out over the soles. Synthetic leather tends to stretch less than natural leather, but it may also be hotter. Usually, additional mesh areas are built in to provide the necessary breathability.

Shoes that support the bones of the arch allow the ligaments that tie the bones together to relax. Shoes that don't support the arch stress the ligaments and tire the supporting muscles.

Feet with significant mechanical or structural abnormalities, such as very high arches, flat feet, or feet that tend to pronate (roll in) or supinate (roll out), often need more support than ordinary shoes can provide. In addition to making your feet ache, these

SHOE SHOPPING CHECKLIST

- Shop late in the day, when your feet are their largest. Feet tend to swell as the day progresses.

- Let the salesclerk know what type of activity you will be performing, such as high-impact step aerobics or kickboxing.

- Try the shoes on with the socks, inserts, or orthotics you intend to wear when using the shoes. See whether the insole will pull out for easy washing, airing or replacement.

- Try on several different brands. Different brands use different lasts. A last is the mold from which the shoe is constructed. Some lasts are more curved than others. Find the one that fits your foot. The shoe should be comfortable right away—there is no need for a "break-in" period.

- Ask what materials are used for cushioning and shock absorption. Are they quality materials, such as molded compressed EVA, dual density EVA, etc.?

- Relace the shoes starting at the farthest eyelets. Use the lacing system that is appropriate for your feet.

- Wiggle your toes while standing still—all your toes should be free to wiggle if the toe box is high and wide enough.

- Perform some aerobic dance steps, and see whether the shock absorption system feels natural to you as you move.

- Perform some forward and backward jumping motions to make sure your toes do not hit the end of the shoes.

- Check the heel counter by moving side to side and see whether the shoe continues to fit snugly. Your heel should not slide.

- Check to see whether the heel is padded and notched and fits comfortably.

- Stand on your toes and twist or swivel side to side. Make sure the lateral support holds your feet in position.

- Jump from side to side and see whether the lateral support (straps, shanks, wrapped outsole, etc.) holds your feet in position. You should not feel as though you are rolling out over the side of the shoe or sliding from side to side.

- Check for arch support. The arch cookie should be in contact with your arch.

- Check for flexibility by walking normally, standing on the balls of your feet, and jumping up and down on the balls of your feet. The shoe should "break" at the same point as your foot bends. You should also be able to bend the shoe easily so that you can roll down from the balls of your feet. Look for outersole grooves and flex points.

- Make sure there is adequate ventilation for your feet. Mesh breathes more than leather. Look for air holes.

- Check the price. Quality shoes will cost more, but they last longer. Ask about the difference between last year's model and this year—you may be able to save money buying last year's model if the changes are primarily cosmetic.

---

abnormalities can cause impact vibrations to be sent up the legs on an angle. Vibrations repeatedly striking the knee at an angle can cause irritation on the inside or outside of the knee. Shinsplints, hip pain, and even lower back pain can originate from problems with the feet.

If you think your feet need extra support, consult a podiatrist. You may need orthotics—custom-made plastic insoles that slip inside your shoe to provide form-fitting support. If you are being fit for orthotics, be sure to tell the podiatrist you intend to use them for exercise, because sports orthotics are more flexible than others. Orthotics are relatively expensive, but they are as indispensable to bad feet as eyeglasses are to bad eyes.

Finally, be sure to replace your shoes when they start to wear out. Simply because a shoe *looks* like it is still good does not guarantee that it has not worn out. See the When to Replace Your Aerobics Shoes box for tips on when it's time to get new aerobics shoes.

OTHER CLOTHING

SOCKS AND FOOT CARE

Socks prevent blisters and calluses by reducing the friction between your shoes and the skin on your feet. To prevent soreness when you are breaking in a new pair of shoes, place bandages or tape over sensitive

WHEN TO REPLACE YOUR AEROBICS SHOES

It's time to replace your aerobics shoes when:

- you have worn them for 3–6 months, depending on how often you exercise in them and how sturdy their construction is

- you experience any foot pain or chronic injury symptoms that you don't normally experience, such as shinsplints, knee soreness, etc.

- the shoe has stretched and become loose on your foot

- the heels are rolling over

- the shoe allows you to pronate (roll your ankle inward)

- the tread has become too smooth

---

areas such as the back of your heels and the outside of your little toes. If you have sensitive feet or are planning a long day at a workshop or competition, you can further reduce friction by wearing two pairs of socks (the inner pair should be thinner), putting baby powder between your pairs of socks, or applying petroleum jelly to your feet.

Socks also absorb perspiration, thus keeping your feet dry and helping to prevent itching, cracking, and athlete's foot. Basic cotton socks absorb moisture well but do not wick it away. The newer blend socks effectively wick moisture away from the skin, which keeps your feet dryer and cooler. White socks are recommended over colored socks because the dye in the latter may irritate the skin when sweat-soaked. People with diabetes should take extra good care of their feet and see a physician immediately if problems occur.

DANGEROUS CLOTHING

Rubber or plastic suits (or regular sweats worn in warm/hot conditions) prevent normal body cooling; dehydration and dangerous heat stress may result. The large weight losses observed after exercising in this type of outfit can be attributed to large fluid losses. As soon as the body is properly rehydrated, the weight will return. No positive health benefits are achieved by the use of these suits. Plastic wraps (cellophane) trap heat the same way rubber suits do and should be avoided for the same reasons. Warm clothing should be removed following the warm-up.

Avoid restrictive clothing that interferes with breathing. Exercise demands oxygen and causes deeper, faster breathing. Tight belts, tight-fitting shorts, or other tight clothing may result in shallow, inadequate breathing and can lead to fainting. Restrictive clothing also limits your ability to perform an exercise through its full range of motion; this will limit the benefits you will achieve from your exercise.

EQUIPMENT

Equipment will generally be provided for you. Different types of classes use different equipment. Mats and positional aids will be described here; other equipment, including pedometers, heart-rate monitors, exercise bands, stability balls, weights, and step benches, are described within the appropriate chapters.

MATS

Exercise mats come in a variety of thicknesses. Pilates and yoga mats are generally ⅛- or ¼- inch thick. You can also purchase thicker mats so that you "feel the floor" less. Most mats roll or fold up for easy carrying. Some people prefer to bring their own mat or a towel to place on top of a mat to ensure cleanliness.

POSITIONAL AIDS

When you are performing certain stretches, you may need to extend your reach. Special yoga/pilates straps or a simple towel can be wrapped around a limb and then pulled to create the desired stretch. For some examples of positional aids, see Chapter 7. Pillows, wedges, blocks, bolsters, and towels are also used to add comfort during exercise positions. The most commonly used are foam or wooden blocks in yoga and a step bench during a step class. For example, persons who are too inflexible to place their hands on the floor during a standing forward lunge can place their hands on the blocks or straddle the step bench and place hands on top of the step (Figure 7.24c).

Internet Resources

Health and Wellness

American Medical Association
www.ama-assn.org

Centers for Disease Control and Prevention
www.cdc.gov

CNN Health
www.cnn.com/HEALTH

Go Ask Alice! Columbia University's Health Q & A
Internet Service
www.goaskalice.columbia.edu/Cat3.html

Healthfinder
www.healthfinder.gov

Healthy People 2000/Healthy People 2010/Healthy
People 2020
http://odphp.osophs.dhhs.gov/pubs/hp2000
www.healthypeople.gov
www.healthypeople.gov/HP2020

Mayo Clinic
www.mayoclinic.com

National Center for Chronic Disease Prevention
www.cdc.gov/nccdphp

National Health Information Center (NHIC)
www.health.gov/nhic

National Women's Health Information Center
www.4women.gov

New York Online Access to Health (bilingual Spanish
and English site)
www.noah-health.org

Physical Fitness

Aerobics and Fitness Association of America (AFAA)
www.afaa.com

American Alliance for Health, Physical Education,
Recreation, and Dance (AAHPERD)
www.aahperd.org

American College of Sports Medicine (ACSM)
www.acsm.org

American Council on Exercise (ACE)
www.acefitness.org

American Diabetes Association
www.diabetes.org/exercise

Internet Fitness Resource
www.netsweat.com

The Fitness Partner Connection Jumpsite
http://primusweb.com/fitnesspartner

Turnstep.com (Step Aerobics)
www.turnstep.com

Aerobic (Cardiorespiratory) Endurance

American Heart Association
www.americanheart.org

Cardiovascular Institute of the South
www.cardio.com

National Heart, Lung, and Blood Institute
www.nhlbi.nih.gov

Muscular Strength and Endurance

Human Anatomy On-line
   www.innerbody.com/htm/body.html

National Academy of Sports Medicine (NASM)
   www.nasm.org

National Strength and Conditioning Association
   www.nsca-cc.org

Flexibility

NIH Back Pain Fact Sheet
   www.ninds.nih.gov/health_and_medical/
   disorders/backpain_doc.htm

Southern California Orthopedic Institute
   www.scoi.com

Nutrition, Weight Control, and Body Composition

American Heart Association
   www.americanheart.org
   www.deliciousdecisions.org

American Dietetic Association
   www.eatright.org

Arbor Nutrition Guide
   http://arborcom.com

California Dietetic Association
   http://dietitian.com

Calorie Control Council
   www.caloriecontrol.org

Cancer Information Service
   http://cis.nci.nih.gov

Center for Nutrition Policy and Promotion, USDA
   www.usda.gov/cnpp

Fast Food Facts—Interactive Food Finder
   www.foodfacts.info

Food and Drug Administration
   www.fda.gov

National Osteoporosis Foundation
   www.nof.org

United States Department of Agriculture,
MyPyramid.gov
   www.mypyramid.gov

Veggies Unite!
   www.vegweb.com

Injury Prevention and Care

National Athletic Trainers' Association
   www.nata.org

WORKSHEET 1: HEALTH AND FITNESS LOG

PERSONAL INFORMATION

Name: _____ Phone: _____

Address: _____

Age: _____ Height: _____ Weight: _____ % Fat: _____

Class Time: _____ Days of the Week: _____

HEALTH HISTORY

CHECK THE APPROPRIATE BOXES:	NEVER HAD	HAVE HAD	PRESENTLY HAVE	FAMILY HISTORY
Heart Disease				
Chest Pain w/Exertion				
Difficulty Breathing				
High Blood Pressure				
Low Blood Pressure				
Pulmonary Lung Disease				
Diabetes				
Epilepsy				
Thyroid Disease				
Hypoglycemia				
Asthma				
Arthritis				
Persistent Headaches				
Dizzy Spells				
Bursitis				
Varicose Veins				
Obesity				
Allergies				
Bulimia				
Anorexia Nervosa				
Other:				

List any muscle injuries you have had (include dates): _____
_____

List any bone or joint injuries you have had (include dates): _____
_____

List any muscle, bone, or joint pain you are presently experiencing: _____
_____

Continued on next page

215

Specify any medications you are presently taking: _____
_____

Specify any activities you have been advised by a physician to avoid: _____
_____

Specify any activities about which you must be cautious: _____
_____

Do you smoke?   Yes   No   If yes, how much? _____

Are you pregnant or have you had a baby within the last six months?   Yes   No

Do you have any other health condition that might limit your participation in this aerobics class?
_____

PHYSICAL FITNESS HISTORY

In your estimation, how physically fit are you right now?

        Unfit   Below Average   Average   Above Average   Very Fit

Have you been exercising regularly?   Yes   No

If no, how long has it been since you did? _____

If yes, describe your exercise program below.

ACTIVITY	FREQUENCY (TIMES/WEEK)	DURATION (TIME/SESSION)	INTENSITY (DIFFICULTY)

Briefly describe why you signed up for this course: _____
_____
_____
_____

WORKSHEET 2: SUMMARY RECORD SHEET

Name: _____ Age: _____ Height: _____ Weight: _____

% Fat: _____ Healthy Weight: _____ THR: _____ beats/minute, _____ beats/10 seconds

Fitness Goals

1. _____

   _____

2. _____

   _____

3. _____

   _____

Cardiorespiratory Fitness Tests

STEP TEST (12-INCH)

	Date _____	Date _____	Date _____
1 min. Post-Exercise HR:	_____	_____	_____
Fitness Rating:	_____	_____	_____

12-MINUTE WALK/RUN

Distance:	_____	_____	_____
Fitness Rating:	_____	_____	_____

1.5-MILE RUN

Time:	_____	_____	_____
Fitness Rating:	_____	_____	_____

Flexibility Tests

(Mark "P" for pass, "F" for fail.)

TRUNK FORWARD FLEXION TEST (SIT-AND-REACH)

	Date _____	Date _____	Date _____
Score:	_____	_____	_____
Fitness Rating:	_____	_____	_____

Neck Test:	_____		_____		_____	
Shoulder Test I:	R _____ L _____		R _____ L _____		R _____ L _____	
Shoulder Test II:	R _____ L _____		R _____ L _____		R _____ L _____	
Shoulder Test III:	_____		_____		_____	
Trunk Test:	_____		_____		_____	
Hip Flexor Test:	R _____ L _____		R _____ L _____		R _____ L _____	
Alternate Hip Flexor Test:	R _____ L _____		R _____ L _____		R _____ L _____	
Hip Abduction Test:	R _____ L _____		R _____ L _____		R _____ L _____	
Hamstring Test:	R _____ L _____		R _____ L _____		R _____ L _____	
Quadriceps Test:	R _____ L _____		R _____ L _____		R _____ L _____	
Calf Test:	R _____ L _____		R _____ L _____		R _____ L _____	

Continued on next page

Muscular Endurance Tests

Date _____ Date _____ Date _____

CURL-UPS

Number Completed: _____ _____ _____
Fitness Rating: _____ _____ _____

PUSH-UPS

Number Completed: _____ (reg./mod.) _____ (reg./mod.) _____ (reg./mod.)
Fitness Rating: _____ _____ _____

BODY MEASUREMENTS

DIRECTIONS FOR TAKING BODY MEASUREMENTS Keep the tape measure level, and bring the ends together with a light tension. To measure the upper arms, shoulders, buttocks, and hips, find the area of largest girth. To measure the upper leg, find the midpoint between the top of the hip and the knee. To measure the waist, find the area of least girth. Measure the chest at nipple height.

Date _____ Date _____ Date _____

		Date 1		Date 2		Date 3	
Women:	Ankle (optional):	R _____	L _____	R _____	L _____	R _____	L _____
	Calf:	R _____	L _____	R _____	L _____	R _____	L _____
	Thigh:	R _____	L _____	R _____	L _____	R _____	L _____
	Buttocks:	_____		_____		_____	
	Hips:	_____		_____		_____	
	Waist:	_____		_____		_____	
	Chest:	_____		_____		_____	
	Upper Arm:	R _____	L _____	R _____	L _____	R _____	L _____
Men:	Ankle (optional):	R _____	L _____	R _____	L _____	R _____	L _____
	Calf:	R _____	L _____	R _____	L _____	R _____	L _____
	Thigh:	R _____	L _____	R _____	L _____	R _____	L _____
	Buttocks:	_____		_____		_____	
	Abdomen:	_____		_____		_____	
	Chest (relaxed):	_____		_____		_____	
	Chest (expanded):	_____		_____		_____	
	Upper Arm (relaxed):	R _____	L _____	R _____	L _____	R _____	L _____
	Upper Arm (flexed):	R _____	L _____	R _____	L _____	R _____	L _____
	Shoulders:	_____		_____		_____	
	Neck (optional):	_____		_____		_____	

Weight Management/Body Composition Tests

Date _____ Date _____ Date _____

Body Mass Index (BMI): _____ _____ _____
Waist/Hip Ratio: _____ _____ _____
Skin-Fold Measurements:
Site: _____ _____ mm _____ mm _____ mm
Site: _____ _____ mm _____ mm _____ mm
Site: _____ _____ mm _____ mm _____ mm
TOTAL: _____ mm _____ mm _____ mm
BODY FAT: _____ % _____ % _____ %

WORKSHEET 3: CALCULATING YOUR TARGET HEART RATE

Maximum Heart-Rate Formula (Zero to Peak Formula)

(Refer to Chapter 4, pages 35–36.)

STEP ONE
Find your maximum heart rate (MHR).

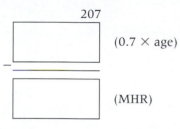

207

(0.7 × age)

(MHR)

EXAMPLE:
The MHR of a 20-year-old.

$$\begin{array}{r} 207 \\ -\ 14 \\ \hline 193 \end{array} \quad (0.7 \times 20)$$

STEP TWO
Find the lower end of your THR in beats/minute.

(MHR)

× 0.7

(beats/minute)

EXAMPLE:

$$\begin{array}{r} 193 \\ \times\ \ 0.7 \\ \hline 135.10 \end{array}$$

STEP THREE
Find the upper end of your THR in beats/minute.

(MHR)

× 0.85

(beats/minute)

EXAMPLE:

$$\begin{array}{r} 193 \\ \times\ 0.85 \\ \hline 965 \\ 15440 \\ \hline 165.05 \end{array}$$

My target heart-rate range is _____ to _____ beats/minute.
                          (lower)   (upper)

EXAMPLE: My THR is 135 to 165 beats/minute.

Continued on next page

STEP FOUR
Find the lower end of your THR in beats/10 seconds.

$$6\overline{)\boxed{\text{Step 2 Answer}}} = \underline{\hspace{2cm}} \text{ beats/10 seconds}$$

EXAMPLE:

$$\begin{array}{r} 22.5 \\ 6\overline{)135} \\ \underline{12} \\ 15 \\ \underline{12} \\ 30 \\ \underline{30} \\ 0 \end{array}$$

STEP FIVE
Find the upper end of your THR in beats/10 seconds.

$$6\overline{)\boxed{\text{Step 3 Answer}}} = \underline{\hspace{2cm}} \text{ beats/10 seconds}$$

EXAMPLE:

$$\begin{array}{r} 27.58 \\ 6\overline{)165} \\ \underline{12} \\ 45 \\ \underline{42} \\ 35 \\ \underline{30} \\ 50 \\ \underline{48} \\ 2 \end{array}$$

My target heart-rate range is _____ to _____ beats/10 seconds.
                                  (lower)   (upper)

EXAMPLE: My THR is 23 to 28 beats/10 seconds.

WORKSHEET 4: CALCULATING YOUR TARGET HEART RATE

Karvonen Formula

(Refer to Chapter 4, page 36.)

First find your average resting heart rate by counting your pulse for 1 minute while you are still lying in bed. Do this on three consecutive mornings.

Resting heart rate on the first morning: _____ beats/minute
Resting heart rate on the second morning: _____ beats/minute
Resting heart rate on the third morning: _____ beats/minute
Average Resting Heart Rate (RHR): _____ beats/minute

STEPS ONE AND TWO

Find your maximum heart rate and heart-rate reserve.

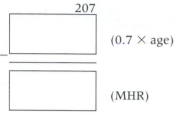

207
(0.7 × age)

(MHR)

(RHR)

(HRR)

EXAMPLE:

A 20-year-old with an RHR of 75.

```
    207
 −   14     (0.7 × 20)
 ─────
    193
 −   75     (RHR)
 ─────
    118     (HRR)
```

STEPS THREE AND FOUR

For the lower limit of the THR, calculate 60% of the HRR and add the RHR to the answer.

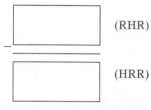

(HRR)

× 0.6

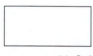

(RHR)

+

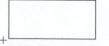

Lower end of THR
in beats/minute

EXAMPLE:

```
    118     (HRR)
 ×  0.6
 ─────
   70.8
 + 75.0     (RHR)
 ─────
  145.8
```

Continued on next page

STEPS FIVE AND SIX

For the upper limit of the THR, calculate 80% of the HRR and add the RHR to the answer.

EXAMPLE:

```
    118      (HRR)
×   .08
_____
   94.4
+  75.0      (RHR)
_____
  169.4
```

┌──────────┐
│   │ (HRR)
└──────────┘
     × 0.8
────────────
┌──────────┐
│   │
└──────────┘

┌──────────┐
│   │ (RHR)
+└──────────┘
────────────
┌──────────┐
│   │ Upper end of THR
└──────────┘ in beats/minute

My target heart-rate range is _____ to _____ beats/minute.
                    (lower)   (upper)

EXAMPLE: My THR is 146 to 169 beats/minute.

STEPS SEVEN AND EIGHT

Divide both ends of the THR in beats/minute by 6 to obtain a THR in beats per 10 seconds.

EXAMPLE:

```
      24.3
   _____
6 | 146
    12
   ____
    26
    24
   ____
    20
    18
   ____
     2
```

EXAMPLE:

```
      28.1
   _____
6 | 169
    12
   ____
    49
    48
   ____
    10
     6
```

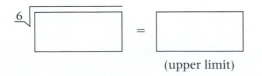

┌──────────┐   ┌──────────┐
6| │   =   │   │
└──────────┘   └──────────┘
                   (lower limit)

┌──────────┐   ┌──────────┐
6| │   =   │   │
└──────────┘   └──────────┘
                   (upper limit)

My target heart-rate range is _____ to _____ beats/10 seconds.
                    (lower)   (upper)

EXAMPLE: My THR is 24 to 28 beats/10 seconds.

WORKSHEET 5: HEART-RATE CHART

DIRECTIONS:

EHR = exercise heart rate
RHR = resting heart rate
PreHR = pre-exercise heart rate
RecHR = recovery heart rate

1. On the other side of this worksheet, draw two thick horizontal lines on the graph to represent the lower and upper limits of your THR.

2. Prior to exercise, take your PreHR and plot it on the chart.

3. During aerobic exercise, take your EHR several times. Plot the highest one.

4. One minute after the aerobic portion of class, take and plot your RecHR.

5. To see heart-rate trends, connect all the PreHR dots, connect all the EHR dots, and connect all the RecHR dots. (See Figure 4.4 on page 39 for an example of this procedure.)

6. Each month, take your RHR for a full minute while still lying down three mornings in a row, and record your daily counts and averages in beats per minute on the chart below.

	MONTH	RHR 1	RHR 2	RHR 3	AVERAGE
1.					
2.					
3.					
4.					
5.					
6.					

Add the average resting heart rates to the graph on page 224 for a visual record. Watch to see if your RHR drops as your aerobic fitness improves. (An upward trend in RHR may be a sign of overtraining.)

Continued on next page

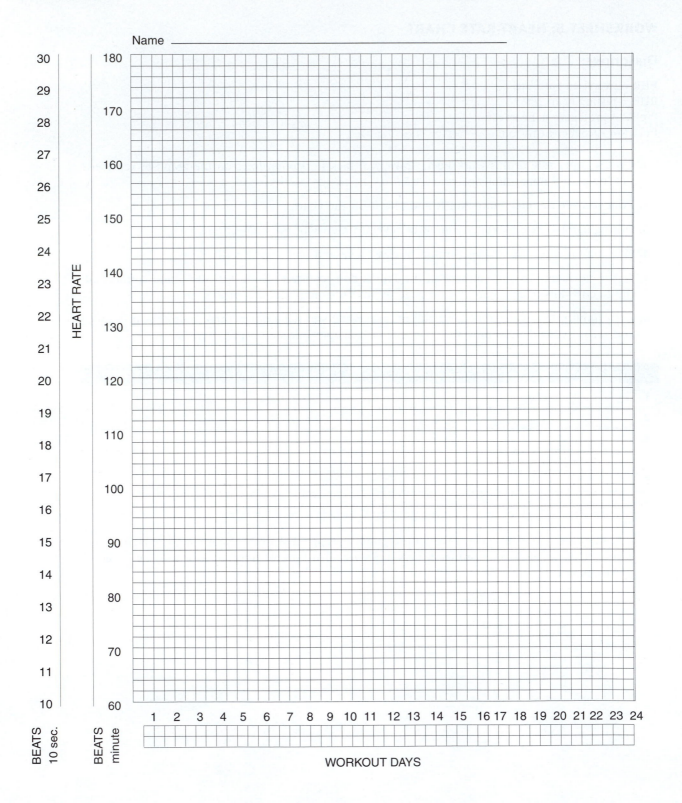

Name

HEART RATE

BEATS 10 sec.

BEATS minute

WORKOUT DAYS

WORKSHEET 6: GOAL SETTING/BEHAVIOR CHANGE

1. You have read about the benefits of regular exercise. List here any of the benefits you think you would like to pursue. In other words, what do you want to get out of your exercise program?

_____

_____

_____

2. Look at your wish list in #1 and pick the one that is most important to you right now. (Because you are enrolled in an exercise course, you may be able to accomplish more than one, depending on your goals. Do not, however, choose too many and risk failure from overcommitment.)

_____

_____

_____

3. Identify a way to assess your present status (fitness, body composition, calorie intake, etc.) and a way to track your progress.

_____

_____

_____

4. Pretest now to assess where you are in terms of your selected goal. (See fitness test worksheets or ask your instructor for additional assessment tools, such as skin-folding, computerized diet analysis, etc.)

_____

_____

_____

5. List the type of exercise(s) or activities that will help you attain your goal. Include any activities you would consider doing outside of class.

_____

_____

_____

_____

6. Determine a realistic timetable for reaching your goal. Establish a date for a follow-up assessment. Example: I will retest my hamstring flexibility in 6 weeks.

_____

_____

_____

_____

7. State your goal in terms as specific as possible. Example: I want to _____ using _____ over a period of _____ and assessed by _____.

_____

_____

_____

_____

Continued on next page

8. Identify at least two sources of motivation you can tap into to keep you focused on this goal. Consider both intrinsic and extrinsic sources of motivation.

a. _____

_____

b. _____

_____

9. Make a plan now for how you will maintain progress toward your goal during vacation time and when the course ends.

_____

_____

_____

10. During the course, or when the course ends, what types of things are most apt to interfere with your ability to maintain your goal behavior? What do you see as barriers to continued success?

_____

_____

_____

_____

11. What strategies can you use to prevent the barriers you listed in #10 from interrupting your goal behavior?

_____

_____

_____

_____

12. Illness, vacations, family emergencies, and so on can disrupt even the most established wellness behaviors. Consider making a plan now for how you will get yourself restarted if, and when, you stop doing your goal behavior.

_____

_____

_____

WORKSHEET 7: FITNESS LOGS

The fitness log is a place where you can record your participation in any type of physical activity that leads toward fitness. Keeping a record helps you identify trends as well as improvements. For example, you may discover that you feel better, or are more apt to exercise, if you do it in the morning as opposed to the afternoon or evening. Or you may discover that you are getting plenty of aerobic workout, but not as much muscular workout as you would like. You can track increases in your frequency, intensity, and duration if your goal is to increase your fitness. The comments section acts as a mini-journal, allowing you to gain insight over time about how you "feel" during and after exercise. If trends aren't positive, or aren't leading toward your fitness goals, you can reevaluate your choice of activities rather than simply dropping out. If the trends are good and you are enjoying yourself, this record serves as positive reinforcement for what you are doing. Your log can, but does not have to, include your aerobic dance class. Below are some examples of how a log entry might appear. Blank logs follow on pages 228 and 229.

DATE	TIME OF DAY	ACTIVITY	INTENSITY	DURATION/DISTANCE	COMMENTS
1/23	9:00 AM	aerobic dance	moderate (70% maximum heart rate)	30 min.	feeling more comfortable with the steps
1/23	9:40 AM	muscle toning	moderate (10 reps to exhaustion)	10 min.	able to complete all repetitions today
1/24	6:15 AM	wt. training	light (60% of RM)	30 min.	too easy, time to increase weight
1/25	6:30 PM	distance swim	high (170 bpm)	20 min. or no. of laps	invigorating
1/26	1:00 PM	cleaning	light to moderate	2 hours	arms tired, feel organized

You may want to keep a more detailed record of your resistance training, one that includes the amount of resistance, the number of repetitions and sets, and how long you rest between exercises or sets. You may also want to keep a log of how you feel during workouts. Here is an example:

EXERCISES	Squats (barbell)	Curl-ups (ball)	Biceps curl (dumbbells)	Wall sit (isometric)	Seated row (band)					
DATE	LOAD (wt.) Reps / Sets	LOAD (wt.) Reps / Sets	LOAD (wt.) Reps / Sets	LOAD (wt.) Reps / Sets	LOAD (wt.) Reps / Sets	LOAD (wt.) Reps / Sets	LOAD (wt.) Reps / Sets	LOAD (wt.) Reps / Sets	Rest between Sets	COMMENTS
2/12	20 lbs. 12 / 1	body wt. 15 / 2	5 lbs. 10 / 2	body wt. 30 sec. hold	light 10 / 2				30 sec.	a little sore
2/14	30 lbs. 8 / 1	body wt. 10 / 1	5 lbs. 8 / 3	—	—				2 min.	felt sluggish
2/16	35 lbs. 12 / 1	body wt. 15 / 2	5 lbs. 10 / 2	body wt. 45 sec. hold	medium 10 / 2				1 min.	ate well; feeling good; energized!

Note: This chart represents examples using various forms of resistance and different numbers of repetitions and sets. It is not a program to follow. Fill in your own choice of exercises.

Continued on next page

NAME: _____

DATE	TIME OF DAY	ACTIVITY	INTENSITY	DURATION/DISTANCE	COMMENTS

Continued on next page

NAME: _____

EXERCISES / DATE	LOAD (wt.) Reps / Sets	LOAD (wt.) Reps / Sets	LOAD (wt.) Reps / Sets	LOAD (wt.) Reps / Sets	LOAD (wt.) Reps / Sets	LOAD (wt.) Reps / Sets	LOAD (wt.) Reps / Sets	LOAD (wt.) Reps / Sets	Rest between Sets	COMMENTS

NAME: _____

EXERCISES	DATE	LOAD (wt.) Reps / Sets	LOAD (wt.) Reps / Sets	LOAD (wt.) Reps / Sets	LOAD (wt.) Reps / Sets	LOAD (wt.) Reps / Sets	LOAD (wt.) Reps / Sets	LOAD (wt.) Reps / Sets	LOAD (wt.) Reps / Sets	Rest between Sets	COMMENTS

WORKSHEET 8: GOAL TRACKING WITH A PEDOMETER

Record your baseline steps for 8 days. Consecutive days work the best so that your baseline measure includes all the days of the week. It is important to capture information about weekdays and weekends because activity levels may fluctuate depending on what you typically do on these days. If you have an unusual day (walk/run for charity, illness, etc.), you many want to eliminate that day and average without it (divide by 7) or substitute it with an additional typical day count.

_____   _____   _____   _____   _____   _____   _____   _____

Day 1   Day 2   Day 3   Day 4   Day 5   Day 6   Day 7   Day 8

Baseline average of the 8 days =_____ steps/day   Example: 6500 steps

10% of the baseline average =_____   Example: 6500 × .10 = 650

Baseline + 10% = 1st step goal   Example: 6500 + 650 = 7150

If you are successfully reaching your daily step goal, in 2 weeks add 10% again.

Repeat every 2 weeks until you are at your final goal level (i.e., 10,000 steps/day).

_____ (1st step goal) + 10% =_____ New 2nd daily step goal   Example: 7150 × .10 = 715

7150 × 715 = 7865

_____ (2nd step goal) + 10% =_____ New 3rd daily step goal

_____ (3rd step goal) + 10% =_____ New 4th daily step goal

_____ (4th step goal) + 10% =_____ New 5th daily step goal

TRACK YOUR PROGRESS

WEEK	DAILY STEP GOAL	MON (# OF STEPS)	TUES (# OF STEPS)	WED (# OF STEPS)	THURS (# OF STEPS)	FRI (# OF STEPS)	SAT (# OF STEPS)	SUN (# OF STEPS)
1.								
2.								
3.								
4.								
5.								

Continued on next page

TRACK YOUR PROGRESS

WEEK	DAILY STEP GOAL	MON (# OF STEPS)	TUES (# OF STEPS)	WED (# OF STEPS)	THURS (# OF STEPS)	FRI (# OF STEPS)	SAT (# OF STEPS)	SUN (# OF STEPS)

WORKSHEET 9: CARDIORESPIRATORY FITNESS

YMCA Step Test (12-inch)

EQUIPMENT:

1. bench 12" high—a step aerobics bench will work (a bleacher 16¼" high can be substituted, and the norms will still be reasonably accurate)

2. stopwatch

3. metronome or other means of establishing the cadence

4. pencil or pen

DIRECTIONS:

1. Practice taking your heart rate. If you will be working with a partner, practice taking your partner's heart rate.

2. Warm up and stretch.

3. Face the bench and practice the stepping pattern: Up, Up, Down, Down.

   Up—step up on the bench with your right foot.

   Up—bring your left foot up on the bench.

   Down—step down to the floor with your right foot.

   Down—step down to the floor with your left foot.

4. Rest until your breathing is back to normal.

5. Set the cadence (rate at which you will step) to 96 beats/minute (24 step/cycles per minute).

6. With the start of the stopwatch, begin the stepping pattern and continue stepping for 3 minutes. If you cannot complete the whole 3 minutes (too tired to keep cadence), stop and record the amount of time you were able to complete: _____ minutes _____ seconds.

7. Stop and find your pulse. Begin counting the pulse within 5 seconds after you stop stepping. Count for an *entire minute*.
   _____ recovery heart rate (RecHR) in beats/minute

8. Look at the chart on the following page to determine your fitness rating.

   My fitness rating is _____.

9. Stretch your legs to prevent muscle soreness.

Continued on next page

Fitness ratings for a 3-minute step test.

FITNESS RATING	% RANKING	18–25 YEARS OLD		26–35 YEARS OLD		36–45 YEARS OLD		46–55 YEARS OLD	
		1-MINUTE POST-EXERCISE HEART RATE							
		M	F	M	F	M	F	M	F
	100	50	52	51	58	49	51	56	63
	95	71	75	70	74	70	77	77	85
Excellent	90	76	81	76	80	76	84	82	91
	85	79	85	79	85	80	89	87	95
	80	82	89	83	89	84	92	89	98
Good	75	84	93	85	92	88	96	93	101
	70	88	96	88	95	92	100	95	104
	65	90	98	91	98	95	102	99	107
Above Average	60	93	102	94	101	98	104	101	110
	55	95	104	96	104	100	107	103	113
	50	97	108	100	107	101	109	107	115
Average	45	100	110	102	110	105	112	111	118
	40	102	113	104	113	108	115	113	120
	35	105	116	108	116	111	118	117	121
Below Average	30	107	120	110	119	113	120	119	124
	25	111	122	114	122	116	124	121	126
	20	114	126	118	126	119	128	124	128
Poor	15	119	131	121	129	124	132	126	132
	10	124	135	126	134	130	137	131	137
	5	132	143	134	141	138	142	139	143
Very Poor	0	157	169	161	171	163	169	159	171

Note: This test presents fitness ratings based on percentiles. If you are in the 95th percentile, you are more fit than 95 out of 100 people. Another way to say this would be to say you are in the top 5%. For basic health-fitness, you do not need to be in the highest categories. If you score in the poor or fair category, you may want to begin with a walking program or equivalent. Those who score as average or higher should have sufficient cardiorespiratory capacity to start out in a regular beginner's program or, if in the higher categories, work out using a program commensurate with their fitness rating.

Source: Adapted from "YMCA of the USA Physical Fitness Evaluation Profile," from the *YMCA Fitness Testing and Assessment Manual*, 4th ed., 2000, 200–11.

WORKSHEET 10: CARDIORESPIRATORY FITNESS

12-Minute Walk/Run Test

Note: This is a maximum-effort test. It is recommended that you exercise regularly for 6 to 8 weeks prior to taking this test.

EQUIPMENT:

1. stopwatch
2. track or other measured course
3. pencil or pen

DIRECTIONS:

1. Warm up with light jogging and stretching.
2. Run/walk as far as possible in 12 minutes. This is best achieved by maintaining a steady pace. Be sure to keep track of how far you run. You may want to do this with a partner so that you can count laps for each other.
3. Record the distance you covered: _____ miles.
4. Cool down with light jogging and stretching.
5. Consult the chart below to determine your fitness rating. My fitness rating is _____.

Distance (miles) covered in 12-minute walk/run test.

		AGE (YEARS)					
FITNESS CATEGORY		**13–19**	**20–29**	**30–39**	**40–49**	**50–59**	**60+**
I. Very Poor	(men)	<1.30*	<1.22	<1.18	<1.14	<1.03	<.87
	(women)	<1.0	<.96	<.94	<.88	<.84	<.78
II. Poor	(men)	1.30–1.37	1.22–1.31	1.18–1.30	1.14–1.24	1.03–1.16	.87–1.02
	(women)	1.00–1.18	.96–1.11	.95–1.05	.88–.98	.84–.93	.78–.86
III. Fair	(men)	1.38–1.56	1.32–1.49	1.31–1.45	1.25–1.39	1.17–1.30	1.03–1.20
	(women)	1.19–1.29	1.12–1.22	1.06–1.18	.99–1.11	.94–1.05	.87–.98
IV. Good	(men)	1.57–1.72	1.50–1.64	1.46–1.56	1.40–1.53	1.31–1.44	1.21–1.32
	(women)	1.30–1.43	1.23–1.34	1.19–1.29	1.12–1.24	1.06–1.18	.99–1.09
V. Excellent	(men)	1.73–1.86	1.65–1.76	1.57–1.69	1.54–1.65	1.45–1.58	1.33–1.55
	(women)	1.44–1.51	1.35–1.45	1.30–1.39	1.25–1.34	1.19–1.30	1.10–1.18
VI. Superior	(men)	>1.87	>1.77	>1.70	>1.66	>1.59	>1.56
	(women)	>1.52	>1.46	>1.40	>1.35	>1.31	>1.19

*< means "less than"; > means "more than."

Source: "1.5 Mile Run Tests" and "12-Minute Walk/Run Test" from *The Aerobics Program for Total Well-Being* by Kenneth H. Cooper, M.D., M.P.H. Copyright © 1982 by Kenneth H. Cooper. Used by permission of Random House, Inc.

WORKSHEET 11: CARDIORESPIRATORY FITNESS

1.5-Mile Timed Run Test

Note: This is a maximum-effort test. It is recommended that you exercise regularly for 6 to 8 weeks prior to taking this test.

EQUIPMENT:

1. stopwatch
2. measured course
3. pencil or pen

DIRECTIONS:

1. Warm up and stretch.
2. On the start signal, run/walk the 1.5-mile course as quickly as possible. (An even pace throughout the course is recommended.)
3. Check your time at the end of the course: _____ minutes.
4. Consult the chart below to find your fitness rating. My fitness rating is _____.

Time in minutes for 1.5-mile run test.

		AGE (YEARS)					
FITNESS CATEGORY		13–19	20–29	30–39	40–49	50–59	60+
I. Very Poor	(men)	>15:31*	>16:01	>16:31	>17:31	>19:01	>20:01
	(women)	>18:31	>19:01	>19:31	>20:01	>20:31	>21:01
II. Poor	(men)	12:11–15:30	14:01–16:00	14:44–16:30	15:36–17:30	17:01–19:00	19:01–20:00
	(women)	16:55–18:30	18:31–19:00	19:01–19:30	19:31–20:00	20:01–20:30	20:31–21:00
III. Fair	(men)	10:49–12:10	12:01–14:00	12:31–14:45	13:01–15:35	14:31–17:00	16:16–19:00
	(women)	14:31–16:54	15:55–18:30	16:31–19:00	17:31–19:30	19:01–20:00	19:31–20:30
IV. Good	(men)	9:41–10:48	10:46–12:00	11:01–12:30	11:31–13:00	12:31–14:30	14:00–16:15
	(women)	12:30–14:30	13:31–15:54	14:31–16:30	15:56–17:30	16:31–19:00	17:31–19:30
V. Excellent	(men)	8:37–9:40	9:45–10:45	10:00–11:00	10:30–11:30	11:00–12:30	11:15–13:59
	(women)	11:50–12:29	12:30–13:30	13:00–14:30	13:45–15:55	14:30–16:30	16:30–17:30
VI. Superior	(men)	<8:37	<9:45	<10:00	<10:30	<11:00	<11:15
	(women)	<11:50	<12:30	<13:00	<13:45	<14:30	<16:30

*< means "less than"; > means "more than."

Source: "1.5 Mile Run Tests" and "12-Minute Walk/Run Test" from *The Aerobics Program for Total Well-Being* by Kenneth H. Cooper, M.D., M.P.H. Copyright © 1982 by Kenneth H. Cooper. Used by permission of Random House, Inc.

WORKSHEET 12: FLEXIBILITY

Trunk Forward Flexion Tests

EQUIPMENT:

1. flexometer (Modified Wells and Dillon)[1]
2. partner
3. pencil or pen

Note: Be sure to take this test under the same conditions each time you take it. For example, if you take the test before working out in the afternoon, take it again at the same time of day, after you warm up, but before you exercise.

DIRECTIONS:

1. Perform a warm-up that includes slow static stretching of the lower back and posterior thighs prior to taking this test (modified hurdle stretch held for 20 seconds repeated twice on each leg).
2. Remove your shoes and sit on the floor with your legs fully extended and the soles of your feet placed flat against the flexometer. Have your partner adjust the flexometer so that the balls of your feet rest against the upper crossboards. Place the inner edge of the soles of your feet 2 centimeters (cm) from the edge of the scale.
3. Keeping your knees fully extended, your arms evenly stretched, and your palms down, bend and reach forward (without jerking), pushing the sliding marker along the scale with your fingertips as far forward as possible. **Note:** Lowering your head will help you reach farther.
4. Hold the position of maximum flexion (stretch) for approximately 2 seconds.
5. DO NOT count the attempt if the knees bend. Your partner should watch for knee bend, but not try to hold your knees down.
6. Take the test twice. Record your scores to the nearest 0.5 cm.
7. Record your maximum score: _____ cm.
8. Consult the chart below to determine your fitness rating. My fitness rating is: _____.

Norms by age groups and gender for trunk forward flexion (cm).[*]

FITNESS RATING	AGE (YEARS)											
	15–19		20–29		30–39		40–49		50–59		60–69	
	M	F	M	F	M	F	M	F	M	F	M	F
Excellent	≥39	≥43	≥40	≥41	≥38	≥41	≥35	≥38	≥35	≥39	≥33	≥35
Very Good	34–38	38–42	34–39	37–40	33–37	36–40	29–34	34–37	28–34	33–38	25–32	31–34
Good	29–33	34–37	30–33	33–36	28–32	32–35	24–28	30–33	24–27	30–32	20–24	27–30
Fair	24–28	29–33	25–29	28–32	23–27	27–31	18–23	25–29	16–23	25–29	15–19	23–26
Needs Improvement	≤23	≤28	≤24	≤27	≤22	≤26	≤17	≤24	≤15	≤24	≤14	≤23

[*]Based on data from the Canada Fitness Survey, 1981.
Source: The Canadian Physical Activity, Fitness and Lifestyle Appraisal: CSEP's Plan for Healthy Active Living. 2nd ed.
© 1998. Reprinted by permission from the Canadian Society for Exercise Physiology.

---

1. For directions on how to construct a Modified Wells and Dillon flexometer, along with a drawing showing how to use it, please refer to the instructor's manual.

Continued on next page

MODIFIED TRUNK FORWARD FLEXION TEST

Note 1: This test can be performed without a flexometer. It may be a little less accurate, but, if done carefully, will still supply a good working estimate of flexibility. Please note that the fitness ratings on the previous page were developed using a Modified Wells and Dillon flexometer. Use of those ratings with this test may not be fully accurate. Following the directions carefully each time you take this test will help ensure a good estimate of flexibility.

Note 2: Be sure to take this test under the same conditions each time you take it. For example, if you take the test before working out in the afternoon, take it again at the same time of day, after you warm up, but before you exercise.

EQUIPMENT:

1. meterstick
2. two partners
3. pencil or pen

DIRECTIONS:

1. Perform a warm-up that includes slow static stretching of the lower back and posterior thighs prior to taking this test (modified hurdle stretch held for 20 seconds, repeated twice on each leg).
2. Remove your shoes and sit on the floor with your legs fully extended. Have another person sit opposite you in the same position so that the soles of your feet are against those of the other person. All toes should point directly toward the ceiling throughout the test (Figure A). A one-legged version can also be performed (Figure B). An imbalance in hamstring flexibility can be noted this way.
3. The measurer (third person) holds the meterstick just above your toes with the number 26 cm even with the bottom of the soles of your feet. If you wish to keep your shoes on, place the 26-cm mark where the soles of your feet would be, rather than at the bottom of the soles of the shoes. The number 1 on the meterstick should be close to you, number 39 away from you.
4. Place one hand over the other, palms down, so that your fingertips are even. Then with your knees fully extended, and your arms evenly stretched, slide your fingers as far down the meterstick as possible. Use a smooth, sustained motion. **Note:** Lowering your head will help you reach farther.
5. Hold the position of maximum flexion (stretch) for approximately two seconds.
6. DO NOT count the attempt if the knees bend. Your partner should watch for knee bend, but should not try to hold your knees down.

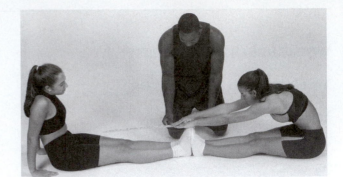

Figure A

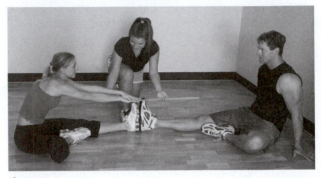

Figure B

7. Take the test twice. Record your scores to the nearest 0.5 cm.
8. Record your maximum score: _____ cm.
9. Consult the chart on the previous page for an approximate fitness rating. My fitness rating is _____.

TRUNK FLEXION WALL TEST

Note: This is a quick and easy check for flexibility that you can perform anywhere there is a wall with sitting space in front of it.

DIRECTIONS:

1. Warm up with 5 to 10 minutes of light cardio work followed by some static stretches of the lower back and posterior thighs.
2. Place your feet flat against a wall.
3. Reach forward with both hands and try to touch the wall.

FITNESS CATEGORY:

Poor	Can't touch the wall.
Good	Can touch the wall with your fingertips.
Very Good	Can touch the walls with your knuckles (hands in fists).
Excellent	Can place both palms flat on the wall.

WORKSHEET 13: QUICK CHECK FLEXIBILITY TESTS

The following 12 tests are pass/fail. They are quick and easy to perform and require only a yardstick and a partner. Because flexibility is joint specific, a variety of tests is provided. Check for imbalances from one side of the body to the other and between paired muscles or muscle groups.

If you would like to keep a record of your flexibility and then check for improvement in 6 to 8 weeks, draw a stick figure indicating the angle of your joint for each test on the record sheets on pages 243–244. If you have a protractor you can measure and record the angle. Another way to measure the angle is to use a simple tool you can create by fastening together two straightedges (for example, plastic rulers or pieces of stiff cardboard) at one end using a paper fastener. Hold your tool near or against your partner's body and open or close the straightedges until the angle of the tool matches the angle of the joint you are measuring. Then move the tool to your record sheet and trace the angle. Be sure to measure both limbs or sides of the body as appropriate.

Neck Test

Stand or sit with your back straight and your face looking forward. Drop your chin to your chest. If you are able to press your chin against an open hand placed on your chest, give yourself a passing grade. If not, measure and record the distance between your chin and hand.

Shoulder Test I

Stand up straight with your arms at your side, palms touching your leg. Raise one arm *forward* and up overhead. If you reach 180 degrees (directly overhead) or more give yourself a passing grade. If not, measure and record the angle between your body and your raised arm.

Shoulder Test II

Stand up straight with your arms at your side, palms touching your leg. Raise one arm *out to the side* and up overhead. If you reach 180 degrees (by your ear), give yourself a passing grade. If not, measure and record the angle between the side of your body and your arm.

Shoulder Test III

Stand up straight and attempt to touch your fingertips by reaching one arm over the shoulder and one arm up the middle of your back. If you can touch your hands, give yourself a passing grade. If not, have a partner measure and record the distance between your fingertips.

Trunk Test

Sit in a chair with your feet flat on the floor. Turn your upper body while keeping your hips square to the front. If you are able to twist 90 degrees or more (shoulders will be square to the side) give yourself a passing grade. If not, have a partner measure and record the angle of rotation. (If you are turning right, measure the angle your left shoulder moved away from dead front.) It will be easier to see whether you have succeeded if you place your hands on your shoulders while you twist.

Lower Back Test

Lie on your back with both knees bent, feet off the floor, and head and lower back touching the floor. Grasp your legs underneath your knees and pull gently toward your shoulders (if you have to pull hard you fail the test). To pass, touch both knees to their respective shoulders or lay your thighs flat along your torso with your lower back and head still touching the floor. If you are unable to, measure the angle between your thighs and your torso.

Hip Flexor Test

Lie on your back on the floor with both legs straight. Keeping one leg straight and along the ground, draw the knee of the other leg up toward your chest. Place your hand on the back of your thigh underneath your knee and pull gently. Give yourself a passing grade if your thigh touches your torso and your other leg remains straight. If not, have your partner measure and record the angle between your torso and thigh.

ALTERNATE TEST:
Lie on your back on a knee-high firm surface, such as a folded mat, bleacher, or table. Bend your knees over

Continued on next page

the edge and put your feet flat on the floor. Draw one knee to your chest while trying to keep the opposite foot flat on the floor. If you can do this comfortably, give yourself a passing grade. If your heel lifts up, have your partner measure and record the distance between your heel and the floor.

Hip Abduction Test

Either standing straight or lying on the ground, move one leg sideways as far from the other leg as possible. If the angle between the legs measures 45 degrees or more, give yourself a passing grade. If not, have your partner measure and record the angle.

Hamstring Test

Lie on your back with both legs straight. Keeping both legs straight, lift the one up and as far toward your head as possible. Give yourself a passing grade if you were able to reach a 90-degree angle (straight up) or more. If not, have your partner measure and record the angle between the floor and your raised leg.

Quadriceps Test

Lie prone on the floor with your head turned to one side. Bend one knee and grasp the ankle. Without forcing it, draw your ankle toward your buttocks. Give yourself a passing grade if your heel touches your buttocks or your lower leg rests against your upper leg. If not, have your partner measure and record the angle behind your knee made by your lower and upper leg.

Calf Test

Sit on the floor with your legs extended straight in front of you. Flex one ankle as much as you can. Give yourself a passing grade if the angle between the sole of your shoe and your shin is 80 to 90 degrees or less. If not, have a partner measure and record the angle.

ALTERNATE POSITION:

Stand with your weight on one foot and the heel of the other foot on the ground. Dorsiflex the ankle of the unweighted foot by drawing the toes toward the shin. Measure the angle created between the floor and the sole of the foot. A passing score is a 10- to 20-degree angle.

NAME _____   DATE _____

Quick Flexibility Test Record

Test	Passing	Your Results			
		Date:	Date:	Date:	Date:
Neck Test	0 inches	___ inches between hand and chin	___ inches between hand and chin	___ inches between hand and chin	___ inches between hand and chin
Shoulder Test I	180 degrees	Left arm ___ deg. Right arm ___ deg.	Left arm ___ deg. Right arm ___ deg.	Left arm ___ deg. Right arm ___ deg.	Left arm ___ deg. Right arm ___ deg.
Shoulder Test II	180 degrees	Left arm ___ deg. Right arm ___ deg.	Left arm ___ deg. Right arm ___ deg.	Left arm ___ deg. Right arm ___ deg.	Left arm ___ deg. Right arm ___ deg.
Shoulder Test III	0 inches (fingers touching)	Right arm up: ___ inches between fingertips Left arm up: ___ inches between fingertips	Right arm up: ___ inches between fingertips Left arm up: ___ inches between fingertips	Right arm up: ___ inches between fingertips Left arm up: ___ inches between fingertips	Right arm up: ___ inches between fingertips Left arm up: ___ inches between fingertips
Trunk Test	90 degrees*	___ degrees of rotation	___ degrees of rotation	___ degrees of rotation	___ degrees of rotation
Lower Back Test	Thighs touching chest (0 degrees)	___ deg.	___ deg.	___ deg.	___ deg.

* For clarity, only 45 degrees is shown. Continue to 90 degrees.

Continued on next page

243

Test	Passing	Your Results			
		Date:	Date:	Date:	Date:
Hip Flexor Test	Thigh touching chest (0 degrees)	left leg: ___ deg. right leg: ___ deg.	left leg: ___ deg. right leg: ___ deg.	left leg: ___ deg. right leg: ___ deg.	left leg: ___ deg. right leg: ___ deg.
Alternate Hip Flexor Test	0 inches	right leg ___ inches between heel and floor left leg ___ inches between heel and floor	right leg ___ inches between heel and floor left leg ___ inches between heel and floor	right leg ___ inches between heel and floor left leg ___ inches between heel and floor	right leg ___ inches between heel and floor left leg ___ inches between heel and floor
Hip Abduction Test	45 degrees	left leg: ___ deg. right leg: ___ deg.	left leg: ___ deg. right leg: ___ deg.	left leg: ___ deg. right leg: ___ deg.	left leg: ___ deg. right leg: ___ deg.
Hamstring Test	90 degrees	left leg: ___ deg. right leg: ___ deg.	left leg: ___ deg. right leg: ___ deg.	left leg: ___ deg. right leg: ___ deg.	left leg: ___ deg. right leg: ___ deg.
Quadriceps Test	Heel touching buttocks (0 degrees)	left leg: ___ deg. right leg: ___ deg.	left leg: ___ deg. right leg: ___ deg.	left leg: ___ deg. right leg: ___ deg.	left leg: ___ deg. right leg: ___ deg.
Calf Test	80 to 90 degrees	left ankle: ___ deg. right ankle: ___ deg.	left ankle: ___ deg. right ankle: ___ deg.	left ankle: ___ deg. right ankle: ___ deg.	left ankle: ___ deg. right ankle: ___ deg.

WORKSHEET 14: MUSCULAR ENDURANCE

Partial Curl-Up Test

Note: A person who suffers from lower back or neck ailments should not perform this test.

EQUIPMENT:

1. gym mat with tape, string, wire, or Velcro markers as indicated below
2. metronome or cassette player and tape with a recorded beat
3. metric ruler
4. pen or pencil
5. carpenter's square, or book, or piece of paper
6. partner

MAT SETUP:

On a gym mat use tape, string, wire, or strips of Velcro and a metric ruler to lay out the diagram below. You can also set this up so that the edge of the mat is the 10-centimeter (cm) mark.

Guidelines for tape and string/Velcro placement on gym mat

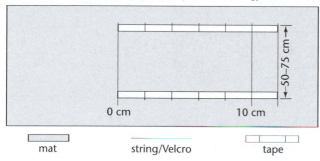

DIRECTIONS:

1. Lie on your back with your head on the mat, arms straight and parallel to your trunk, palms flat on the mat, and the middle fingertip of both hands at the zero mark.

   With the soles of your feet touching the mat, bend your knees at a 90-degree angle. Your partner can use the corner of a textbook or standard piece of paper to check your knee angle.

   Have your partner place a strip of tape under your heels to mark where your heels are to stay in contact with the mat.

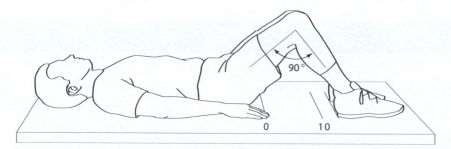

2. Turn on the metronome to 50 beats per minute (or cassette tape recording of the same). You will be curling up on one beat and down on the next at a rate of 25 curl-ups per minute.

Continued on next page

3. Curl up by first flattening out your lower back region (pelvic tilt) and then slowly curling up your upper spine. Slide your palms in contact with the mat along the tape until they touch the string or Velcro at the 10-cm mark. During the curl-up, the palms and heels must remain in contact with the mat. Anchoring of the feet is not permitted. Breathe normally throughout, exhaling as you curl up.

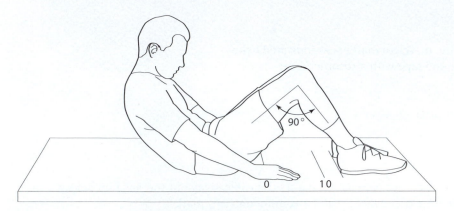

4. Return to your starting position—lying flat, head down, fingertips at the zero mark on the string or Velcro. Practice twice, making sure that you take an equal amount of time to curl in each direction. Use continuous and well-controlled movements.

5. Perform continuous curl-ups until you reach a maximum of 25. Stop sooner if you experience severe discomfort or pain, if you fall 2 repetitions behind cadence, or if your partner indicates that you have lost proper technique over 2 consecutive repetitions as outlined below:

- moving your seat (changing your knee angle)
- lifting or sliding your heels
- bending your elbows or lifting your palms off the mat
- sliding your fingers short of, or beyond, the 10-cm mark
- pausing between movements at either the top or bottom of the curl-up
- getting ahead of or behind the cadence

6. Stretch your abdominal and leg muscles.

7. Record the number of curl-ups you completed: _____

8. Consult the chart below and determine your fitness level. Be sure to look under the appropriate age and gender.

My fitness rating is: _____.

Norms and health benefits by age groups and gender for partial curl-up.

	AGE (YEARS)											
	15–19		**20–29**		**30–39**		**40–49**		**50–59**		**60–69**	
FITNESS RATING	M	F	M	F	M	F	M	F	M	F	M	F
Excellent	25	25	25	25	25	25	25	25	25	25	25	≥18
Very Good	23–24	23–24	23–24	23–24	23–24	23–24	22–24	21–24	20–24	16–24	16–24	11–17
Good	21–22	21–22	21–22	19–22	21–22	16–21	16–21	13–20	20–24	16–24	16–24	11–17
Fair	16–20	16–20	13–20	13–18	13–20	11–15	11–15	6–12	9–13	4–8	4–9	2–5
Needs Improvement	≤15	≤15	≤12	≤12	≤12	≤10	≤10	≤5	≤8	≤2	≤3	≤1

Source: The Canadian Physical Activity, Fitness and Lifestyle Appraisal: CSEP's Plan for Healthy Active Living. 2nd ed.
© 1998. Reprinted by permission from the Canadian Society for Exercise Physiology.

WORKSHEET 15: MUSCULAR ENDURANCE

Push-Up Test

EQUIPMENT:

1. partner
2. mat or towel (for knees during modified push-ups)
3. pencil or pen

IMPORTANT NOTES:

1. A person who suffers from any lower back ailment should not perform this test.
2. The norms for this test are based on women performing modified push-ups and men performing regular push-ups. If, however, a woman wishes to perform regular push-ups, she can with the understanding that the norms are based on men. Similarly, men who lack the upper-body strength to do regular push-ups can begin with modified push-ups and record their progress.

DIRECTIONS FOR THE MODIFIED PUSH-UP:

1. Warm up and stretch, especially your arms and chest.
2. Lie on your stomach, legs together. Position your hands under your shoulders with fingers pointing forward. Push up from the mat by fully extending your elbows and using your knees as the pivot point. The upper body must be kept in a straight line. Return to the starting point, chin to the mat. The stomach should not touch the mat. The lower legs remain in contact with the mat, ankles plantar-flexed (extended), and feet in contact with the mat. Exhale when you push up and inhale as you lower down.
3. Perform as many consecutive push-ups as you are able. There is no time limit. The test stops when you have to strain forcibly or are unable to maintain the proper push-up technique over 2 consecutive repetitions.

4. Record the number of correct push-ups you completed: _____.
5. Consult the normative chart and determine your fitness level: _____. (Fill in an "x" if there are no gender-appropriate norms for the test you performed.)
6. Stretch your arms and chest muscles to prevent soreness.

DIRECTIONS FOR THE REGULAR PUSH-UP:

1. Warm up and stretch, especially your arms and chest.
2. Lie on your stomach, legs together. Position your hands under your shoulders with fingers pointing forward. Push up from the mat by fully extending your elbows and using your toes as the pivot point. The upper body must be kept in a straight line. Return to the starting point touching only the chin, not the stomach or the thighs. Exhale when you push up, and inhale as you lower down.
3. Perform as many consecutive push-ups as you are able. There is no time limit. The test stops when you have to strain forcibly or are unable to maintain the proper push-up technique over 2 consecutive repetitions.
4. Record the number of correct push-ups you completed: _____.
5. Consult the normative chart and determine your fitness level: _____. (Fill in an "x" if there are no gender-appropriate norms for the test you performed.)
6. Stretch your arms and chest muscles to prevent soreness.

Continued on next page

Norms by age groups and gender for push-ups.[*]

FITNESS RATING	AGE (YEARS)											
	15–19		20–29		30–39		40–49		50–59		60–69	
	M	F	M	F	M	F	M	F	M	F	M	F
Excellent	≥39	≥33	≥36	≥30	≥30	≥27	≥22	≥24	≥21	≥21	≥18	≥17
Above Average	29–38	25–32	29–35	21–29	22–29	20–26	17–21	15–23	13–20	11–20	11–17	12–16
Average	23–28	18–24	22–28	15–20	17–21	13–19	13–16	11–14	10–12	7–10	8–10	5–11
Below Average	18–22	12–17	17–21	10–14	12–16	8–12	10–12	5–10	7–9	2–6	5–7	1–4
Poor	≤17	≤11	≤16	≤9	≤11	≤7	≤9	≤4	≤6	≤1	≤4	≤1

[*]Based on data from the Canada Fitness Survey, 1981.
Source: The Canadian Physical Activity, Fitness and Lifestyle Appraisal: CSEP's Plan for Healthy Active Living. 2nd ed.
© 1998. Reprinted by permission from the Canadian Society for Exercise Physiology.

WORKSHEET 16: HEALTHY WEIGHT

WAIST/HIP RATIO

1. Measure, or have a partner measure, your waist at the point of noticeable waist narrowing (approximately at your navel). If there is no noticeable narrowing, feel for the twelfth (bottom or floating) rib and take the measurement just below it. Pull the tape enough to maintain its position but not so much that it indents the skin. Be sure the tape is horizontal all the way around your body. Record the measurement to the nearest eighth of an inch ($\frac{1}{8} = .13$, $\frac{2}{8} = .25$, $\frac{3}{8} = .38$, $\frac{4}{8} = .50$, $\frac{5}{8} = .63$, $\frac{6}{8} = .75$, $\frac{7}{8} = .88$).

   Waist measurement: _____ inches

2. Measure, or have a partner measure, your hips at the greatest circumference to the nearest eighth of an inch.

   Hip measurement: _____ inches

3. Calculate the waist/hip ratio:

   _____ ÷ _____ = _____
   waist   hip   ratio

4. A waist-to-hip ratio greater than 1.0 for men and 0.8 for women indicates an increased cardiac risk.

   ___ I **do not** have an increased risk.

   ___ I **do** have an increased risk.

BODY MASS INDEX (BMI)

Note: Be sure to read the discussion in the text about BMI. Muscular individuals can be incorrectly classified.

1. Weigh yourself without shoes. If your weight is in pounds, convert it to kilograms.

   _____(pounds) ÷ 2.2 = _____ kilograms

2. Determine your height. If your height is in inches, convert it to meters.

   _____ inches ÷ 39 = _____ meters

3. Calculate BMI:

   $$\frac{weight}{height \times height} = \underline{\hspace{2cm}} \text{ BMI}$$

OR

1. Multiply your weight in pounds (no shoes) by 703.

2. Divide the answer by your height (in inches, no shoes).

3. Divide the answer again by your height (in inches, no shoes).

   _____ I am normal weight.   BMI = 18.5–24.9

   _____ I am overweight.   BMI = 25–29.9[*]

   _____ I am obese.   BMI = 30 or greater

[*]Individuals who are overweight should try not to gain weight. Individuals who are overweight and have two or more risk factors for heart disease and/or have a high waist measurement should try to lose weight. Individuals who are obese should try to lose weight gradually with a $\frac{1}{2}$- to 2-pound loss per week.

Source: Clinical Guidelines on the Identification, Evaluation, and Treatment of Overweight and Obesity in Adults, National Heart, Lung, and Blood Institute, in cooperation with the National Institute of Diabetes and Digestive and Kidney Diseases, National Institutes of Health, June 1998.

Continued on next page

Healthy Weight Calculated Using Known Percent Fat

(See page 182, Chapter 12.)

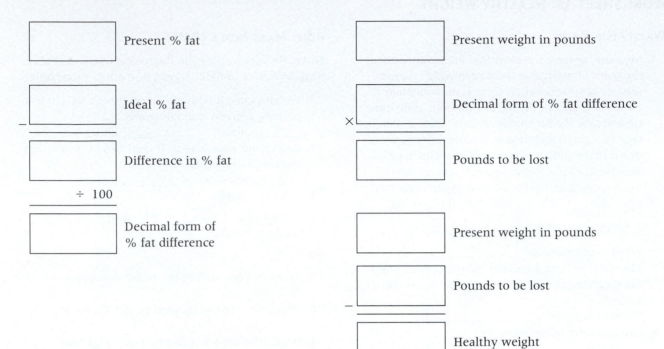

WORKSHEET 17: NUTRITION AWARENESS

Weekday

Record what you eat during one **weekday**.   Date: _____

MEAL:	FOODS ──────▶	FOOD GROUPS	──▶ AMOUNTS/SERVINGS
Breakfast: Time _____	_____ ▶	_____	▶ _____
Time spent eating _____	_____ ▶	_____	▶ _____
Location _____	_____ ▶	_____	▶ _____
_____	_____ ▶	_____	▶ _____
_____	_____ ▶	_____	▶ _____
_____	_____ ▶	_____	▶ _____
Lunch: Time _____	_____ ▶	_____	▶ _____
Time spent eating _____	_____ ▶	_____	▶ _____
Location _____	_____ ▶	_____	▶ _____
_____	_____ ▶	_____	▶ _____
_____	_____ ▶	_____	▶ _____
_____	_____ ▶	_____	▶ _____
Dinner: Time _____	_____ ▶	_____	▶ _____
Time spent eating _____	_____ ▶	_____	▶ _____
Location _____	_____ ▶	_____	▶ _____
_____	_____ ▶	_____	▶ _____
_____	_____ ▶	_____	▶ _____
_____	_____ ▶	_____	▶ _____
Snacks: Time(s) _____	_____ ▶	_____	▶ _____
Time spent eating _____	_____ ▶	_____	▶ _____
Location _____	_____ ▶	_____	▶ _____
_____	_____ ▶	_____	▶ _____
_____	_____ ▶	_____	▶ _____
_____	_____ ▶	_____	▶ _____
Alcohol: Time(s) _____	_____ ▶	_____	▶ _____
Time spent drinking _____	_____ ▶		

Compare your diet to the recommended portions for each food group using the MyPyramid guidelines. Remember that MyPyramid uses a variety of pyramids, individualized for different calorie levels. Figure 12.1 on page 175 provides information based on a 2000-calorie diet. To find the amounts that are right for you, go to www.MyPyramid.gov. To assist you in identifying serving sizes, refer to Figure 12.3 on page 178.

Note: You may also want to keep a journal that tracks what you are doing and how you are feeling when you eat.

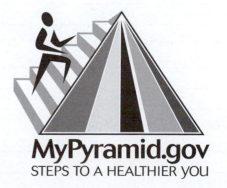

MyPyramid.gov
STEPS TO A HEALTHIER YOU

Continued on next page

Look over your **weekday** food log and try to answer the following questions.

1. Did you eat the appropriate number of servings for each food group? If not, can you think of a food you would consider eating that would fulfill the requirements of a food group?

   _____

2. Did you drink 6 to 8 glasses of water (any fluid not containing alcohol)? _____

3. List in separate columns your complex (and natural sugar) carbohydrates and the simple carbohydrates you ate. Were the vast majority complex carbohydrates?

   _____

   _____

   _____

4. When during the day did you eat the most food? When did you eat the highest-calorie foods? Thinking about your schedule for the past week, is this pattern the same?

   _____

   _____

   _____

5. Do you usually eat your meals at the same time each day? What implications might this have?

   _____

   _____

   _____

6. If you could start the day over and pick one thing to do differently concerning diet, what would it be?

   _____

   _____

   _____

7. Is there one thing concerning diet that you would keep the same (e.g., a moment you were proud of such as exchanging an empty calorie snack for a nutritious one, getting all your vegetable servings)?

   _____

   _____

   _____

8. If you are trying to or would like to lose weight, can you identify any triggers (things that encouraged you) to eat high-fat, high-cholesterol, or high-sugar foods on this particular day? Can you think, now, how you might have avoided or resisted the trigger?

   _____

   _____

   _____

9. How do your weekend eating habits compare to your weekday eating habits?

   _____

   _____

   _____

10. Other comments or observations?

   _____

   _____

   _____

WORKSHEET 18: NUTRITION AWARENESS

Weekend Day

Record what you eat during one **weekend day**.   Date: _____

MEAL:	FOODS ⟶	FOOD GROUPS ⟶	AMOUNTS/SERVINGS
Breakfast: Time _____	_____ ➡	_____	➡ _____
Time spent eating _____	_____ ➡	_____	➡ _____
Location _____	_____ ➡	_____	➡ _____
_____	_____ ➡	_____	➡ _____
_____	_____ ➡	_____	➡ _____
	_____ ➡	_____	➡ _____
Lunch: Time _____	_____ ➡	_____	➡ _____
Time spent eating _____	_____ ➡	_____	➡ _____
Location _____	_____ ➡	_____	➡ _____
_____	_____ ➡	_____	➡ _____
_____	_____ ➡	_____	➡ _____
	_____ ➡	_____	➡ _____
Dinner: Time _____	_____ ➡	_____	➡ _____
Time spent eating _____	_____ ➡	_____	➡ _____
Location _____	_____ ➡	_____	➡ _____
_____	_____ ➡	_____	➡ _____
_____	_____ ➡	_____	➡ _____
	_____ ➡	_____	➡ _____
	_____ ➡	_____	➡ _____
Snacks: Time(s) _____	_____ ➡	_____	➡ _____
Time spent eating _____	_____ ➡	_____	➡ _____
Location _____	_____ ➡	_____	➡ _____
_____	_____ ➡	_____	➡ _____
_____	_____ ➡	_____	➡ _____
Alcohol: Time(s) _____	_____ ➡	_____	➡ _____
Time spent drinking _____	_____ ➡	_____	➡ _____

Compare your diet to the recommended portions for each food group using the MyPyramid guidelines. Remember that MyPyramid uses a variety of pyramids, individualized for different calorie levels. Figure 12.1 on page 175 provides information based on a 2000-calorie diet. To find the amounts that are right for you, go to www.MyPyramid.gov. To assist you in identifying serving sizes, refer to Figure 12.3 on page 178.

Note: You may also want to keep a journal that tracks what you are doing and how you are feeling when you eat.

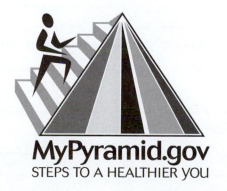

MyPyramid.gov
STEPS TO A HEALTHIER YOU

Continued on next page

Look over your **weekend day** food log and try to answer the following questions:

1. Did you eat the appropriate number of servings for each food group? If not, can you think of a food you would consider eating that would fulfill the requirements of a food group?

_____

2. Did you drink 6 to 8 glasses of water (any fluid not containing alcohol)? _____

3. List in separate columns your complex (and natural sugar) carbohydrates and the simple carbohydrates you ate. Were the vast majority complex carbohydrates?

_____

_____

_____

4. When during the day did you eat the most food? When did you eat the highest-calorie foods? Thinking about your schedule for the past week, is this pattern the same?

_____

_____

_____

5. Do you usually eat your meals at the same time each day? What implications might this have?

_____

_____

_____

6. If you could start the day over and pick one thing to do differently concerning diet, what would it be?

_____

_____

_____

7. Is there one thing concerning diet that you would keep the same (e.g., a moment you were proud of such as exchanging an empty calorie snack for a nutritious one, getting all your vegetable servings)?

_____

_____

_____

8. If you are trying to or would like to lose weight, can you identify any triggers (things that encouraged you) to eat high-fat, high-cholesterol, or high-sugar foods on this particular day? Can you think, now, how you might have avoided or resisted the trigger?

_____

_____

_____

9. How do your weekday eating habits compare to your weekend eating habits?

_____

_____

_____

10. Other comments or observations?

_____

_____

_____

Glossary

active stretch A flexibility exercise in which the muscle or muscle groups that oppose the target muscle(s) (one being stretched) are contracted with the effect of relaxing the target muscle(s).

adenosine triphosphate (ATP) The high-energy phosphate molecule used to make cellular energy. Muscle cells use ATP to fuel contraction.

aerobic Living, active, or occurring only in the presence of oxygen.

aerobic exercise Exercise that demands a large and continuous supply of oxygen and that ultimately results in the improvement of the oxygen carrying and delivery systems. Exercise that involves continuous rhythmic large-muscle movements.

aerobic glycolysis The metabolic process of breaking down carbohydrate in the presence of oxygen.

aerobic system The metabolic processes of breaking down carbohydrate, fat, and protein in the presence of oxygen to produce energy (ATP).

aerobic target zone The fitness target zone for aerobic activity. *See* fitness target zone.

aerobics Any physical activity that requires oxygen for a prolonged amount of time.

agonist A muscle that is undergoing contraction.

anaerobic Without or in the absence of oxygen.

anaerobic glycolysis *See* lactic acid system.

anaerobic system The metabolic processes that produce energy (ATP) in the absence of oxygen. *See* phosphagen system *and* lactic acid system.

anorexia nervosa An eating disorder characterized by a continual desire to lose weight because of fear of being fat. Unless treated, individuals suffering from this disease can starve themselves to death.

antagonist A muscle working in opposition to the agonist. When the agonist contracts, the antagonist relaxes.

antagonist stretching A type of stretching in which the agonist is contracted to aid the stretch and relaxation of the antagonist. Works on the principle of reciprocal innervation.

antioxidants Chemical compounds that neutralize cell-damaging free radicals that are created when oxygen is used inside the body's cells.

aqua aerobics A low-impact form of aerobic conditioning performed in water using water resistance to enhance training. (*Synonym:* water aerobics)

arteriosclerosis Hardening of the arteries. *See* atherosclerosis.

artery A vessel that carries blood away from the heart.

assisted stretch *See* passive stretching.

atherosclerosis A specific form of arteriosclerosis characterized by the formation of fatty deposits (plaque) along the walls of the arteries.

ATP *See* adenosine triphosphate.

autogenic training A psychophysiological technique of using visual metaphors to relax the body.

ballistic stretching A technique used to develop flexibility. It is characterized by a series of bouncing or pulsing movements that alternately stretch and then relax the muscle. These movements may elicit the stretch reflex. (Opposite of static stretching.)

binge-eating disorder A type of eating disorder characterized by episodes of uncontrolled excessive and rapid overeating without purging.

blood pressure The amount of pressure the blood exerts against the walls of the arteries during ventricular contraction (systolic pressure) and ventricular relaxation (diastolic pressure). It is generally represented as a fraction: systolic/diastolic pressure.

body alignment The positioning of the body's segments in relationship to each other.

body composition The relative amounts of lean body mass and fat in the body.

body mass index (BMI) A measure of weight in relation to height which is used to estimate healthy weight and determine health risk.

body posture The position of the body in space (e.g., sitting, standing, lying down).

bulimia An eating disorder characterized by binge-and-purge behavior. Purging may be accomplished through self-induced vomiting or use of diuretics or laxatives.

CAD *See* coronary artery disease.

calorie Common usage form of the word *kilocalorie*. A measure of the value of foods to produce heat and energy in the human body. One calorie is equal to the amount of heat required to raise the temperature of 1 gram of water 1°C.

capillaries The smallest blood vessels in the body. They supply blood (oxygen) to the tissues.

carbohydrates Compounds such as sugars and starches that are made up of carbon, hydrogen, and oxygen. Carbohydrates serve as the primary source of energy for the body. They are broken down and transported in the blood as glucose and stored in the liver and muscles as glycogen. Dietary sources include complex carbohydrates (e.g., grains and beans) and simple carbohydrates (e.g., refined sugars and natural sugars).

cardiac output The amount of blood pumped by the heart in 1 minute.

cardiorespiratory endurance The ability to perform large-muscle movements over a sustained period of time. Also, the ability of the lung-heart system to deliver oxygen for sustained energy production. (*Synonyms:* cardiovascular fitness *or* endurance; cardiorespiratory fitness)

carotid artery An artery that runs close to the surface of the skin just to either side of the larynx. This artery is commonly used for counting the pulse.

cellulite Fat stored under the skin where it is separated into little compartments by connective fibers.

CHD *See* coronary heart disease.

cholesterol A fatty substance in the blood and body tissues that is naturally synthesized by the body and is also contained in certain foods. High levels of cholesterol in the blood are associated with atherosclerosis.

CIA *See* combination high-/low-impact aerobics.

circuit training A method of aerobic or resistance training that involves moving through a series of exercise stations with short or no breaks between stations.

combination high-/low-impact aerobics (CIA) A form of aerobic dance exercise that uses both low- and high-impact movements in one class. (*Synonyms:* hi-/lo-impact, combo-impact)

combo-impact *See* combination high-/low-impact aerobics.

concentric contraction A muscle contraction during which the muscle is shortening.

cool-down Movements performed after the aerobic workout that systematically decrease in intensity so that the body can return to a near resting level.

core training The use of resistance exercises to develop the muscles that support the middle of the body, especially the spine.

core warm-up *See* general warm-up.

coronary arteries The arteries that supply the heart with oxygen.

coronary artery disease (CAD) Narrowing or blockage of the coronary arteries resulting in reduced blood supply, and therefore, reduced oxygen supply to the heart muscle.

coronary heart disease (CHD) The major form of cardio-vascular disease, or a disease of the heart or blood vessels. It is the single largest leading cause of death in the United States.

diabetes mellitus A group of metabolic diseases in which the body is unable to produce sufficient insulin (type I), or effectively use the insulin it does produce (type II).

diastolic pressure The pressure exerted by the blood in the arteries when the ventricles are filling. Diastolic pressure is represented by the denominator in the blood pressure fraction.

duration The length of a single exercise session.

dynamic contraction A muscle contraction taken over a range of motion. It is used to increase strength throughout a movement.

dynamic flexibility Ranges of motion achieved with exercises that use the speed of the movement to assist in stretching muscles through a range of motion; smooth controlled movements are used, rather than ballistic ones.

dynamic stretching A type of stretching that uses the pull of a muscle or group of muscles and the body's momentum to move through a full range of motion.

dynamic warm-up A series of exercises that include general mobility exercises, dynamic stretching, and balance and coordination movements.

eccentric contraction A muscle contraction during which the muscle is lengthening.

EHR *See* exercise heart rate.

energy balance A state in which caloric intake is equal to caloric expenditure. No weight change occurs during energy balance.

exercise ball *See* stability ball.

exercise band A form of resistance training equipment that consists of a band of stretchable material. This may be a stretch cable, specialized exercise/therapeutic band, surgical tubing, or heavy duty rubber band.

exercise heart rate (EHR) The number of times the heart beats per minute (or per 10 seconds) during an exercise session.

extrinsic motivation Motivation that has its source outside the individual.

failure The point during a resistance exercise when proper technique is lost or when an additional repetition of the exercise cannot be performed.

fat One of the six essential nutrients. This energy-rich compound made up of glycerol and fatty acids serves as a source of energy for the body, particularly during aerobic activity. It is stored as adipose tissue.

fatty acid oxidation An aerobic metabolic process that produces energy (ATP) through the breakdown of fatty acids.

fiber A general term for food substances that the body can't fully digest. (*Synonym:* roughage)

FIT An acronym for the three variables involved in overload: frequency, intensity, and time. (Also called FITT, where the last T stands for "type of activity.")

fitness target zone The optimal range of exercise, defined by frequency, intensity, and time (duration) and performed with the purpose of maintaining or improving physical fitness. The lower limit of the zone is called the threshold of training. The upper limit is the maximum amount of exercise that is beneficial.

FITT principle An exercise principle describing the frequency, intensity, time, and type of activity.

flexibility The ability to move a joint or series of joints through its full range of motion.

free weights Resistance equipment that is not part of a machine, for example, dumbbells, barbells, and medicine balls.

frequency The number of times a person exercises per week.

general warm-up A series of easy, active large muscle movements that increase blood circulation and raise the core temperature 1 to 2 degrees.

glucose The simplest form of sugar. Carbohydrate is broken down into glucose before being absorbed into the bloodstream and taken to the cell for energy production.

glycogen A form of carbohydrate stored in the muscle.

group fitness The popular term for exercise classes, such as aerobic dance and group cycling, that emphasize working out as a group.

hatha yoga The physical aspect of yoga; what most Americans call yoga. Uses a variety of poses, breathing techniques, and meditation. *See also* yoga.

HDL *See* high-density lipoprotein.

heart rate (HR) The number of times the heart beats per minute.

heart-rate reserve (HRR) The maximum heart rate minus the resting heart rate.

HIA *See* high-impact aerobics.

hi-/lo-impact aerobics *See* combination high-/low-impact aerobics.

high-density lipoprotein (HDL) A complex of lipids (fat) and proteins that picks up cholesterol in the blood and carries it to the liver. (Often called HDL-C when carrying cholesterol.) Exercise increases the amount of HDL in the blood.

high-impact aerobics (HIA) A style of aerobics in which both feet may temporarily leave the floor at the same time when performing moves such as jogging, jumping, and hopping.

homeostasis State of balance or dynamic equilibrium. The energy demand is being met by energy production.

HRR *See* heart-rate reserve.

hydrostatic weighing A method of estimating body fat. (*Synonym:* underwater weighing)

hypertension A higher than normal blood pressure.

hypertrophy An increase in size. In exercise this usually refers to an increase in muscle size.

intensity The level of exertion during exercise.

interval training A method of conditioning that alternates short, high-intensity exercise bouts with short rest periods or lower-intensity bouts.

intrinsic motivation Motivation that arises from within a person; self-motivation.

isokinetic contractions A muscle contraction in which the speed of movement is controlled and the force applied is met with an equal resistence. Especially good for rehabilitation.

isometric contraction A muscle contraction in which there is tension but no movement. It is used to increase strength in one position.

isotonic contraction Muscular strength and endurance exercises in which the tension of the muscle remains the same throughout the range of the motion.

Karvonen formula A method of calculating the intensity target range for aerobic work using a percentage of the heart-rate reserve.

lactic acid A by-product of high-intensity anaerobic exercise. Accumulation of lactic acid is associated with muscle fatigue and "burn."

lactic acid system The metabolic process of breaking down carbohydrates in the absence of oxygen to produce energy (ATP).

LDL *See* low-density lipoprotein.

lean body mass (LBM) All the tissues of the body except fat. LBM includes bone, muscle, water, organs, connective tissue, etc., and is used to determine body composition.

LIA *See* low-impact aerobics.

ligament The fibrous tissue that connects bones to bones.

low-density lipoprotein (LDL) A complex of lipids and proteins that carries cholesterol and deposits it along the walls of the arteries. (Often called LDL-C when carrying cholesterol.) High concentrations of LDL are associated with an increased risk of heart disease.

low-impact aerobics (LIA) A type of aerobics in which the participant keeps one foot on the floor at all times. It is often characterized by moderately paced movements involving a full range of motion with a lot of upper-body work.

maximum heart rate (MHR) The highest heart rate obtainable with exertion.

maximum heart-rate formula A method of estimating the intensity range for an aerobic workout using a percentage (70 to 85%) of the maximum heart rate. (*Synonym:* zero to peak formula)

mental imagery A cognitive (thought-based) technique to enhance task performance. Uses mental rehearsal/practice.

MHR *See* maximum heart rate.

MIA *See* moderate-impact aerobics.

minerals Inorganic compounds that are essential to normal body function.

moderate-impact aerobics (MIA) A form of aerobic dance in which the center of gravity is raised and lowered (all the way up on and off the balls of the feet) while using steps that keep one foot on the floor at all times.

muscular endurance The ability of a muscle, or group of muscles, to apply force repeatedly or to sustain a muscular contraction for a period of time.

muscular strength The maximum force a muscle, or group of muscles, can exert against a resistance.

obese Being more than 30% fat for women and 25% fat for men.

one repetition maximum To exert one maximal force.

overfat A condition in which the percentage of body weight that is fat weight is too high.

overweight An amount of weight above the average as determined by a standard height/weight chart or body mass index.

oxygen consumption The rate at which oxygen is used to produce energy, measured in liters per minute or milliliters per kilogram of body weight per minute. (*Synonym:* oxygen uptake)

passive stretching Flexibility exercise in which the stretch (lengthening) of the muscle is created by an outside source such as a partner, gravity, or body part not involved in the stretch.

phosphagen system An anaerobic system that rapidly produces energy through the breakdown and resynthesis of high-energy phosphagens (not carbohydrate). This system can supply only a few seconds of energy.

physical fitness The physical aspects of a person's well-being that enable a person to function at an optimal level.

physioball *See* stability ball.

phytochemicals Food components, "plant chemicals," that ward off cancer, cardiovascular diseases, diabetes, and hypertension.

pilates A method of mental and physical conditioning that aims to develop strength balanced with flexibility.

PNF stretching A method of stretching that uses proprioceptive neuromuscular facilitation (PNF). First the muscle is isometrically contracted, and then it is stretched.

pre-exercise heart rate (PreHR) The rate at which the heart is beating prior to exercise.

PreHR *See* pre-exercise heart rate.

principle of individuality An exercise principle that states that any two people can react differently to the same exercise.

principle of overload An exercise principle stating that a physiological system or organ of the body repeatedly subjected to greater than normal stress will adapt to the stress. A proper amount of overload will result in positive adaptations.

principle of overuse An exercise principle that states that too much stress over a period of time can result in fatigue and injury.

principle of progression An exercise principle that states that the gradual increase (or overload) of the intensity, frequency, or duration of exercise will improve physical fitness.

principle of reversibility An exercise principle stating that a physiological system or organ that is not repeatedly stressed but is instead subjected to less than normal amounts of stress will adapt by deconditioning. (*Synonyms:* use/disuse principle; principle of regularity)

principle of specificity An exercise principle stating that physiological adaptations are specific to the systems that are overloaded through exercise.

progressive relaxation A physiolgoical method of systematically relaxing skeletal muscles with the belief that this will reduce tension throughout the body. Muscles are alternately contracted and relaxed.

proprioceptive neuromuscular facilitation stretching
See PNF stretching.

protein A compound made up of amino acids that is found in certain foods. It is primarily used to build and repair body tissues but may also serve as a source of energy.

psychoneuroimmunology An area of neurology that studies how the psyche (brain) influences the immune system.

pulse The wave of pressure felt in the arteries when the heart beats.

radial artery An artery that runs close to the surface of the skin on the inside of the wrist. This artery is commonly used for counting the pulse.

ratings of perceived exertion (RPE) A method of estimating the intensity of an exercise session that uses a scale of numbers with brief qualifiers developed by Gunnar Borg.

RecHR *See* recovery heart rate.

recovery heart rate (RecHR) The rate at which the heart beats following exercise. Usually counted 1 or 2 minutes after exercise is stopped.

repetition maximum To exert a maximal force over 1 repetition (1 RM).

resistance ball *See* stability ball.

resting heart rate (RHR) The rate at which the heart beats when the body is at rest.

RHR *See* resting heart rate.

RICE An acronym for immediate first aid for injuries such as sprains, strains, and contusions: rest, ice, compression, elevation.

RPE *See* ratings of perceived exertion.

set point theory A genetic-based theory that asserts that the body seeks to maintain a preset level of fat.

shinsplints A general term for pain on the front or side of the shin. A common overuse injury in aerobic activity.

skin-fold technique A method of estimating a person's percentage of body fat. Subcutaneous fat is measured using a skin-fold caliper.

spot reducing One of the all-time greatest myths that states an individual can take fat off a specific part of the body by exercising that specific part. A person actually can lose fat throughout the body only by exercising aerobically and eating a proper diet.

sprain Overstretching or tearing a ligament or joint capsule resulting in swelling, discoloration, and pain.

stability ball A large inflated rubber, vinyl, or solid foam ball used to perform resistance and/or core training exercises using an unstable environment.

static contraction *See* isometric contraction.

static stretching A technique of developing flexibility that places the muscle in a stretch position and then holds that stretch without moving. (Opposite of *ballistic stretching*.)

step aerobics A form of aerobic dance exercise in which you step up and down on a bench to the beat of the music at a rate of 118 to 122 bpm (beginners), maximum 128 bpm (advanced).

strain Overstretching or tearing a muscle or tendon, resulting in swelling, discoloration, and pain.

strength *See* muscular strength.

stretch reflex The automatic muscular contraction that occurs when a muscle is suddenly stretched.

stroke volume The amount of blood the heart pumps in 1 beat.

supersetting A method of resistance training in which an exercise for one muscle is immediately followed by an exercise for the opposing muscle. (Sometimes the definition also includes performing two exercises for the same muscle group one immediately after another.)

Swiss ball *See* stability ball.

systolic pressure The pressure exerted by the blood in the arteries when the ventricles are contracting. Systolic pressure is represented by the numerator in the blood pressure fraction.

tapless step A type of step aerobics that makes transitions from one lead leg to another without using a tap change.

target heart-rate zone *See* training heart-rate range.

TC *See* total cholesterol.

tendinitis Inflammation of a tendon. This is a common overuse injury.

tendon Fibrous tissue that connects muscle to bone.

THR *See* training heart-rate range.

threshold of aerobic training The lower limit of the aerobic target zone. It is usually described by a percentage of the maximum volume of oxygen consumed, the maximum heart rate, or the heart-rate reserve. *See* threshold of training.

threshold of training The minimum amount and intensity of exercise that must be performed for an individual to make physical fitness gains.

time The length of a single exercise session.

total cholesterol The sum of HDL and LDL.

training heart-rate range (THR) The optimum intensity range for aerobic exercise using the exercise heart rate as the indicator of intensity. Training within the range improves cardiorespiratory endurance. (*Synonym:* target heart-rate zone)

***trans* fats** Fats artificially produced from liquid unsaturated fats into solid fats. Linked to higher cholesterol levels and greater risk of coronary heart disease.

underwater weighing *See* hydrostatic weighing.

use/disuse principle *See* principle of reversibility.

vein A vessel that carries blood toward the heart.

venous pump Action of the muscles that helps to massage blood up the veins against gravity.

vitamins Organic compounds that help release energy from food and act as metabolic regulators. Vitamins A, D, E, and K are fat soluble; the rest are water soluble.

VO₂max The largest amount of oxygen the body can consume in 1 minute, measured in liters per minute or milliliters per kilogram of body weight per minute. (*Synonym:* maximum oxygen uptake *or* MOU)

warm-up The period of time in which individuals prepare the body for vigorous activity by performing easy movements through a range of motion, thus raising the core temperature of the body and stretching out and lubricating muscles and joints. Leading into the aerobic workout, it is a gradual increase in activity level that allows the heart and lungs to make a smooth transition into exercise.

warm-up stretch A series of gentle flexibility exercises to prepare the body for vigorous movement.

water aerobics A low-impact form of aerobic conditioning performed in water using water resistance to enhance training. (*Synonym:* aqua aerobics)

wellness A way of being that involves taking responsibility for one's own well-being and practicing lifestyle habits that promote physical, social, emotional, mental, and spiritual health.

yoga An ancient Eastern Indian philosophy with an ultimate goal of reaching self-realization. Embraces living in harmony and achieving an inner peace. *See also* hatha yoga.

zero to peak formula *See* maximum heart-rate formula.

Index

Page references followed by *f* indicate figure; by *t* indicate table; by *b* indicate box.